Classification and Examples of Differential Equations and their Applications

Mathematics and Physics for Science and Technology
Series Editor: L.M.B.C. Campos
Director of the Center for Aeronautical
and Space Science and Technology
Lisbon University

Volumes in the series

Topic A – Theory of Functions and Potential Problems

Volume I (Book 1) – Complex Analysis with Applications to Flows and Fields
L.M.B.C. Campos

Volume II (Book 2) – Elementary Transcendentals with Applications to Solids and Fluids
L.M.B.C. Campos

Volume III (Book 3) – Generalized Calculus with Applications to Matter and Forces
L.M.B.C. Campos

Topic B – Boundary and Initial-Value Problems

Volume IV – Ordinary Differential Equations with Applications to Trajectories and Vibrations
L.M.B.C. Campos

Book 4 – Linear Differential Equations and Oscillators
L.M.B.C. Campos

Book 5 – Non-Linear Differential Equations and Dynamical Systems
L.M.B.C. Campos

Book 6 – Higher-order Differential Equations and Elasticity
L.M.B.C. Campos

Book 7 – Simultaneous Differential Equations and Multi-Dimensional Vibrations
L.M.B.C. Campos

Book 8 – Singular Differential Equations and Special Functions
L.M.B.C. Campos

Book 9 – Classification and Examples of Differential Equations and their Applications
L.M.B.C. Campos

For more information about this series, please visit: https://www.crcpress.com/Mathematics-and-Physics-for-Science-and-Technology/book-series/CRCMATPHYSCI

Mathematics and Physics for Science and Technology

Volume IV

Ordinary Differential Equations with Applications to Trajectories and Vibrations

Book 9

Classification and Examples of Differential Equations and their Applications

By

L.M.B.C. Campos

Director of the Center for Aeronautical and Space Science and Technology

Lisbon University

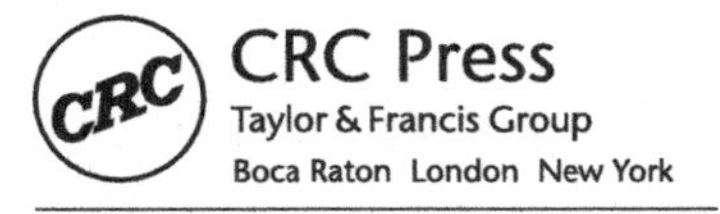

CRC Press is an imprint of the
Taylor & Francis Group, an **informa** business

CRC Press
Taylor & Francis Group
6000 Broken Sound Parkway NW, Suite 300
Boca Raton, FL 334 87-2742

Printed on acid-free paper

International Standard Book Number-13: 978-0-367-13724-3 (Hardback)

DOI: 10.1201/9780429060816

Visit the Taylor & Francis Web site at
http://www.taylorandfrancis.com

and the CRC Press Web site at
http://www.crcpress.com

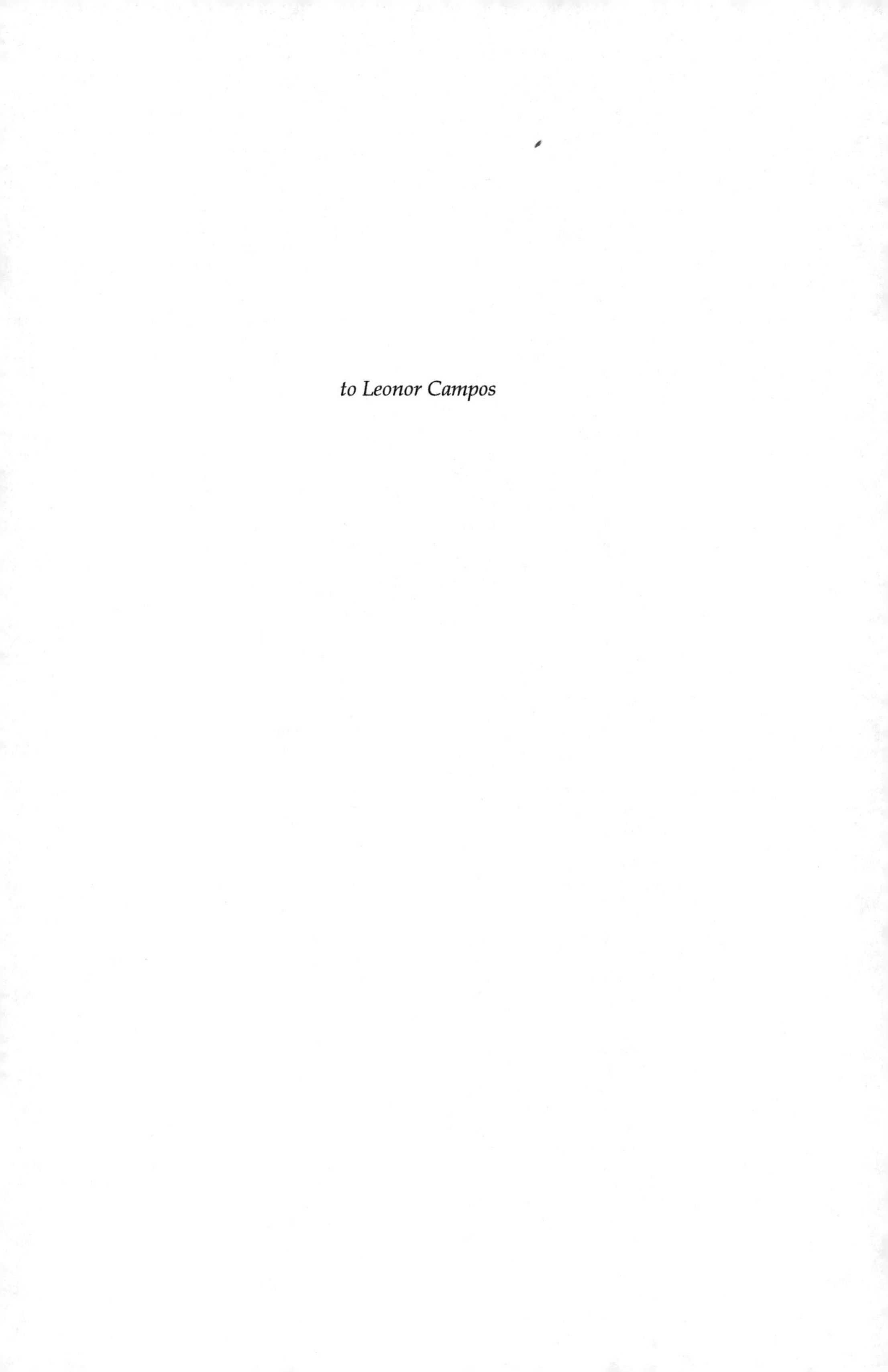

to Leonor Campos

Contents

List of Classifications and Tables

Classifications

Tables

Preface

Volume IV (*Ordinary Differential Equations with Applications to Trajectories and Oscillations*) is organized like the preceding three volumes of the series *Mathematics and Physics Applied to Science and Technology*: (volume III) *Generalized Calculus with Applications to Matter and Forces*; (volume II) *Transcendental Representations with Applications to Solids and Fluids*; (volume I) *Complex Analysis with Applications to Flows and Fields*. The present book, *Classifications of Differential Equations and Examples of their Applications*, is the sixth and last book of volume IV and the ninth book of the series. This book consists of chapter 10 of volume IV, containing 20 examples related to the preceding five books and chapters 1 to 9. This book includes two recollections—the first details a classification of differential equations into 500 standards and the second provides a list of 500 applications. The examples and classifications cover the ensemble of the first five books of volume IV, which correspond to books 4 to 8 of the series, namely: (i) Book 4—*Linear Differential Equations and Oscillators*; (ii) Book 5—*Non-Linear Differential Equations and Dynamical Systems*; (iii) Book 6—*Higher-Order Differential Equations and Elasticity*; (iv) Book 7—*Simultaneous Differential Equations and Multi-Dimensional Vibrations*; (v) Book 8—*Singular Differential Equations and Special Functions*. The aggregate of contents is summarized next.

Organization of the Contents

Volume IV consists of ten chapters: (i) the odd-numbered chapters present mathematical developments; (ii) the even-numbered chapters contain physical applications; (iii) the last chapter is a set of 20 detailed examples of (i) and (ii). The chapters are divided into sections and subsections, for example, chapter 9, section 9.1, and subsection 9.1.1. Chapter 10 contains 20 examples, Example 10.1 to Example 10.20, some with subsections, such as E10.1.2. The formulas are numbered by chapters in curved brackets, for example, (10.2) is equation 2 of chapter 10. When referring to volume I the symbol I is inserted at the beginning, for example: (i) chapter I.36, section I.36.1, subsection I.36.1.2; (ii) equation (I.36.33a). The final part of each chapter includes: (i) a conclusion referring to the figures as a kind of visual summary; (ii) the notes, lists, tables, diagrams, and classifications as additional support. The latter (ii) apply at the end of each chapter, and are numbered within the chapter (for example, classification—Classification 10.2, table—Table 10.3); if there is more than one note, list, table, diagram, or classification, they are numbered sequentially (for example, Table 10.1 to Table 10.4). The chapter starts with an introductory preview, and related topics may be mentioned in the notes at the end. The "Series Preface" and "Mathematical Symbols" from the first book of volume IV are not repeated in this book and "Bibliography" is not added to this book. The "Physical Quantities," "References," and "Index" in this book cover all six books of the volume IV to account for the close relationship among them.

Summary of Volume IV

Following the three volumes on complex, transcendental, and generalized functions, this fourth volume is the first volume on boundary and initial value problems, and concerns ordinary differential equations with a variety of applications, including trajectories and oscillations. The differential equations are classified in 500 standards indicating their properties, methods of solution, and examples, and include: linear and non-linear ordinary differential equations and simultaneous systems; in particular, linear equations with constant coefficients having a characteristic polynomial, and linear equations with variable coefficients leading to 23 special functions. The applications consist of 500 problems with physical formulation, mathematical solutions, and interpretation of results; the problems include linear and non-linear oscillators with one or several degrees-of-freedom, with or without damping, and forcing including ordinary, parametric, multiple, and non-linear resonance. Other applications include trajectories, orbits, electromechanical systems, and chains with deterministic and chaotic behavior; also included are deformations and buckling of elastic beams, membranes, and plates. Included in the contents are:

- Ordinary differential equations of first, second, and higher orders, and simultaneous systems;
- Linear differential and finite difference equations and simultaneous systems with characteristic polynomials;
- Linear differential equations with variable coefficients and 23 associated special functions, such as generalized Bessel, hypergeometric, etc.;
- Non-linear differential equations, bifurcations, and dynamical and chaotic systems;
- Existence, unicity, uniformity, robustness, and stability theorems;
- Applications to trajectories, dynamos, and other electromechanical systems and chains;

- Linear and non-linear oscillators with one or several degrees-of-freedom, with damping and forcing;
- Linear, non-linear, multiple, and parametric resonance of mechanical and electrical systems;
- Torsional, longitudinal, and bending deformations and buckling of rods, membranes, and plates.

Acknowledgments

The fourth volume of the series justifies renewing some of the acknowledgments also made in the first three volumes, to those who contributed more directly to the final form of the volume: Ms. Ana Moura, L. Sousa, and S. Pernadas for help with the manuscripts; Mr. J. Coelho for all the drawings; and at last, but not least, to my wife as my companion in preparing this work.

About the Author

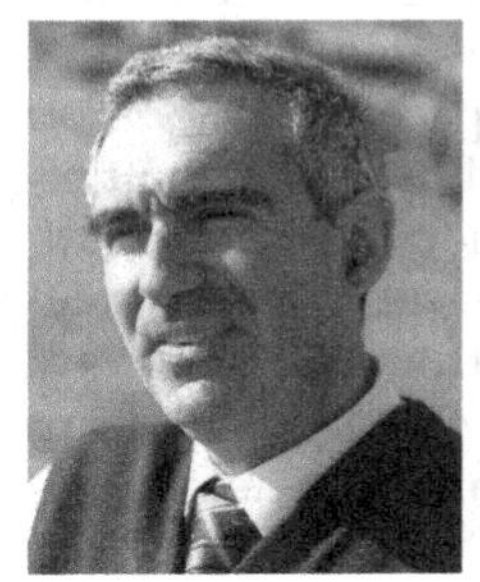

L.M.B.C. Campos was born on March 28, 1950, in Lisbon, Portugal. He graduated in 1972 as a mechanical engineer from the Instituto Superior Tecnico (IST) of Lisbon Technical University. The tutorials as a student (1970) were followed by a career at the same institution (IST) through all levels: assistant (1972), assistant with tenure (1974), assistant professor (1978), associate professor (1982), chair of Applied Mathematics and Mechanics (1985). He has served as the coordinator of undergraduate and postgraduate degrees in Aerospace Engineering since the creation of the programs in 1991. He is the coordinator of the Scientific Area of Applied and Aerospace Mechanics in the Department of Mechanical Engineering. He is also the director and founder of the Center for Aeronautical and Space Science and Technology.

In 1977, Campos received his doctorate on "waves in fluids" from the Engineering Department of Cambridge University, England. Afterwards, he received a Senior Rouse Ball Scholarship to study at Trinity College, while on leave from IST. In 1984, his first sabbatical was as a Senior Visitor at the Department of Applied Mathematics and Theoretical Physics of Cambridge University, England. In 1991, he spent a second sabbatical as an Alexander von Humboldt scholar at the Max-Planck Institut fur Aeronomic in Katlenburg-Lindau, Germany. Further sabbaticals abroad were excluded by major commitments at the home institution. The latter were always compatible with extensive professional travel related to participation in scientific meetings, individual or national representation in international institutions, and collaborative research projects.

Campos received the von Karman medal from the Advisory Group for Aerospace Research and Development (AGARD) and Research and Technology Organization (RTO). Participation in AGARD/RTO included serving as a vice-chairman of the System Concepts and Integration Panel, and chairman of the Flight Mechanics Panel and of the Flight Vehicle Integration Panel. He was also a member of the Flight Test Techniques Working Group. Here he was involved in the creation of an independent flight test capability, active in Portugal during the last 30 years, which has been used in national and international projects, including Eurocontrol and the European Space Agency. The participation in the European Space Agency (ESA) has afforded Campos the opportunity to serve on various program boards at the levels of national representative and Council of Ministers.

His participation in activities sponsored by the European Union (EU) has included: (i) 27 research projects with industry, research, and academic institutions; (ii) membership of various Committees, including Vice-Chairman of the Aeronautical Science and Technology Advisory Committee; (iii) participation on the Space Advisory Panel on the future role of EU in space. Campos has been a member of the Space Science Committee of the European Science Foundation, which works with the Space Science Board of the National Science Foundation of the United States. He has been a member of the Committee for Peaceful Uses of Outer Space (COPUOS) of the United Nations. He has served as a consultant and advisor on behalf of these organizations and other institutions. His participation in professional societies includes member and vice-chairman of the Portuguese Academy of Engineering, fellow of the Royal Aeronautical Society, Astronomical Society and Cambridge Philosophical Society, associate fellow of the American Institute of Aeronautics and Astronautics, and founding and life member of the European Astronomical Society.

Campos has published and worked on numerous books and articles. His publications include 10 books as a single author, one as an editor, and one as a co-editor. He has published 152 papers (82 as the single author, including 12 reviews) in 60 journals, and 254 communications to symposia. He has served as reviewer for 40 different journals, in addition to 23 reviews published in *Mathematics Reviews*. He is or has been member of the editorial boards of several journals, including *Progress in Aerospace Sciences, International Journal of Aeroacoustics, International Journal of Sound and Vibration*, and *Air & Space Europe*.

Campos's areas of research focus on four topics: acoustics, magnetohydrodynamics, special functions, and flight dynamics. His work on acoustics has concerned the generation, propagation, and refraction of sound in flows with mostly aeronautical applications. His work on magnetohydrodynamics has concerned magneto-acoustic-gravity-inertial waves in solar-terrestrial and stellar physics. His developments on special functions have used differintegration operators, generalizing the ordinary derivative and primitive to complex order; they have led to the introduction of new special functions. His work on flight dynamics has concerned aircraft and rockets, including trajectory optimization, performance, stability, control, and atmospheric disturbances.

The range of topics from mathematics to physics and engineering fits with the aims and contents of the present series. Campos's experience in university teaching and scientific and industrial research has enhanced his ability to make the series valuable to students from undergraduate level to research level.

Campos's professional activities on the technical side are balanced by other cultural and humanistic interests. Complementary non-technical interests include classical music (mostly orchestral and choral), plastic arts (painting, sculpture, architecture), social sciences (psychology and biography), history (classical, renaissance and overseas expansion) and technology (automotive, photo, audio). Campos is listed in various biographical publications, including *Who's Who in the World* since 1986, *Who's Who in Science and Technology* since 1994, and *Who's Who in America* since 2011.

Physical Quantities

The location of first appearance is indicated, for example "2.7" means "section 2.7," "6.8.4" means "subsection 6.8.4," "N8.8" means "note 8.8," and "E10.13.1" means "example 10.13.1."

1 Small Arabic Letters

a — acceleration: 2.1.1
— amplitude of oscillation: 2.2.11
— moment arm: 4.7.3
a_i — acceleration vector: 6.8.3
a_n — coefficients of a series: 4.4.10
b — stiffness dispersion parameter of an elastic bar: N6.12
— width of a water channel: N7.12
$\bar{b}$ — stiffness dispersion parameter for an elastic plate: N6.10
c — speed of light *in vacuo*: 2.1.9
— phase speed of waves: N5.13, N6.14, N8.1
c_1, c_2 — speed of transversal waves in the directions of principal stress of an anisotropic elastic membrane: N6.7
c_e — speed of transversal waves in an elastic string: N6.3
— speed of transversal waves in an isotropic elastic membrane: N6.4
c_{em} — speed of electromagnetic waves: 2.1.11
c_ℓ — speed of longitudinal waves in an elastic rod: N6.6
c_r — isothermal sound speed: 5.5.24
c_s — adiabatic sound speed: 5.5.14
c_t — speed of torsional waves along an elastic rod: N6.5
c_w — speed of water waves along a channel: N7.13
$\vec{e}_i$ — non-unit base vector: N8.8
e_{ijk} — three-dimensional permutation symbol: 6.8.4
f — forcing function: 2.1.8
$\vec{f}$ — force vector per unit area: 6.5.4
f_i — force vector per unit volume: 6.8.3
f_r — reduced external force: 8.2.1

g — acceleration of gravity: 6.3.14
— determinant of the covariant metric tensor: N8.8
g_ℓ — reduced modal force: 8.1.1
g_{ij} — covariant metric tensor: N8.8
g^{ij} — contravariant metric tensor: N8.8
h — friction force: 2.1.1
— amplitude of excitation of parametric resonance: 4.3.2
— thickness of a plate: 6.5.4
— depth of water channel: N7.12
h_i — friction force vector: 8.1.1
— scale factors: N8.8
j — restoring force: 2.1.1
— electric current: 2.1.6
$\vec{j}$ — convective electric current vector: 2.1.9
j_i — restoring force vector: 8.1.1
k — resilience of a point translational spring: 2.1.2
— Boltzmann constant: 5.5.16
— transversal wavenumber: N5.14
— curvature: 6.1.11
— wavenumber: N7.25, N8.2
k' — differential resilience of a distributed spring: 6.3.1
$\bar{k}$ — resilience of a point rotational spring: 6.2.6
k_1, k_2 — principal curvatures: 6.7.2
k_{ij} — matrix of curvatures and cross-curvatures: 6.7
k_{rs} — resilience matrix: 8.1.2
ℓ — lengthscale for horns: N7.28
m — mass of a particle or body: 2.1.1
m_{rs} — mass matrix: 8.2.1
n — number of degrees of freedom of a molecule: 5.5.21
$\vec{n}$ — unit vector normal to a curve: 6.9.7
p — pressure: 5.5.4, 6.5.1
— buckling parameter: 6.1.2
q — electric charge: 2.1.6
— non-linearity parameter for pendular motion: 4.7.13
q_ℓ — modal coordinates: 8.2.4
s — arc length: 6.1.1

t — time: 2.1.1
— time of reception: 2.1.11
t_0 — time of emission: 2.1.11
u — longitudinal displacement of a bar: 6.4.1
$\vec{u}$ — displacement vector: 6.4.1, 6.8.5
v — velocity: 2.1.1
$\vec{v}$ — velocity vector: 5.2.1
w — group velocity: N6.16
x — independent variable in ordinary differential equation: 1.1.1
— Cartesian coordinate: 2.1.1
$\vec{x}$ — position vector of observer: 2.1.11
y — dependent variable in ordinary differential equation: 1.1.1
— Cartesian coordinate: 2.1
$\vec{y}$ — position vector of source: 2.1.11
z — Cartesian coordinate: 6.1.1
— specific impedance: N7.47

2 Capital Arabic Letters

A — Activity or power: 2.1.4
— anharmonic factor: 4.4.10
— cross-sectional area of a horn: N7.16
— admittance: 8.9.1
— Avogadro number: 5.5.17
A_n — modal amplitudes: 8.8.5
$\vec{A}$ — vector magnetic potential: 2.1.10
A_{ab} — elastic compliance matrix: 6.8.10
$\vec{B}$ — magnetic induction vector: 2.1.9
B_{mn} — terms in the modal matrix: 8.8.5
C — constant of integration: 1.1.1
— capacity of an electric condenser: 2.1.6
— torsional stiffness of an elastic rod: N6.4
$\vec{C}$ — bending vector: 6.7.8
C_p — specific heat at constant pressure: 5.5.12

C_v — specific heat at constant volume: 5.5.12
C_{ab} — elastic stiffness matrix: 6.8.7
$C_{ijk\ell}$ — elastic stiffness tensor: 6.8.6
D — drag force: 4.8.13
— bending stiffness of an elastic plate: 6.7.2
$\bar{D}$ — generalized bending stiffness: 6.8.14
D_2 — relative area change: 6.5.5
D_3 — relative volume change: 6.5.1
$\vec{D}$ — electric displacement vector: 2.1.9
E — Young modulus of elasticity: 6.4.1, 6.5.1
E_0, E_1 — coefficients in the non-uniform Young modulus: 6.4.4
$\vec{E}$ — electric field vector: 2.1.9
$\bar{E}_b$ — elastic energy per unit area of in-plane deformation: 6.9.4
$\bar{\bar{E}}_b$ — total elastic energy of in-plane deformation: 6.9.5
E_c — elastic energy per unit area for the deflection of an elastic membrane: 6.6.2
$\bar{E}_c$ — total elastic energy of deflection for a membrane: 6.6.2
$\bar{\bar{E}}_c$ — total elastic energy of deflection for a plate: 6.9.5
E_d — elastic energy per unit volume for a plate: 6.7.8
$\bar{\bar{E}}_d$ — total elastic energy for a plate: 6.7.8
$\tilde{E}_d$ — elastic energy per unit length along the boundary of a plate: 6.8.16
$\hat{E}_d$ — total elastic energy along the boundary of a plate: E10.13.1
E_e — electric energy: 2.1.7
E_{em} — electromagnetic energy: 2.1.7
E_m — magnetic energy: 2.1.7
E_t — total energy: 2.1.4
E_v — kinetic energy: 2.1.4, 6.8.5
F — force: 3.9.11
— free energy: 5.5.8
— longitudinal force in a bar: 6.4.1
$\vec{F}$ — force vector: 6.5.4
F_e — electromotive force: 2.1.6
F_m — mechanical force: 2.1.1
F_ℓ — reduced external force: 8.2.1
G — free enthalpy: 5.5.8
G_ℓ — modal forces: 8.2.9

H — friction force on a belt: 2.5.1
— enthalpy: 5.5.8
$\vec{H}$ — magnetic field vector: 2.1.9
I — moment of inertia: 4.7.3
$\overline{I}$ — deformation vector: 6.7.9
J — electric current: 4.7.1
— heat flux: 6.4.2
$\vec{J}$ — electric current vector: 2.1.9
$J^{\pm}$ — invariants of acoustic horns: N7.28
K — longitudinal wavenumber: N5.14
— curvature quadratic form: 6.7.3
— reduced wavenumber: N7.29
$\vec{K}$ — enhanced wavenumber: N7.33
L — induction of a coil or self: 2.1.6, 4.4.7.1
— lift force: 4.8.13
— lengthscale of variation of wave speed: N5.19
L_A — lengthscale of variation of the cross-sectional area: N7.17
L_b — lengthscale of variation of the width of a water channel: N7.12
L_c — lengthscale of variation of the torsional stiffness: N7.10
L_E — lengthscale of change of the Young modulus: N7.11
L_T — lengthscale of change of tension: N7.9
L_ε — lengthscale of variation of the dielectric permittivity: N7.15
L_μ — lengthscale of variation of the magnetic permeability: N7.15
M — friction moment on a cam: 2.5.4
— molecular mass: 5.5.17
— moment of the inertia forces: N6.4
$\vec{M}$ — moment of forces: 6.8.4
M_1, M_2 — principal bending moments: 6.7.2
M_a — applied axial moment: N6.4
M_n — normal stress coupled: 6.8.16
— mass of n-th element of a radioactive disintegration chain: 8.7.1
M_x, M_y — stress couples: 6.7.4
M_{xy} — twist couple: 6.7.4
M_{rs} — modal matrix: 8.2.13
N — number of particles: 5.5.17

$\vec{N}$ — unit outer normal to a surface: 5.5.1
— turning moment: 6.7.6
N_n — normal turning moment: 6.8.16
$\bar{N}_n$ — augmented normal turning moment: 6.9.5
N_x, N_y — turning moments: 6.7.6
N_{rs} — undamped modal matrix: 8.2.14
P — reduced pressure perturbation spectrum: N7.23
P_{2N} — dispersion polynomial: 8.2.2
P_{ij} — dispersion matrix: 8.2.2
Q — heat: 3.9.11
— heat source: 6.4.2
— concentrated torque: E10.10.1
$Q_{r\ell}$ — transformation matrix: 8.2.7
R — electrical resistance: 2.1.6, 4.7.1, 8.9.2
— perfect gas constant: 5.5.17
— radius of curvature: 6.1.1
— reflection coefficient: N7.47
S — entropy: 3.9.11
— dynamo parameter: 4.7.3
— strain: 6.4.1
— surface adsorption coefficient: N7.48
S_a — row of components of the strain tensor: 6.8.7
S_{ij} — strain tensor: 6.5.1, 6.8.8
— scattering matrix: N7.53
T — temperature: 3.9.11
— thrust: 4.8.13
— tangential tension along an elastic string: 6.1.1
— transmission coefficient: N7.51
$\bar{T}$ — effective axial tension: 6.3.12
$\vec{T}$ — stress vector: 6.6.2, 6.8.3
T_a — row of components of the stress tensor: 6.8.7
T_{ij} — stress tensor: 6.5.1, 6.8.3
$\overset{o}{T}_{ij}$ — residual stresses: 6.8.6
U — internal energy: 3.9.11

V — specific volume: 5.5.4
— reduced velocity perturbation spectrum: N7.23
W — work: 2.2.2, 3.9.11, 5.5.4
— weight: 4.8.13
W_b — work of deformation: 6.8.5
W_v — work of the inertia force: 6.8.5
Y — inductance: 8.9.1
Z — impedance: 4.7.2, 8.9.1
$\tilde{Z}$ — overall impedance: N7.52
Z_0 — impedance of a plane sound wave: N7.47

3 Small Greek Letters

α — phase of an oscillator: 2.2.1
— angle of cylindrical helix: 3.9.5
— coefficient of the cubic term of the quartic potential: 4.5.1
— diffusivity: N8.1
α_e — ohmic electrical diffusivity: 2.1.11
β — coefficient of the quartic term in the biquadratic potential: 4.4.4
— amplification/attenuation factor: N7.50
— potential: N8.1
χ — thermal conductivity: 6.4.2
— stiffness ratio parameter: 6.8.16
— damping parameter: 6.8.14
δ_{ij} — identity matrix: 6.5.1, 6.8.4, 8.1.4
ε — dielectric permittivity: 2.1.9
$\varphi_\pm$ — phase of waves propagating in opposite directions: N6.14
γ — dimensionless non-linearity parameter: 4.4.8
— adiabatic exponent: 5.5.12
λ — damping: 2.1.8
λ_ℓ — modal dampings: 8.2.5
λ_{rs} — damping matrix: 8.2.1
μ — kinematic friction coefficient: 2.1.3, N6.10
— magnetic permeability: 2.1.9

μ_{rs} — kinematic friction matrix: 8.1.3
ν — number of particles per unit volume: 5.5.17
— resilience of distributed translational spring: N6.10
ν_n — disintegration rate of the mass of the n-th element in a chain: 8.7.1
θ — angle of inclination of a string or a beam: 6.1.11
— temperature: 6.4.2
ρ — mass density per unit volume: 5.8.11
ρ_1 — mass density per unit length: N6.3
ρ_2 — mass density per unit area: N6.4
σ — Ohmic electrical conductivity: 2.1.9
— Poisson ratio: 6.5.1
— mass density per unit length: N7.8
τ — period of oscillation 2.1.12
— twist: 6.7.13
— torsion: N6.5
$\overline{\tau}$ — decay rate: 2.1.12
ω_0 — natural frequency: 2.1.8
ω_1 — fundamental natural frequency: N6.13
ω_n — natural frequency of n-th harmonic: N6.13
ω_ℓ — modal frequencies: 8.2.4
$\overline{\omega}$ — oscillation frequency: 2.3.3, 2.4.1
$\overline{\omega}_n$ — oscillation frequency of n-th harmonic: N6.17
$\overline{\omega}_\ell$ — oscillation frequencies of modes: 8.2.6
$\tilde{\omega}$ — average of applied and natural frequencies: 2.7.5
ω_a — applied frequency of sinusoidal forcing: 2.7.1
ω_e — excitation frequency of parametric resonance: 4.3.2
ω_r — natural frequency for rotary spring: N6.10
ω_t — natural frequency for translational spring: N6.10
ω_{r1}, ω_{r2} — natural frequencies for a vector rotary spring: N6.10
ω_{rs}^2 — oscillation matrix: 8.2.1
ψ — non-linearity parameter for a quartic potential: 4.6.1
ζ — transverse deflection of a string, beam, membrane or plate: 6.1.1

4 Capital Greek Letters

Φ — primal wave variable: N7.19

Φ_e — scalar electric potential: 2.1.10

Φ_m — mechanical potential energy: 2.1.4, 8.1.2

ϑ — resilience of a rotary spring in one dimension: N6.10

$\bar{\vartheta}$ — resilience vector of a rotary spring in two dimensions: N6.10

Θ — stress function: 6.5.5

Ω — angular velocity of rotation: 4.7.1

Ω_{ij} — rotation bivector: 6.8.6

Ψ — dual wave variable: N7.19

Ψ_e — dissipation by electrical resistance: 2.1.7

Ψ_m — dissipation by mechanical friction: 2.1.4, 8.1.2

10

Examples 10.1 to 10.20

EXAMPLE 10.1 One Finite Difference (Two Differential) Equation(s) with the Same Characteristic Polynomial

Solve two linear forced third-order differential equations with constant (homogeneous) coefficients [E10.1.1 (E10.1.2)] and the same characteristic polynomial as a linear forced third-order finite difference equation with constant coefficients (E10.1.3).

E10.1.1 Linear Differential Equation with Constant Coefficients

Consider the forced linear third-order differential equation with constant coefficients:

$$\begin{aligned} y''' + y'' - 2y = x^2 + x + 1 + e^{3x} + e^x + \sinh(2x) \\ + e^{-2x}\cosh x + e^{2x}\sin x + e^{-x}\cos x + e^x \sin x \end{aligned} \tag{10.1}$$

and obtain the complete integral. The linear third-order ordinary differential equation (10.1) has characteristic polynomial (10.2a–c) of ordinary derivatives (10.2d):

$$P_3(D) = D^3 + D^2 - 2 = (D-1)(D^2 + 2D + 2) = (D-1)(D+1-i)(D+1+i), \tag{10.2a–c}$$

$$D \equiv \frac{d}{dx}: \qquad P_3'(D) = 3D^2 + 2D = D(3D+2); \tag{10.2d, e}$$

the roots (10.3a) of (10.2c) specify the general integral (10.3b) of the unforced equation:

$$D = 1, -1 \pm i: \qquad y(x) = A e^x + e^{-x}(B\cos x + C\sin x), \tag{10.3a, b}$$

where A, B, C are arbitrary constants of integration. The polynomial forcing term has a particular integral specified by the inverse polynomial of derivatives:

$$\begin{aligned}\frac{1}{P_3(D)}\left(x^2+x+1\right)&=-\frac{1}{2}\frac{1}{1-D^2(1+D)/2}\left(x^2+x+1\right)\\&=-\frac{1}{2}\left\{1+\frac{D^2}{2}+O\left(D^3\right)\right\}\left(x^2+x+1\right)=-\frac{x^2}{2}-\frac{x}{2}-1.\end{aligned}\tag{10.4}$$

The remaining particular integrals in (10.1) correspond to the following cases:

$$\begin{aligned}&y(x)-Ax-\frac{1}{x}\left(B\cos x+C\sin x\right)+\frac{x^2}{2}+\frac{x}{2}+1\\&\quad=\frac{e^{3x}}{P_3(3)}+\frac{xe^{x}}{P_3'(1)}+\frac{1}{2}\left[\frac{e^{2x}}{P_3(2)}-\frac{e^{-2x}}{P_3(-2)}\right]+\frac{1}{2}\left[\frac{e^{-x}}{P_3(-1)}+\frac{e^{-3x}}{P_3(-3)}\right]\\&\quad+\operatorname{Im}\left[\frac{e^{(2+i)x}}{P_3(2+i)}\right]+\operatorname{Re}\left[\frac{xe^{(i-1)x}}{P_3'(i-1)}\right]+\operatorname{Im}\left[\frac{e^{(1+i)x}}{P_3(1+i)}\right],\end{aligned}\tag{10.5}$$

because; (i) the exponential $\exp(3x)$ is non-resonant (1.129a, b); (ii) the exponential $\exp(x)$ is resonant (1.134a, b); (iii) the hyperbolic sine $\sinh(2x)$ is non-resonant (1.147a, b); (iv) the product of exponential $\exp(-2x)$ and hyperbolic cosine $\cosh(x)$ is not resonant (1.165a, b); (v) the product of the exponential $\exp(2x)$ and circular sine $\sin(x)$ is also non-resonant (1.173a, b); (vi) the product of the exponential $\exp(-2x)$ by the circular cosine $\cos x$ is resonant (1.174a–c); (vii) the product of the exponential $\exp(x)$ by the circular cosine $\cos(x)$ is non-resonant (1.176a, b). The characteristic polynomial (10.2b) and its first-order derivative (10.2e) evaluate the coefficients (10.6a–i) in (10.5):

$$\frac{1}{P_3(3)}=\frac{1}{34},\quad\frac{1}{P_3'(1)}=\frac{1}{5},\quad\frac{1}{P_3(2)}=\frac{1}{10},\quad\frac{1}{P_3(-2)}=-\frac{1}{6},\tag{10.6a–d}$$

$$\frac{1}{P_3(-1)}=-\frac{1}{2},\quad\frac{1}{P_3(-3)}=-\frac{1}{20},\quad\frac{1}{P_3(2+i)}=\frac{1}{3(1+5i)}=\frac{1-5i}{78},\tag{10.6e–g}$$

$$\frac{1}{P_3'(i-1)}=-\frac{1}{2(1+2i)}=-\frac{1-2i}{10},\qquad\frac{1}{P_3(1+i)}=\frac{1}{4(i-1)}=-\frac{1+i}{8},\tag{10.6h, i}$$

Substitution of (10.6a–i) in (10.5) leads to the complete integral (10.7) of (10.1):

$$\bar{y}(x) = Ae^{x} + e^{-x}(B\cos x + C\sin x) - \frac{x^2 + x + 2}{2} + \frac{e^{3x}}{34}$$

$$+\frac{xe^{x}}{5} + \frac{e^{2x}}{20} + \frac{e^{-2x}}{12} - \frac{e^{-x}}{4} - \frac{e^{-3x}}{40} + \frac{e^{2x}}{78}(\sin x - 5\cos x) \tag{10.7}$$

$$-\frac{xe^{-x}}{10}(\cos x + 2\sin x) - \frac{e^{x}}{8}(\sin x + \cos x),$$

where (A, B, C) are arbitrary constants of integration.

E10.1.2 Linear Differential Equation with Homogeneous Coefficients

Consider the forced linear third-order differential equation with homogeneous coefficients:

$$x^3y''' + 4\,x^2y'' + 2xy' - 2y = \log^2 x + \log x + 1 + x^3 + x$$

$$+\sinh(2\log x) + \frac{\cosh(\log x)}{x^2} + x^2\sin(\log x) + \frac{\cos(\log x)}{x} \tag{10.8}$$

$$+\,x\sin(\log x),$$

and obtain the complete integral. The characteristic polynomial (10.9b–d) of homogeneous derivatives (10.9a):

$$\delta \equiv x\frac{d}{dx}: \qquad P_3(\delta) = \delta(\delta-1)(\delta-2) + 4\delta(\delta-1) + 2\delta - 2$$

$$= (\delta-1)[\delta(\delta+2)+2] = (\delta-1)(\delta^2+2\delta+2), \tag{10.9a–d}$$

coincides with (10.9d) ≡ (10.2c). Thus, the substitutions (10.10a, b), which imply (10.10c, d):

$$e^{x} \leftrightarrow x, \quad x \leftrightarrow \log x: \qquad e^{ax} \leftrightarrow x^{a}, \qquad x^{n} \leftrightarrow \log^{n} x, \tag{10.10a–d}$$

interchange the complete integrals (10.7) [(10.11)]:

$$y(x) = Ax + \frac{B\cos(\log x) + C\sin(\log x)}{x} - \frac{\log^2 x + \log x + 2}{2} + \frac{x^3}{34} + \frac{x\log x}{5}$$

$$+\frac{x^2}{20} - \frac{1}{12x^2} - \frac{1}{4x} - \frac{1}{40x^3} + \frac{x^2}{78}[\sin(\log x) - 5\cos(2\log x)] \tag{10.11}$$

$$-\frac{\log x}{10x}[\cos(\log x) + 2\sin(2\log x)] - \frac{x}{8}[\cos(\log x) + \sin(\log x)],$$

of the forced linear third-order differential equations with constant (10.1) [homogeneous (10.8)] coefficients.

E10.1.3 Linear Finite Difference Equation with Constant Coefficients

Consider the forced linear third-order finite difference equation with constant coefficients:

$$y_{n+3} + y_{n+2} - 2y_n = 3^n + 2^{n-1} + (-2)^{n-1} + \frac{(-)^n}{2} + \frac{(-3)^n}{2}, \tag{10.12}$$

and obtain the complete solution. The characteristic polynomial of forward finite differences (10.13a) of (10.12) is (10.13b) ≡ (10.9d) ≡ (10.2c):

$$\Delta y_n = y_{n+1}: \qquad P_3(\Delta) = \Delta^3 + \Delta^2 - 2; \quad y(x) \leftrightarrow y_n, \; y^{(k)}(x) \leftrightarrow y_{n+k}, \; e^{ax} \leftrightarrow a^n, \tag{10.13a–e}$$

the changes (10.13c–e) imply:

$$\begin{aligned} e^{(a+ib)x} \leftrightarrow (a+ib)^n &= \left\{ \left|a^2+b^2\right|^{1/2} \exp\left[i \arctan(b/a)\right] \right\}^n \\ &= \left|a^2+b^2\right|^{n/2} \exp\left[i n \arctan(b/a)\right], \end{aligned} \tag{10.13f, g}$$

for example:

$$\begin{aligned} e^{-x \pm ix} \leftrightarrow (-1 \pm i)^n &= \left(\sqrt{2}\, e^{\pm i 3\pi/4}\right)^n = 2^{n/2} e^{\pm i 3\pi n/4} \\ &= 2^{n/2}\left[\cos(3\pi n/4) \pm i \sin(3\pi n/4)\right], \end{aligned} \tag{10.13h, i}$$

and also:

$$\begin{aligned} \cos, \sin(ax) = \frac{e^{iax} \pm e^{-iax}}{\{2, 2i\}} &\leftrightarrow \frac{(ia)^n \pm (-ia)^n}{\{2, 2i\}} = a^n \frac{\left(e^{i\pi/2}\right)^n \pm \left(e^{-i\pi/2}\right)^n}{\{2, 2i\}} \\ &= a^n \frac{e^{in\pi/2} \pm e^{-in\pi/2}}{\{2, 2i\}} = a^n \cos, \sin(n\pi/2). \end{aligned} \tag{10.13j–m}$$

Use of the relations (10.13a–c, h, i) transforms: (i) the differential equation (10.1) with the fourth, sixth, and seventh terms on the right-hand side (r.h.s.) to the finite difference equation (10.12); (ii) the corresponding terms of the complete integral (10.7) to solution (10.14):

$$y_n = A + 2^{n/2}\left[B \cos\left(\frac{\pi n}{4}\right) + C \sin\left(\frac{\pi n}{4}\right)\right] + \frac{3^n}{34} + \frac{2^{n-2}}{5} - \frac{(-2)^{n-2}}{3} - \frac{(-)^n}{4} - \frac{(-3)^n}{40}. \tag{10.14}$$

The solution (10.14) [complete integral (10.11)] of the linear finite difference (differential) equation (10.12) [(10.8)]: (i) have been obtained using the transformations (10.13a–m) [(10.10a–d)] applied to the equivalent linear differential equation with constant coefficients (10.1) and its complete integral (10.7); (ii) can be confirmed using directly the methods in the section(s) 1.9 (1.7–1.8).

EXAMPLE 10.2 Energies, Dissipation, and Power of an Oscillation

For a linear harmonic oscillator, obtain the exact (a) time dependences and (b) average over a period starting at any time of: (i) the potential, kinetic, and total energies and the dissipation for free damped subcritical oscillations, and check the agreement with the particular case of weak damping (E10.2.1–E10.2.2); (ii) the potential, kinetic, and total energies and the power of the applied force for the undamped forcing with resonance, and check the agreement with the particular case of slow amplitude growth in a period (E10.2.3–E10.2.4).

E10.2.1 Potential, Kinetic, and Total Energies

Omitting the phase shift (10.15a), the potential, kinetic, and total energies of the harmonic oscillator with subcritical damping (2.106b, c) are given, respectively, by (10.15b–d) using (2.105d):

$$\alpha = 0: \quad \Phi(t) = \frac{k}{2}\left[x(t)\right]^2 = \frac{ka^2}{2} e^{-2\lambda t} \cos^2(\bar{\omega} t) = \frac{ka^2}{4} e^{-2\lambda t}\left[1 + \cos(2\bar{\omega} t)\right], \tag{10.15a, b}$$

$$\begin{aligned} E_v(t) &= \frac{1}{2} m\left[\dot{x}(t)\right]^2 = \frac{ka^2}{2\,\omega_0^2} e^{-2\lambda t}\left[\bar{\omega}\sin(\bar{\omega} t) + \lambda\cos(\bar{\omega} t)\right]^2 \\ &= \frac{ka^2}{2\omega_0^2} e^{-2\lambda t}\left[\bar{\omega}^2 \sin^2(\bar{\omega} t) + \lambda^2\cos^2(\bar{\omega} t) + 2\lambda\bar{\omega}\cos(\bar{\omega} t)\sin(\bar{\omega} t)\right] \qquad (10.15c) \\ &= \frac{ka^2}{4} e^{-2\lambda t}\left[1 + \frac{2\lambda\bar{\omega}}{\omega_0^2}\sin(2\bar{\omega} t) + \frac{\lambda^2 - \bar{\omega}^2}{\omega_0^2}\cos(2\bar{\omega} t)\right], \end{aligned}$$

$$E(t) = \Phi(t) + E_v(t) = \frac{ka^2}{2} e^{-2\lambda t}\left[1 + \frac{\lambda\bar{\omega}}{\omega_0^2}\sin(2\bar{\omega} t) + \frac{\lambda^2}{\omega_0^2}\cos(2\bar{\omega} t)\right]. \tag{10.15d}$$

The exact average values over a period starting at an arbitrary time t and ending at $t+\overline{\tau}_1$ are given by:

$$\langle\Phi(t)\rangle, \langle E_v(t)\rangle, \langle E(t)\rangle$$
$$= \frac{ka^2}{4}\left\{I_0 + I_+,\quad I_0 + \frac{2\lambda\overline{\omega}}{\omega_0^2}I_- + \frac{\lambda^2 - \overline{\omega}^2}{\omega_0^2}I_+,\quad 2I_0 + \frac{2\lambda\overline{\omega}}{\omega_0^2}I_- + \frac{2\lambda^2}{\omega_0^2}I_+\right\}, \tag{10.16a–c}$$

involving the integrals:

$$I_0 = \frac{1}{\overline{\tau}}\int_t^{t+\overline{\tau}} e^{-2\lambda t}dt = \frac{\overline{\omega}}{2\pi}\left[\frac{e^{-2\lambda t}}{-2\lambda}\right]_t^{t+2\pi/\overline{\omega}} = \frac{\overline{\omega}}{4\pi\lambda}e^{-2\lambda t}\left(1 - e^{-4\pi\lambda/\overline{\omega}}\right), \tag{10.17a}$$

$$I_\pm = \frac{1}{\overline{\tau}}\int_t^{t+\overline{\tau}} e^{-2\lambda t}\cos,\sin(2\overline{\omega}t)dt = \frac{\overline{\omega}}{2\pi}\mathrm{Re},\mathrm{Im}\left\{\int_t^{t+2\pi/\overline{\omega}} e^{-2\lambda t + i2\overline{\omega}t}\,dt\right\}$$
$$= -\frac{\overline{\omega}}{4\pi}\mathrm{Re},\mathrm{Im}\left\{\frac{1}{\lambda - i\overline{\omega}}\left[e^{-2(\lambda - i\overline{\omega})t}\right]_t^{t+2\pi/\overline{\omega}}\right\} \tag{10.17b}$$
$$= \frac{\overline{\omega}}{4\pi}\mathrm{Re},\mathrm{Im}\left\{\frac{\lambda + i\overline{\omega}}{\lambda^2 + \overline{\omega}^2}e^{-2(\lambda - i\overline{\omega})t}\left(1 - e^{-4\pi\lambda/\overline{\omega}}\right)\right\};$$

the latter splits into:

$$\{I_+, I_-\} = \frac{\overline{\omega}}{4\pi}\frac{1 - e^{-4\pi\lambda/\overline{\omega}}}{\omega_0^2}e^{-2\lambda t}$$
$$\times\left\{\lambda\cos(2\overline{\omega}t) - \overline{\omega}\sin(2\overline{\omega}t),\ \lambda\sin(2\overline{\omega}t) + \overline{\omega}\cos(2\overline{\omega}t)\right\}. \tag{10.18a, b}$$

Substituting (10.17a; 10.18a, b) in (10.16a–c) specifies the exact average over a period (10.19a) of, respectively. (10.19b/c/d) the potential (10.15b), kinetic (10.15c). and total energies (10.15d) of a subcritically damped harmonic oscillator:

$$(t, t+\overline{\tau}) \equiv (t, t+2\pi/\overline{\omega}): \qquad \langle\Phi(t)\rangle, \langle E_v(t)\rangle, \langle E(t)\rangle = \frac{ka^2}{16\pi}e^{-2\lambda t}\left(1 - e^{-4\pi\lambda/\overline{\omega}}\right)$$
$$\times\left\{\frac{\overline{\omega}}{\lambda} + \frac{\lambda\overline{\omega}}{\omega_0^2}\cos(2\overline{\omega}t) - \frac{\overline{\omega}^2}{\omega_0^2}\sin(2\overline{\omega}t),\ \frac{\overline{\omega}}{\lambda} + \frac{\overline{\omega}\lambda}{\omega_0^2}\cos(2\overline{\omega}t)\right.$$
$$\left. + \frac{\overline{\omega}^2}{\omega_0^2}\sin(2\overline{\omega}t),\ 2\frac{\overline{\omega}}{\lambda} + \frac{2\overline{\omega}\lambda}{\omega_0^2}\cos(2\overline{\omega}t)\right\}. \tag{10.19a–d}$$

The total energy decays for strong (E10.2.1) or weak (E10.2.2) damping.

E10.2.2 Strong Subcritical or Weakly Damped Oscillations

The dissipation (10.20a) is related to the kinetic energy (10.15c) by (10.20b):

$$\Psi(t) = -\mu\left[\dot{x}(t)\right]^2 = -\frac{2\mu}{m}E_v(t) = -4\lambda E_v(t); \tag{10.20a–c}$$

thus, the average of the dissipation over a period (10.19a) is given (10.19c) by (10.21b):

$$\begin{aligned}\langle\Psi(t)\rangle &= -4\lambda\langle E_v(t)\rangle = -\frac{ka^2}{4\pi}e^{-2\lambda t}\left(1-e^{4\pi\lambda/\bar{\omega}}\right)\\ &\times\left[\bar{\omega}+\frac{\bar{\omega}\lambda^2}{\omega_0^2}\cos(2\bar{\omega}t)+\frac{\bar{\omega}^2\lambda}{\omega_0^2}\sin(2\bar{\omega}t)\right].\end{aligned} \tag{10.21a, b}$$

The time derivative of the total energy (10.15d) is balanced by the dissipation (10.20a) at any time in the absence of external forces, that is, $A = 0$ in (2.12); thus, the same relation applies to the time derivative of the average of the total energy over a period (10.19d) that is given (10.20a–c; 10.21a, b) by (10.22a):

$$\begin{aligned}\frac{d\left[\langle E(t)\rangle\right]}{dt} &= \frac{ka^2}{4\pi}e^{-2\lambda t}\left(1-e^{4\pi\lambda/\bar{\omega}}\right)\\ &\times\left[\bar{\omega}+\frac{\bar{\omega}\lambda^2}{\omega_0^2}\cos(2\bar{\omega}t)+\frac{\bar{\omega}^2\lambda}{\omega_0^2}\cos(2\bar{\omega}t)\right] = -\langle\psi(t)\rangle,\end{aligned} \tag{10.22a, b}$$

minus the dissipation (10.21b), both averaged over a period (10.22b). In the case of weak damping (10.23a), substitution of (10.23b) gives (10.23c):

$$\lambda^2 << \omega_0^2 \sim \bar{\omega}^2: \qquad 1-e^{-4\pi\lambda/\bar{\omega}} \sim \frac{4\pi\lambda}{\bar{\omega}} \sim \frac{4\pi\lambda}{\omega_0}. \tag{10.23a–c}$$

Substituting in (10.19b–d) yields, respectively, the mean values over a period of the potential (10.24a), kinetic (10.24b), and total (10.24c, d) energies:

$$\begin{aligned}\langle\Phi(t)\rangle &= \frac{ka^2}{16\pi}e^{-2\lambda t}\frac{4\pi\lambda}{\omega_0}\left[\frac{\omega_0}{\lambda}+\frac{\lambda}{\omega_0}\cos(2\omega_0 t)-\sin(2\omega_0 t)\right]\\ &= \frac{ka^2}{4}e^{-2\lambda t}\left[1-\frac{\lambda}{\omega_0}\sin(2\omega_0 t)+O\left(\frac{\lambda^2}{\omega_0^2}\right)\right],\end{aligned} \tag{10.24a}$$

$$\begin{aligned}\langle E_v(t)\rangle &= \frac{k a^2}{16\pi} e^{-2\lambda t} \frac{4\pi\lambda}{\omega_0}\left[\frac{\omega_0}{\lambda} + \frac{\lambda}{\omega_0}\cos(2\omega_0 t) + \sin(2\omega_0 t)\right] \\ &= \frac{k a^2}{4} e^{-2\lambda t}\left[1 + \frac{\lambda}{\omega_0}\sin(2\omega_0 t) + O\left(\frac{\lambda^2}{\omega_0^2}\right)\right],\end{aligned} \tag{10.24b}$$

$$\lambda^2 << \omega_0^2: \qquad \langle E(t)\rangle = \frac{k a^2}{16\pi} e^{-2\lambda t} \frac{4\pi\lambda}{\omega_0} 2\frac{\omega_0}{\lambda} = \frac{k a^2}{2} e^{-2\lambda t}. \tag{10.24c, d}$$

The further assumption (10.25a) that is met by (10.25b) leads to the equipartition of potential energy and kinetic energy (10.25c–e):

$$\sin(2\omega_0 t) << \frac{\omega_0}{\lambda}: \quad \omega_0 >> \lambda, \quad \frac{k a^2}{4} e^{-2\lambda t} = \langle \Phi(t)\rangle = \langle E_v(T)\rangle = \frac{\langle E(t)\rangle}{2}. \tag{10.25a–e}$$

Thus, for (problem 10) a subcritically damped oscillator (2.106a–c) omitting the phase (10.15a): (i)(ii) the instantaneous value (average over a period) are given by (10.15b/c/d) [(10.19b/c/d)] for the potential/kinetic/total energies and by (10.20a–c) [(10.21a, b)] for the dissipation; (iii) in the case (problem 11) of weak damping (10.24c) the total energy (10.24d) decays at twice the damping rate; (iv) with the further assumption (10.25a) there is equipartition (10.25c–e) of potential and kinetic energies; (v) the assumption (10.25a) is met by (10.25b), which implies negligible damping, except in the exponential term $\exp(-2\lambda t)$*, which is much smaller than unity for* $2t > 1/\lambda$ *but is close to unity for short time* $t << 2/\lambda$.

E10.2.3 Averages over a Period of Energies and Power

In the case of the resonance of an undamped oscillator, the potential (2.177a), kinetic (2.177b), and total (2.177c) energies, should be considered, respectively (10.26a/b/c), and also the activity or power (2.180a) of the applied force (10.26d):

$$\Phi(t) = \frac{k}{2}\left[x_*(t)\right]^2 = \frac{k f_a^2}{8\omega_0^2} t^2 \sin^2(\omega_0 t) = \frac{m f_a^2}{8} t^2 \sin^2(\omega_0 t), \tag{10.26a}$$

$$\begin{aligned}E_v(t) &= \frac{m}{2}\left[\dot{x}_*(t)\right]^2 = \frac{m f_a^2}{8\omega_0^2}\left[\sin(\omega_0 t) + \omega_0 t\cos(\omega_0 t)\right]^2 \\ &= \frac{m f_a^2}{8\omega_0^2}\left[\sin^2(\omega_0 t) + \omega_0 t \sin(2\omega_0 t) + (\omega_0 t)^2\cos^2(\omega_0 t)\right],\end{aligned} \tag{10.26b}$$

$$E(t) = \Phi(t) + E_v(t) = \frac{m}{8} f_a^2\left[t^2 + \frac{t}{\omega_0}\sin(2\omega_0 t) + \frac{1}{\omega_0^2}\sin^2(\omega_0 t)\right], \tag{10.26c}$$

$$A(t) = f(t)\,\dot{x}_*(t) = \frac{m\,f_a^2}{2\,\omega_0}\cos(\omega_0\,t)\left[\sin(\omega_0\,t) + \omega_0\,t\cos(\omega_0\,t)\right]$$
$$= \frac{m\,f_a^2}{4\omega_0}\left[\sin(2\,\omega_0\,t) + 2\,\omega_0\,t\,\cos^2(\omega_0\,t)\right]. \tag{10.26d}$$

The averages over a period starting at time t and ending at time $t+\tau_0$ are given by:

$$\langle\Phi(t)\rangle\,,\,\langle E_v(t)\rangle,\langle E(t)\rangle,\,\langle A(t)\rangle = \frac{m\,f_a^2}{8\,\omega_0^2}$$
$$\times\left\{J_-\,,\frac{1}{2} + J_0 + J_+\,,\,\frac{1}{2} + J_0 + J_+ + J_-\,,\,4\,\omega_0\,J_1\right\}, \tag{10.27a–d}$$

involving besides (2.116c; 2.117a, b) the integrals:

$$\{J_0,\,J_1,J_\pm\} = \frac{1}{\tau_0}\int_t^{t+\tau_0}\left\{\omega_0 t\sin(2\omega_0 t),\omega_0 t\cos^2(\omega_0 t),\omega_0^2\,t^2\cos^2,\,\sin^2(\omega_0 t)\right\}dt\,, \tag{10.28a–d}$$

to be evaluated exactly.

The first integral (10.28a) is evaluated by a single integration by parts:

$$J_0 = -\frac{1}{2\tau_0}\int_t^{t+\tau_0} t\,\frac{d}{dt}\left[\cos(2\omega_0 t)\right]dt$$
$$= -\frac{1}{2\tau_0}\left[t\cos(2\omega_0 t)\right]_t^{t+\tau_0} + \frac{\omega_0}{4\pi}\int_t^{t+2\pi/\omega_0}\cos(2\omega_0 t)\,dt \tag{10.29}$$
$$= -\frac{1}{2}\cos(2\omega_0 t) + \frac{1}{8\pi}\left[\sin(2\omega_0 t)\right]_t^{t+\tau_0} = -\frac{1}{2}\cos(2\omega_0 t).$$

The second integral (10.28b) is also evaluated by parts:

$$J_1 = \frac{1}{2\tau_0}\int_t^{t+\tau_0}\omega_0\,t\,\left[1 + \cos(2\omega_0 t)\right]dt$$
$$= \frac{\omega_0}{4\tau_0}\left[t^2\right]_t^{t+\tau_0} + \frac{1}{4\tau_0}\int_t^{t+\tau_0} t\left\{\frac{d}{dt}\left[\sin(2\omega_0 t)\right]\right\}dt$$
$$= \frac{\omega_0}{4\tau_0}\left[(t+\tau_0)^2 - t^2\right] + \frac{1}{4\tau_0}\left[t\sin(2\omega_0 t)\right]_t^{t+\tau_0} - \frac{1}{4\tau_0}\int_t^{t+\tau_0}\sin(2\omega_0 t)\,dt \tag{10.30}$$
$$= \frac{\omega_0}{4}(2t + \tau_0) + \frac{1}{4}\sin(2\omega_0 t) + \frac{1}{8\tau_0\omega_0}\left[\cos(2\omega_0 t)\right]_t^{t+\tau_0}$$
$$= \frac{\omega_0 t}{2} + \frac{\pi}{2} + \frac{1}{4}\sin(2\omega_0 t)\,,$$

so that only the remaining pair is (10.28c, d).

The last two integrals (10.28c, d) are evaluated by:

$$J_\pm = \frac{1}{2\tau_0}\int_t^{t+\tau_0} (\omega_0 t)^2 \left[1 \pm \cos(2\omega_0 t)\right] dt$$

$$= \frac{\omega_0^2}{6\tau_0}\left[t^3\right]_t^{t+\tau_0} \pm \frac{1}{4\tau_0\omega_0}\int_t^{t+\tau_0} (\omega_0 t)^2 \left\{\frac{d}{dt}\left[\sin(2\omega_0 t)\right]\right\} dt$$

$$= \frac{\omega_0^2}{6\tau_0}\left[\left(t+\tau_0\right)^3 - t^3\right] \pm \frac{1}{8\pi}\left[(\omega_0 t)^2 \sin(2\omega_0 t)\right]_t^{t+\tau_0} \mp \frac{1}{2\tau_0}\int_t^{t+\tau_0} \omega_0 t \sin(2\omega_0 t)\, dt$$

$$= \frac{\omega_0^2}{6}\left(3t^2 + 3t\tau_0 + \tau_0^2\right) \pm \frac{1}{8\pi}\omega_0^2\,\tau_0\left(2t+\tau_0\right)\sin(2\omega_0 t) \pm \frac{1}{4}\cos(2\omega_0 t); \tag{10.31}$$

the last term on the r.h.s. of (10.31) is J_0 in (10.28a), which is specified by (10.29), so that no more integrations by parts are needed:

$$J_\pm = \frac{\omega_0^2 t^2}{2} + \pi\omega_0 t + \frac{2\pi^2}{3} \pm \left(\frac{\omega_0 t}{2} + \frac{\pi}{2}\right)\sin(2\omega_0 t) \pm \frac{1}{4}\cos(2\omega_0 t), \tag{10.32a, b}$$

to obtain the integrals (10.28c, d).

E10.2.4 Balance of Forcing and Fast Amplification

The integrals (10.32a, b) together with (10.29; 10.30) ≡ (10.33a, b):

$$J_0 = -\frac{1}{2}\cos(2\omega_0 t), \qquad J_1 = \frac{\pi}{2} + \frac{\omega_0 t}{2} + \frac{1}{4}\sin(2\omega_0 t), \tag{10.33a, b}$$

substituted in (10.27a–d) yield (10.34a–d):

$$\langle\Phi(t)\rangle,\ \langle E_v(t)\rangle,\langle E(t),\rangle,\ \langle A(t)\rangle = \frac{m f_a^2}{16\omega_0^2}$$

$$\times\Big\{\ \omega_0^2 t^2 + 2\pi\omega_0 t + \frac{4\pi^2}{3} - (\pi + \omega_0 t)\ \sin(2\omega_0 t) - \frac{1}{2}\cos(2\omega_0 t),$$

$$1 + \omega_0^2 t^2 + 2\pi\omega_0 t + \frac{4\pi^2}{3} + (\pi + \omega_0 t)\sin(2\omega_0 t) - \frac{1}{2}\cos(2\omega_0 t),$$

$$1 + 2\omega_0^2 t^2 + 4\pi\omega_0 t + \frac{8\pi^2}{3} - \cos(2\omega_0 t)\,,\ 4\pi\omega_0 + 4\omega_0^2 t + 2\omega_0\sin(2\omega_0 t)\Big\}. \tag{10.34a–d}$$

The activity of the applied forces (10.34d) equals the rate of change of the total energy (10.34c):

$$\frac{d}{dt}\left[\langle E(t)\rangle\right] = \frac{d}{dt}\left\{\frac{f_a^2 m}{16\omega_0^2}\left[2\omega_0^2 t^2 + 4\pi\omega_0 t - \cos(2\omega_0 t)\right]\right\}$$
$$= \frac{f_a^2 m}{16\omega_0^2}\left[4\omega_0^2 t + 4\pi\omega_0 + 2\omega_0 \sin(2\omega_0 t)\right] = \langle A(t)\rangle. \quad (10.35)$$

If has been proved that *an undamped harmonic oscillator (problem 29) corresponds to: (i) the displacement (2.176b) and velocity (2.176c); (ii) the potential energy (2.177a) ≡ (10.26a), the kinetic-energy (2.177b) ≡ (10.26b), and the total energy (2.130) ≡ (10.26c), and the activity (2.180a) ≡ (10.26d) of the applied force; (iii) their exact average over the period from t to* $t + \tau_0$ *is given exactly by (10.34a–d); (iv) the terms growing fastest with time t are:*

$$\langle \Phi(t)\rangle = \langle E_v(t)\rangle = m\left(\frac{f_a t}{4}\right)^2 = \frac{\langle E(t)\rangle}{2}, \quad \langle A(t)\rangle = \frac{m f_a^2 t}{4} = \frac{d}{dt}\left[\langle E(t)\rangle\right], \quad (10.36a–c)$$

in agreement with (2.178a–c; 2.179b) valid for amplitude varying slowly over a wave period; (v) within the latter approximation (iv) there is equipartition of the potential (10.36a) and kinetic (10.36b) energies, whose sum is the total energy (10.36c), growing like the square of time t due to the work of the applied forces growing linearly in time.

EXAMPLE 10.3 Power-Law Forcing of a Harmonic Oscillator

Determine the forced displacement for a one-dimensional, linear, undamped (10.37a) harmonic oscillator with natural frequency ω_0:

$$\lambda = 0: \qquad \ddot{x} + \omega_0^2 x = f_a t^n, \quad f_a t \cos(\omega_a t), \quad (10.37a–c)$$

to which an external force is applied whose dependence on time t is specified by: (i) a power (10.37b); (ii) time multiplied by a sinusoidal function (10.37c) with frequency ω_a. Consider also the forcings:

$$\ddot{x} + 2\lambda\dot{x} + \omega_0^2 x = f_a t, f_a t \cos(\omega_a t), \quad (10.38a, b)$$

in the damped case with damping λ.

E10.3.1 Power-Law Monotonic and Oscillating Forcing

The undamped (10.37a) harmonic oscillator (10.37b, c) corresponds to the characteristic polynomial (10.39a):

$$P_2(D) = D^2 + \omega_0^2: \qquad f_0\, t^n = f_0 \lim_{a\to 0} \frac{\partial^n}{\partial a^n}\left(e^{at}\right), \tag{10.39a, b}$$

and the forcing to (10.37b) ≡ (10.39b). The corresponding response is (problem 39) obtained using the inverse of the characteristic polynomial:

$$\begin{aligned}\lambda = 0: \qquad x_*(t) &= \frac{f_a}{P_2(D)} t^n = \frac{f_a}{\omega_0^2}\left(1+\frac{D^2}{\omega_0^2}\right)^{-1} t^n = \frac{f_a}{\omega_0^2}\sum_{m=0}^{\infty}\frac{(-)^m}{\omega_0^{2m}} D^{2m}\, t^n \\ &= \frac{f_a}{\omega_0^2}\sum_{m=0}^{\le n/2}\frac{(-)^m}{\omega_0^{2m}}\frac{n!}{(n-2m)!} t^{n-2m}.\end{aligned} \tag{10.40a, b}$$

The forcing (10.37c) leads to the response:

$$\begin{aligned} x_*(t) &= \mathrm{Re}\left\{\frac{f_a}{P_2(D)} t\, e^{i\omega_a t}\right\} = \mathrm{Re}\left\{f_a\, e^{i\omega_a t}\frac{1}{P_2(D+i\omega_a)} t\right\} \\ &= \mathrm{Re}\left\{\frac{f_a\, e^{i\omega_a t}}{(D+i\omega_a)^2+\omega_0^2} t\right\} = \mathrm{Re}\left\{\frac{f_a\, e^{i\omega_a t}}{\omega_0^2-\omega_a^2+2i\omega_a D+D^2} t\right\}.\end{aligned} \tag{10.41}$$

This splits into: (i) the non-resonant (10.42a, b) case (problem 40):

$$\begin{aligned}\lambda = 0,\quad \omega_0 \neq \omega_a: \quad x_*(t) &= \frac{f_a}{\omega_0^2-\omega_a^2}\,\mathrm{Re}\left\{e^{i\omega_a t}\left[1+\frac{2i\omega_a D+D^2}{\omega_0^2-\omega_a^2}\right]^{-1} t\right\} \\ &= \frac{f_a}{\omega_0^2-\omega_a^2}\,\mathrm{Re}\left\{e^{i\omega_a t}\left[1-\frac{2i\omega_a D}{\omega_0^2-\omega_a^2}+O\left(D^2\right)\right] t\right\} \\ &= \frac{f_a}{\omega_0^2-\omega_a^2}\,\mathrm{Re}\left\{e^{i\omega_a t}\left(t-\frac{2i\omega_a}{\omega_0^2-\omega_a^2}\right)\right\} \\ &= \frac{f_a}{\omega_0^2-\omega_a^2}\left[t\cos(\omega_a t)+\frac{2\omega_a}{\omega_0^2-\omega_a^2}\sin(\omega_a t)\right],\end{aligned} \tag{10.42a–c}$$

for which the amplitude of the displacement (10.42c) is a linear function of time t like the forcing (10.37c) with time $O(t)$ terms in phase; (ii) in (problem 41) the resonant case (10.43a, b) does not hold (10.42c) and (10.41) leads to (10.43c):

$$\lambda = 0: \quad \omega_0 \equiv \omega_a: \quad x_*(t) = \mathrm{Re}\left\{\frac{f_a\, e^{i\omega_a t}}{D(2i\omega_0 + D)}t\right\} = \mathrm{Re}\left\{\frac{f_a}{2i\omega_0}\frac{e^{i\omega_a t}}{D}\left(1 + \frac{D}{2i\omega_0}\right)^{-1} t\right\}$$

$$= -\mathrm{Re}\left\{\frac{i f_a}{2\,\omega_0}\frac{e^{i\omega_a t}}{D}\left(1 - \frac{D}{2i\omega_0}\right)t\right\} = -\mathrm{Re}\left\{\frac{i f_a}{2\,\omega_0}\frac{e^{i\omega_a t}}{D}\left(t - \frac{1}{2\,i\omega_0}\right)\right\}$$

$$= -\mathrm{Re}\left\{\frac{i f_a}{2\omega_0} e^{i\omega_a t}\left(\frac{t^2}{2} - \frac{t}{2i\omega_0}\right)\right\} = \frac{f_a t^2}{4\omega_0}\sin(\omega_0 t) + \frac{f_a t}{4\omega_0^2}\cos(\omega_0 t), \tag{10.43a–c}$$

showing that the amplitude of the displacement is a quadratic function of time t (10.43c) instead of linear for the forcing (10.37c) and the highest order term $O(t^2)$ in (10.43c) is out-of-phase by $\pi/2$ relative to the forcing (10.37c), that is, $O(t)$. Setting (10.44b) in (10.42c) leads to (10.44d):

$$\lambda = 0,\ \omega_a = 0,\ n = 1: \qquad x_*(t) = \frac{f_a t}{\omega_0^2}, \tag{10.44a–d}$$

which is the same result (10.44d) ≡ (10.40b) for (10.44c). It has been shown that *the undamped (10.37a) harmonic (10.37b) oscillator with forcings (10.37b) [(10.37c)] has displacements (10.40a, b) [(10.42a, c)/(10.43a, c)], respectively, in the [non-resonant/resonant cases]. The non-resonant (resonant) cases differ in that the amplitude of the displacement is a function of time t with the same exponent (exponent one unit higher) than the forcing and the highest powers are in-phase (out-of-phase by $\pi/2$).*

E10.3.2 Forcing of an Undamped and Damped Oscillator

The undamped (damped) harmonic oscillator (10.37a, b)[(10.38a)] has the characteristic polynomial (10.39a) [(10.45a)] and the forcing term in (10.37c) [(10.38a)] is (10.39b) [(10.45b)]:

$$P_2(D) = D^2 + 2\lambda D + \omega_0^2: \qquad f_0\, t = f_0 = \lim_{a \to 0}\frac{\partial}{\partial a}\left(e^{at}\right). \tag{10.45a, b}$$

The forcing of the damped harmonic oscillator by a function linear on time t (10.38a) has response (problem 42):

$$x_*(t) = \frac{f_a}{P_2(D)}t = \frac{f_a}{\omega_0^2 + 2\lambda D + D^2}t = \frac{f_a}{\omega_0^2}\left(1 + \frac{2\lambda D + D^2}{\omega_0^2}\right)^{-1} t$$

$$= \frac{f_a}{\omega_0^2}\left[1 - \frac{2\lambda}{\omega_0^2}D + O\left(D^2\right)\right]t = \frac{f_a t}{\omega_0^2} - \frac{2 f_a \lambda}{\omega_0^4}. \tag{10.46}$$

In the case of $\lambda = 0$ of no damping (10.46) simplifies to (10.44d). The forcing of the damped harmonic oscillator (10.38b) linear on time t with a sinusoidal factor has response (problem 43):

$$
\begin{aligned}
x_*(t) &= \operatorname{Re}\left\{\frac{f_a}{P_2(D)}\, t\, e^{i\omega_a t}\right\} = \operatorname{Re}\left\{\frac{f_a e^{i\omega_a t}}{P_2(D+i\omega_a)}\, t\right\} \\
&= \operatorname{Re}\left\{\frac{f_a\, e^{i\omega_a t}}{\omega_0^2 + 2\lambda(D+i\omega_a) + (D+i\omega_a)^2}\, t\right\} \\
&= \operatorname{Re}\left\{\frac{f_a\, e^{i\omega_a t}}{\omega_0^2 - \omega_a^2 + 2i\lambda\omega_a + 2(\lambda + i\omega_a)D + D^2}\, t\right\} \\
&= \operatorname{Re}\left\{\frac{f_a\, e^{i\omega_a t}}{\omega_0^2 - \omega_a^2 + 2i\lambda\omega_a}\left[1 + \frac{2(\lambda+i\omega_a)D + D^2}{\omega_0^2 - \omega_a^2 + 2i\lambda\omega_a}\right]^{-1} t\right\} \\
&= \operatorname{Re}\left\{f_a\, e^{i\omega_a t}\, \frac{\omega_0^2 - \omega_a^2 - 2i\lambda\omega_a}{\left(\omega_0^2 - \omega_a^2\right)^2 + 4\lambda^2\omega_a^2}\left[1 - \frac{2(\lambda+i\omega_a)D}{\omega_0^2 - \omega_a^2 + 2i\lambda\omega_a}\right] t\right\} \\
&= f_a\, t\, \frac{\left(\omega_0^2 - \omega_a^2\right)\cos(\omega_a t) + 2\lambda\omega_a \sin(\omega_a t)}{\left(\omega_0^2 - \omega_a^2\right)^2 + 4\lambda^2\omega_a^2} \\
&\quad - \frac{2 f_a}{\left[\left(\omega_0^2 - \omega_a^2\right)^2 + 4\lambda^2\omega_a^2\right]^2}\left\{\lambda\left[\left(\omega_0^2 + \omega_a^2\right)^2 - 4\omega_a^2\left(\omega_a^2 + \lambda^2\right)\right]\right. \\
&\quad \left.\cos(\omega_a t) - \omega_a\left[\left(\omega_0^2 - \omega_0^2\right)^2 + 4\lambda^2\omega_0^2\right]\sin(\omega_a t)\right\}.
\end{aligned}
\tag{10.47}
$$

In the last term on the r.h.s. of (10.47) was used:

$$
\begin{aligned}
(\lambda + i\omega_a)\left(\omega_0^2 - \omega_a^2 - 2i\lambda\omega_a\right)^2 &= (\lambda + i\omega_a)\left[\left(\omega_0^2 - \omega_a^2\right)^2 - 4\lambda^2\omega_a^2 - 4i\lambda\omega_a\left(\omega_0^2 - \omega_a^2\right)\right] \\
&= \lambda\left[\left(\omega_0^2 - \omega_a^2\right)^2 - 4\lambda^2\omega_a^2 + 4\omega_a^2\left(\omega_0^2 - \omega_a^2\right)\right] \\
&\quad + i\omega_a\left[\left(\omega_0^2 - \omega_a^2\right)^2 - 4\lambda^2\omega_a^2 - 4\lambda^2\left(\omega_0^2 - \omega_a^2\right)\right] \\
&= \lambda\left[\left(\omega_0^2 + \omega_a^2\right)^2 - 4\omega_a^2\left(\omega_a^2 + \lambda^2\right)\right] \\
&\quad + i\omega_a\left[\left(\omega_0^2 - \omega_a^2\right)^2 - 4\lambda^2\omega_0^2\right].
\end{aligned}
\tag{10.48}
$$

In the resonant (10.49a) case (10.47) simplifies to (10.49b):

$$\omega_a = \omega_0: \qquad x_*(t) = \frac{f_a t}{2\lambda\omega_0}\sin(\omega_0 t) + \frac{f_a}{2\lambda\omega_0}\left[\frac{\cos(\omega_0 t)}{\omega_0} + \frac{\sin(\omega_0 t)}{\lambda}\right]. \qquad (10.49\text{a, b})$$

In (problem 44) the absence (10.42a) of damping (10.47) simplifies to (10.42c). It has been shown that *the damped harmonic oscillator with forcings (10.38a) [(10.38b)] has displacements (10.46)[(10.47)]. The latter (10.47) simplifies to (10.49b) [(10.42c)] in the resonant (10.49a) [undamped (10.42a)] case. The undamped (10.43a) resonant case (10.43b) leads to the displacement (10.43c).*

EXAMPLE 10.4 Five Standards of First-Order Differential Equations

Classify the following five first-order linear differential equations (10.50a–10.54a):

$$\text{L:} \qquad y' = y\log x, \qquad y(x) = C\,e^{-x}x^x, \qquad (10.50\text{a, b})$$

$$\text{LII:} \qquad y' = -\frac{y}{x} + \cos x, \qquad y(x) = \frac{C}{x} + \sin x + \frac{\cos x}{x}, \qquad (10.51\text{a, b})$$

$$\text{LIII, LXIV:} \qquad y' = \frac{y}{x} + \frac{y^2}{x^2}, \qquad y(x) = \frac{x}{C - \log x}, \qquad (10.52\text{a, b})$$

$$\text{LXIV:} \qquad y' = \frac{y^2 - x^2}{xy}, \qquad y(x) = x\sqrt{C - 2\log x} \qquad (10.53\text{a, b})$$

$$\text{LV:} \qquad y' = y - y^2 - \frac{1}{x}; \qquad y(x) = \frac{1}{x} + \frac{e^x}{x^2}\left(C + \int^x \frac{e^\xi}{\xi^2}\,d\xi\right)^{-1}, \qquad (10.54\text{a, b})$$

and use the appropriate method to obtain the respective general integrals (10.50b–10.54b), where C is an arbitrary constant.

The first differential equation (10.50a) is (subsection 3.2.1), separable (standard L) and thus, (10.55a) integrable by quadratures leading to (10.55b) ≡ (10.50b):

$$\int \frac{dy}{y} = \int \log x\,dx, \qquad \log y = \log C + x\log x - x. \qquad (10.55\text{a, b})$$

The second differential equation (10.51a) ≡ (3.28) is (section 3.3) linear forced (standard LII) with coefficients (10.51a, b), leading (3.20a; 3.31a) to (10.51c, d):

$$P=-\frac{1}{x}, \quad Q=\cos x: \qquad X(x)=\exp\left\{-\int^{x}\frac{d\xi}{\xi}\right\}=\exp(-\log x)=\frac{1}{x}, \tag{10.56a–c}$$

$$Y(x)=\int^{x}\xi\cos\xi\,d\xi=x\sin x-\int^{x}\sin\xi\,d\xi=x\sin x+\cos x, \tag{10.56d}$$

where an integration by parts in (10.56d) was performed; substitution of (10.56c, d) in (3.31b) leads to the general integral (10.51b).

The third differential equation (10.52a) is both (section 3.4) of a Bernoulli type (standard LII) and (subsections 3.7.1–3.7.3) homogeneous (standard LXIV). As a Bernoulli type (3.38) it has coefficients (10.57a, b) leading (3.48a, b) to (10.57c, d):

$$P=\frac{1}{x}, Q=\frac{1}{x^2}: \quad X_2(x)=\exp\left\{-\int^{x}\frac{d\xi}{\xi}\right\}=\frac{1}{x}, \quad Y_2(x)=-\int^{x}\frac{d\xi}{\xi}=-\log x; \tag{10.57a–d}$$

the order is (10.58a) leading on substitution of (10.57c, d) in (3.43b) to (10.58b) ≡ (10.52b):

$$n=2: \qquad \frac{1}{y(x)}=\frac{1}{x}(C-\log x). \tag{10.58a, b}$$

Taken as a homogeneous equation (3.127) then (10.52a) involves the function (10.59a) leading (3.133) to (10.59b):

$$f(v)=v+v^2: \qquad x=e^{C}\exp\int^{y/x}\frac{dv}{v^2}=e^{C}\exp\left(-\frac{x}{y}\right), \tag{10.59a, b}$$

which can be solved for y leading to (10.52b) ≡ (10.59b) ≡ (10.58b).

The fourth differential equation (10.53a) is (subsections 3.7.1–3.7.3) homogeneous (standard LXIV) with (3.127) function (10.60a) leading (3.133) to (10.60):

$$f(v)=v-\frac{1}{v}: \qquad e^{-C/2}x=\exp\left\{-\int^{y/x}v\,dv\right\}=\exp\left(-\frac{y^2}{2x^2}\right), \tag{10.60a, b}$$

which when solved for y gives (10.60b). The fifth differential equation (10.54a) is of the Riccati type (standard LV), with (3.58) coefficients (10.61a–c) and a particular integral is (10.61d) leading (3.63a–d) to (10.61e–g):

$$Q=-\frac{1}{x},\ P=1, R=-1:\quad g_1(x)=\frac{1}{x},$$

$$Z(x)=\exp\int^x\left(1-\frac{2}{\xi}\right)d\xi=\frac{e^x}{x^2}=\frac{1}{X(x)},\quad Y(x)=\int^x\frac{e^\xi}{\xi^2}d\xi; \tag{10.61a–g}$$

substitution of (10.61d, e, g) in (3.64b) leads to the general integral (10.54b).

EXAMPLE 10.5 Integrating Factor for the Linear First-Order Differential Equation

Show that the forced linear first-order differential equation has an integrating factor that depends only on the independent variable, and use it to obtain the general integral.

The forced linear first-order differential equation (3.27) corresponds (standard LII) to the first-order differential in two variables (10.62a, b) with coefficients (10.62c, d), which is inexact because the curl (10.62e, f) is not zero (10.62g):

$$0=dy-(Py+Q)\,dx=A\,dx+B\,dy:$$

$$\{A,B\}=\{-Py-Q,1\},\quad \Omega\equiv\frac{\partial B}{\partial x}-\frac{\partial A}{\partial y}=-P\neq 0, \tag{10.62a–g}$$

the condition (3.183a) is met (10.63a, b) and thus, there exists (3.183b) an integrating factor (10.62c, d) depending only on x whose differential is (10.62e):

$$-\frac{\Omega}{B}=-P\equiv f(x):\qquad \lambda(x)=\exp\left\{-\int^x P(\xi)\,d\xi\right\}\equiv\frac{1}{X(x)},\quad d\lambda=-P\lambda dx. \tag{10.63a–e}$$

The integrating factor (10.63c) is the same as for the linear unforced first-order differential equation (3.19a) because it does not depend on Q. The general integral depends on Q and is obtained multiplying the inexact differential (10.62a) by the integrating factor (10.62b) and using its differential (10.63c) leading to an exact differential (10.64a, b):

$$\begin{aligned} 0 &= \lambda\, dy - \lambda(Py + Q)dx = \lambda\, dy + y\, d\lambda - \lambda Q\, dx \\ &= d\left\{\lambda y - \int^x \lambda(\xi) Q(\xi) d\xi\right\}, \end{aligned} \quad (10.64a, b)$$

the general integral is (10.65a, b):

$$\begin{aligned} C &= \lambda(x) y(x) - \int^x \lambda(\xi) Q(\xi) d\xi \\ &= \frac{y(x)}{X(x)} - \int^x \frac{Q(\xi)}{X(\xi)} d\xi, \end{aligned} \quad (10.65a, b)$$

which coincides with (3.31a, b) ≡ (10.65a, b), using (10.63e) ≡ (3.20a).

EXAMPLE 10.6 First-Order Differentials in Two Variables

Classify the following eight first-order differentials in two variables (10.66a–10.73a):

LXVI: $(x^2 + y^2)\, dx + y(y + 2x)\, dy = 0, \qquad x^3 + y^3 + 3xy^2 = C, \qquad (10.66a, b)$

LXVI: $\frac{x}{y^2} dx - \frac{x^2}{y^3} dy = 0, \qquad x^2 = 2Cy^2, \qquad (10.67a, b)$

LXVI: $\cos x \cos y\, dx - \sin x \sin y\, dy = 0, \qquad \sin x \cos y = C, \qquad (10.68a, b)$

LXVII: $dx + \cot x \tan y\, dy = 0, \qquad \cos x \cos y = C, \qquad (10.69a, b)$

LXIX: $2xy\, dx - x^2\, dy = 0, \qquad y = Cx^2, \qquad (10.70a, b)$

LXX: $\frac{2xy}{x+y} dx + (x - y) dy = 0, \qquad 3x^2 y - y^3 = C, \qquad (10.71a, b)$

LXXI: $3xy\, dx + 2x^2\, dx = 0, \qquad x^3 y^2 = C, \qquad (10.72a, b)$

LXXII: $3dx - \frac{2x}{y} dy = 0, \qquad y^2 = C x^3, \qquad (10.73a, b)$

into exact (inexact) followed [sections 3.8 (3.9)] by immediate integration (integration after multiplication by a suitable integrating factor). The roman numerals at the left identify the standard of the differential equation according to the classification 10.1.

E10.6.1 Exact First-Order Differentials in Two Variables

The first three differentials (10.66a–10.68a) have vector of coefficients (10.74a–10.76a) with zero curl (10.74b–10.76b) and thus, are exact (standard LXIV) and immediately integrable (10.74c–10.76c):

$$\{X,Y\}=\{x^2+y^2,y^2+2xy\}: \quad \frac{\partial X}{\partial y}=2y=\frac{\partial Y}{\partial y},$$

$$0=x^2dx+y^2dy+y^2dx+2xy\,dy=d\left(\frac{x^3+y^3}{3}+xy^2\right), \tag{10.74a–c}$$

$$\{X,Y\}=\left\{\frac{x}{y^2},-\frac{x^2}{y^3}\right\}: \quad \frac{\partial X}{\partial y}=-\frac{2x}{y^3}=\frac{\partial Y}{\partial x}, \quad 0=\frac{x\,dx}{y^2}-\frac{x^2}{y^3}dy=d\left(\frac{x^2}{2y^2}\right), \tag{10.75a–c}$$

$$\{X,Y\}=\{\cos x\cos y,-\sin x\sin y\}: \quad \frac{\partial X}{\partial y}=-\cos x\,\sin y=\frac{\partial Y}{\partial x}$$

$$0=\cos x\cos y\,dx-\sin x\sin y\,dy=d(\sin x\cos y), \tag{10.76a–c}$$

leading to the general integrals (10.74c–10.76c) ≡ (10.66b–10.68b).

E10.6.2 Inexact First-Order Differentials in Two Variables

The differentials in two variables (10.69a–10.73a) have a vector of coefficients (10.77a–10.81a) with non-zero curl (10.77b–10.81b) and hence, are inexact:

$$\{X,Y\}=\{1,\cot x\tan y\}: \quad \Omega=-\csc^2 x\,\tan y, \quad \lambda(x,y)=\sin x\cos y, \tag{10.77a–c}$$

$$\lambda(X\,dx+Y\,dy)=\sin x\cos y\,dy+\cos x\sin y\,dy=-\,d(\cos x\cos y); \tag{10.77d}$$

$$\{X,Y\}=\{2xy,-x^2\}: \quad \Omega=-4x, \quad \lambda(y)=\frac{1}{y^2}: \tag{10.78a–c}$$

$$0=\frac{2xy\,dx-x^2\,dy}{y^2}=\frac{2x}{y}dx-\frac{x^2}{y^2}dy=d\left(\frac{x^2}{y}\right); \tag{10.78d}$$

$$\{X,Y\} = \left\{\frac{2xy}{x+y}, x-y\right\}: \qquad \Omega = 1 - \frac{2x^2}{(x+y)^2}, \quad \lambda(x,y) = x+y: \tag{10.79a–c}$$

$$0 = (x+y)\left[\frac{2xy}{x+y}dx + (x-y)dy\right] = 2xy\,dy + x^2dy - y^2\,dy = d\left(x^2y - \frac{y^2}{3}\right); \tag{10.79d}$$

$$\{X,Y\} = \{3xy, 2x^2\}: \qquad \Omega = x, \quad \lambda(xy) = xy: \tag{10.80a–c}$$

$$0 = xy(3xy\,dx + 2x^2\,dy) = 3x^2y^2\,dx + 2x^3y\,dy = d(x^3y^2); \tag{10.80d}$$

$$\{X,Y\} = \left\{3, -\frac{2x}{y}\right\}: \qquad \Omega = -\frac{2}{y}, \quad \lambda(x,y) = \frac{x^2}{y^2}: \tag{10.81a–c}$$

$$0 = \frac{x^2}{y^2}\left(3dx - \frac{2x}{y}dy\right) = \frac{3x^2}{y^2}dx - \frac{2x^3}{y^3}dy = d\left(\frac{x^3}{y^2}\right); \tag{10.81d}$$

multiplication by the integrating factor (10.77c–10.81c) transforms the inexact differentials (10.69a–10.73a) to the exact differentials (10.77d–10.81d) and specifies the general integrals (10.77d–10.81d) ≡ (10.69b–10.73b). The integrating factors for inexact differentials are considered next (E10.6.3).

E10.6.3 Integrating Factors for Inexact Differentials

The integrating factor (10.77c) for the (standard LXVII) inexact differential (10.69a) is found by inspection leading to (10.77d) ≡ (10.69b). The inexact differential (10.70a) with coefficients (10.78a, b) and curl (10.78c) meets (standard LXIX) the condition (3.184a) for (10.82a, b) the existence of an integrating factor (10.82c, d) ≡ (10.78d) depending only on y:

$$\frac{\Omega}{X} = -\frac{2}{y} = g(y): \qquad \lambda(y) = \exp\left\{-2\int^y \frac{d\xi}{\xi}\right\} = \frac{1}{y^2}. \tag{10.82a, b}$$

The inexact differential (10.71a) with coefficients (10.79a, b) and curl (10.79c) meets (standard LXX) the condition (3.196a) for the existence (10.83a) of an integrating factor (10.83b) ≡ (10.79d) depending on $x + y$:

$$\frac{\Omega}{X-Y} = \frac{1}{x+y} = h(x+y): \qquad \lambda(x+y) = \exp\left\{\int^{x+y} \frac{d\xi}{\xi}\right\} = x+y. \tag{10.83a, b}$$

The inexact differential (10.72a) with coefficients (10.80a, b) and curl (10.80c) meets (standard LXXI) the condition (3.201a) for the existence (10.84a) of an integrating factor (10.84b) ≡ (10.80d) depending on xy:

$$\frac{\Omega}{Xx - Yy} = \frac{1}{xy} = j(xy): \qquad \lambda(xy) = \exp\left\{\int^{xy} \frac{d\xi}{\xi}\right\} = xy. \tag{10.84a, b}$$

The inexact differential (10.73a) with coefficients (10.81a, b) and curl (10.81c) meets (standard LXXII) the condition (3.206a) for the existence (10.85a) of an integrating factor (1–0.85b) ≡ (10.81d) depending on y/x:

$$\frac{x^2\,\Omega}{Xx + Yy} = -2\frac{x}{y} = k\left(\frac{y}{x}\right): \qquad \lambda\left(\frac{y}{x}\right) = \exp\left\{-2\int^{y/x} \frac{d\xi}{\xi}\right\} = \frac{x^2}{y^2}. \tag{10.85a, b}$$

The general integrals of the five inexact differentials in two variables are obtained using an integrating factor that depends only on: (i) one variable (10.70a; 10.82a, b); (ii–iv) the sum (10.71a; 10.83a, b), the product (10.72a; 10.84a, b), and the ratio (10.73a; 10.85a, b) of two variables; (v) the two variables (10.70a; 10.77c) in a different way from the preceding (ii–iv).

EXAMPLE 10.7 Paths Near a Stagnation Point of the Second Degree

Compare the velocity fields specified [problem 77(78)] by (10.86a, b) [(10.89a, b)], which both have a stagnation point of the second degree at the origin.

E10.7.1 Paths Tangent at a Stagnation Point of the Second Degree

Consider the velocity field:

$$\frac{dx}{dt} = v_x(x, y) = xy, \qquad \frac{dy}{dt} = v_y(x, y) = y^2 - x^2, \tag{10.86a, b}$$

and determine (problem 77) the paths near the stagnation point.

The paths are specified by the ratio of (10.87a), leading to a first-order ordinary differential equation of degree two, which is not included in the cases of first degree in section 4.1:

$$\frac{dy}{dx} = \frac{y^2 - x^2}{xy} = \frac{y}{x} - \frac{x}{y} = f\left(\frac{y}{x}\right): \qquad f(v) = v - \frac{1}{v}; \tag{10.87a, b}$$

the first-order ordinary differential equation (10.87a, b) is homogeneous (section 3.7) and has (3.133) integral (10.87c, d):

$$-\frac{C^2}{2}+\log x=\int^{y/x}\left(-\frac{1}{v}\right)^{-1}dv=-\frac{y^2}{2x^2} \tag{10.87c, d}$$

$$y^2=x^2\left(C^2-2\log x\right).$$

The integral (10.87d) curves (Figure 10.1). (i) are symmetric relative to the y-axis (10.88b) and exist in the interval with boundaries (10.88a) and (10.88 c, d); (ii) pass through the origin (10.88e) and cross (10.88f) the vertical line $x = 1$ at $y = \pm c$:

$$0\le x\left(y\right)=x(-y)\le\exp\left(\frac{C^2}{2}\right)\equiv x_{\max},\ y(0)=0,\ y\left(1\right)=\pm C, \tag{10.88a–f}$$

$$\lim_{x\to 0}\frac{y^2}{x^2}=\lim_{x\to 0}\left(C-\log x\right)=\infty,\quad \lim_{x\to\pm y}\frac{dy}{dx}=0,$$
$$\lim_{x\to 1}\frac{dy}{dx}=\pm C\mp\frac{1}{C}, \tag{10.88g–j}$$

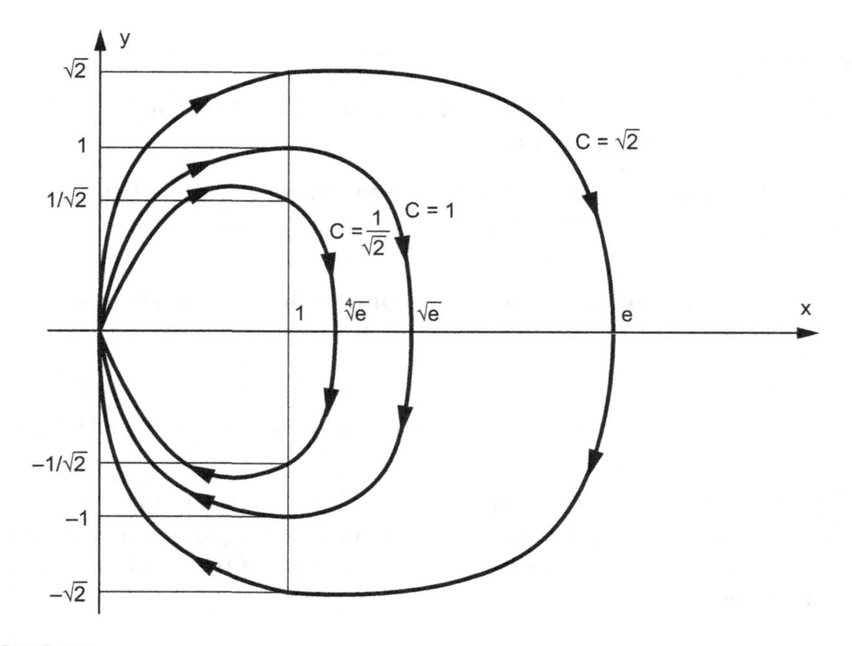

FIGURE 10.1
An example of singular point of a family of curves or streamlines is the point through which all streamlines pass with the same tangent direction.

(iii) the slope is infinite at the origin (10.88g, h) where the tangent is vertical, is zero (10.88i) at the crossing of the diagonal of quadrants and is (10.88j) at the crossing of the vertical line $x = 1$. For example the integral curve: (a) $C = 1$ crosses the x-axis at the ends of the interval $0 \le x \le \sqrt{e} = 1.649$ and has zero slope at $x = 1, y = \pm 1$; (b) $C\sqrt{2}$ crosses the x-axis at the ends of the interval $0 \le x \le e = 2.718$ and has slope $\pm\sqrt{2} \mp 1/\sqrt{2}$ at the points $x = 1, y = \pm\sqrt{2}$; (c) $C = 1/\sqrt{2}$ crosses the x-axis at the ends of the interval $0 \le x \le \sqrt[4]{e} = 1.284$ and has slope $\pm 1/\sqrt{2} \mp \sqrt{2}$ with opposite sign to the case (b) at $x = 1, y = \pm 1/\sqrt{2}$.

E10.7.2 Paths with Three Asymptotes Crossing at a Stagnation Point

Consider (problem 78) the velocity field:

$$\frac{dx}{dt} = v_x(x,y) = -2xy, \qquad \frac{dy}{dt} = v_y(x,y) = y^2 - x^2, \tag{10.89a, b}$$

and compare the paths with the preceding case (E10.7.1).

The ratio (10.90a) of (10.89a, b) specifies the paths that again are not included in (4.9a, b) in section 4.1 and involves (10.90b) one-half of the same homogeneous function as in (10.87b):

$$\frac{dy}{dx} = \frac{1}{2}\frac{x^2 - y^2}{xy} = \frac{1}{2}\left(\frac{x}{y} - \frac{y}{x}\right) = f\left(\frac{y}{x}\right), \quad f(v) = \frac{1}{2}\left(\frac{1}{v} - v\right). \tag{10.90a, b}$$

The integral curves (section 3.7) are specified (3.133) by (10.91a):

$$\log x - \frac{1}{3}\log C = 2\int^{y/x} \frac{v}{1 - 3v}\, dv = -\frac{1}{3}\log\left(1 - 3\frac{y^2}{x^2}\right); \quad x^2 - 3y^2 = \frac{C}{x}. \tag{10.91a, b}$$

The integral curves (10.91b) have asymptotes:

$$0 = \lim_{x\to\infty} \frac{C}{x} = \lim_{x\to\infty}\left(x - y\sqrt{3}\right)\left(x + y\sqrt{3}\right), \quad \infty = \lim_{x\to -0} \frac{1}{3}\left(x^2 - \frac{C}{x}\right) = \lim_{x\to 0} y^2, \tag{10.91c–f}$$

along: (i) the straight lines (10.91c, d) with slopes $\pm 1/\sqrt{3}$ making angles $\pm\pi/6$ with the x-axis; (ii) along the y-axis (10.91e, f) since $y \to \pm\infty$ as $x \to -0$. Thus the asymptotes divide the plane into six angular sectors for $\varphi = \pm\pi/6, \pm\pi/2, \pm 5\pi/6$ that are the only curves passing through the origin (Figure 10.2).

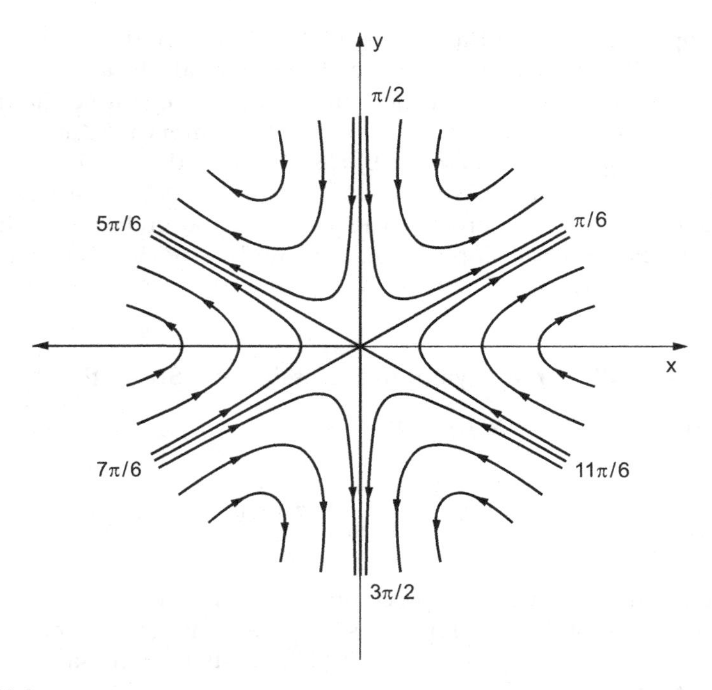

FIGURE 10.2
A different singular point from that in Figure 10.1 is the point through which only six streamlines pass, which are the asymptotes of all other streamlines.

E10.7.3 Comparison of Velocity Fields with a Stagnation Point

The velocity fields (10.86a, b) and (10.89a, b) differ (10.86b) ≡ (10.89b) only by the factor minus two (–2) in (10.86a) ≠ (10.89a), which makes a significant difference, because: (i) the velocity field (10.86a, b) is neither irrotational nor incompressible:

$$\nabla \wedge \vec{v} = \vec{e}_3 \left(\partial v_y / \partial x - \partial v_x / \partial y \right) = -\vec{e}_3 \, 3x, \qquad \nabla . \vec{v} = \partial v_x / \partial x + \partial v_y / \partial y = 3y; \tag{10.92a, b}$$

(ii) the velocity field (10.89a, b) is both:

$$\partial\left(y^2 - x^2\right) / \partial x = -2x = \partial\left(-2xy\right)/y, \quad \partial\left(-2xy\right)/\partial x + \partial\left(y^2 - x^2\right)/\partial y = 0. \tag{10.93a, b}$$

The latter velocity field (10.89a, b) corresponds to the potential flow (section I.12.19) of complex conjugate velocity:

$$f' = v_x - i v_y = -2xy - i\left(y^2 - x^2\right) = i\left(x + iy\right)^2 = iz^2; \tag{10.94a, b}$$

the stream function Ψ, which is the imaginary part of the complex potential:

$$\frac{C}{3} = \operatorname{Im} f = \operatorname{Im}\left(\frac{iz^3}{3}\right) = \operatorname{Im}\left\{\frac{i(x+iy)^3}{3}\right\} = -xy^2 + \frac{x^3}{3}. \qquad (10.95a\text{–}d)$$

specifies the paths (10.95d) ≡ (10.91b) or streamlines. Thus, (10.88a, b) is the velocity field of a potential flow in a corner (I.14.75b) of angle $\theta = \pi/6 = 60°$, so that the stagnation point at the origin is a saddle point with six asymptotes (Figure 10.2), which allow a continuous velocity field on both sides of each asymptote.

EXAMPLE 10.8 First-Order Special Differential Equations

Classify the following four first-order ordinary differential equations (10.96a–10.99a):

$$\text{XCX:} \quad y = y'x + \frac{1}{y'}, \qquad y(x;C) = Cx + \frac{1}{C}; \quad y(x) = 2\sqrt{x}, \qquad (10.96a\text{–}c)$$

$$\text{C:} \quad y = y'^2 x + \frac{y'^3}{3}; \qquad x(p;C) = \frac{C + p^2/2 - p^3/3}{(1-p)^{-2}}, \qquad (10.97a\text{–}c)$$

$$\text{CII:} \quad x = \frac{y}{y'} + y', \qquad y(x;C) = C(x-C); \quad y(x) = \frac{x^2}{4}, \qquad (10.98a\text{–}c)$$

$$\text{CIII:} \quad y'^3 - y'^2 y - 4x^2 y' + 4x^2 y = 0, \quad \left(y - x^2 + C\right)\left(y + x^2 + C\right)\left(y - Ce^x\right) = 0, \qquad (10.99a, b)$$

and obtain the general integrals (10.96b–10.99b) and the special integrals when they exist (10.96c–10.98c). The roman numerals at left identify the standard in the classification of differential equations in the recollection 10.1.

E10.8.1 Cusped Parabola as the Envelope of a Family of Straight Lines

The equation (10.96a) is (standard XCIV) a Clairaut-type (5.29a, b) with (10.100a) and the general integral (5.31c) ≡ (10.100b) ≡ (10.96b):

$$h(p) = \frac{1}{p}: \quad y(x;C) = Cx + \frac{1}{C}: \quad \frac{\partial y}{\partial C} = x - \frac{1}{C^2} = 0, \quad C = \frac{1}{\sqrt{x}}, \quad y(x) = 2\sqrt{x}, \qquad (10.100a\text{–}c)$$

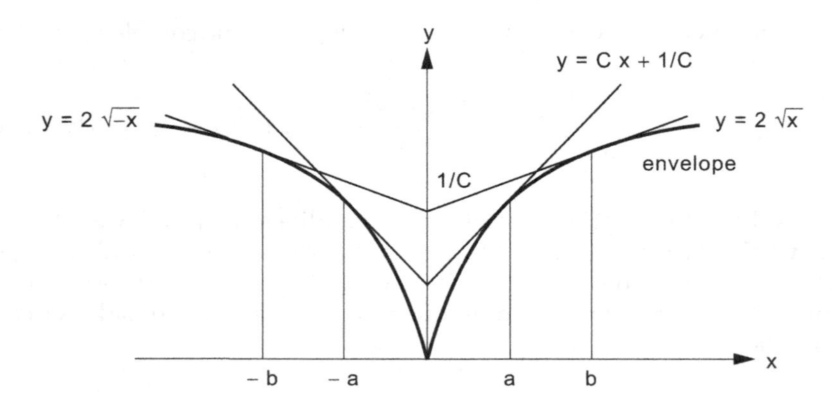

FIGURE 10.3
The cusped parabola is the envelope of a family of straight lines whose ordinate at the origin is the inverse of the slope.

the C-discriminant (10.100c) leads (10.100d) to the special integral (10.100e) ≡ (10.96c). *The integral curves are straight lines (10.100b) of slope C and ordinate 1/C at the origin, tangent to a parabola (10.100e) with a vertical cusp at the origin (Figure 10.3), which is an envelope.*

The equation (10.97a) is (standard C) a D'Alembert-type (5.38a–c) with (10.101a, b):

$$g(p) = p^2, \qquad h(p) = \frac{p^3}{3}: \qquad \varphi(p) = \exp\left\{\int \frac{2}{1-p}\right\} = \frac{1}{(1-p)^2}, \tag{10.101a–d}$$

leading (5.40a) = (10.101c) to (10.101d); the general integral (5.40b) ≡ (10.102) ≡ (10.97b):

$$x(p;C) = \frac{1}{(1-p)^2}\left\{C + \int p(1-p)\,dp\right\} = \frac{C + p^2/2 - p^3/3}{(1-p)^2}. \tag{10.102}$$

The parameter p is eliminated between (10.102) and (10.97a) to specify the integral curves $y\,(x;\,C)$.

E10.8.2 Smooth Parabola as the Envelope of a Family of Straight Lines

The Clairaut (10.96a) [D'Alembert (10.97a)] equation (5.45a, b) is solvable for y, providing an alternate method (subsection 5.4.1) of solution (10.96b, c) [(10.97a, b)]. The equation (10.98a) is (standard CII), solvable for the independent variable (5.47a, b) with (10.103a), and (5.48a) leads to (10.103b):

$$x = \frac{y}{p} + p \equiv g(y,p): \qquad \frac{dp}{dy} = 0; \qquad p = C, \qquad y(x;C) = C(x - C), \tag{10.103a–d}$$

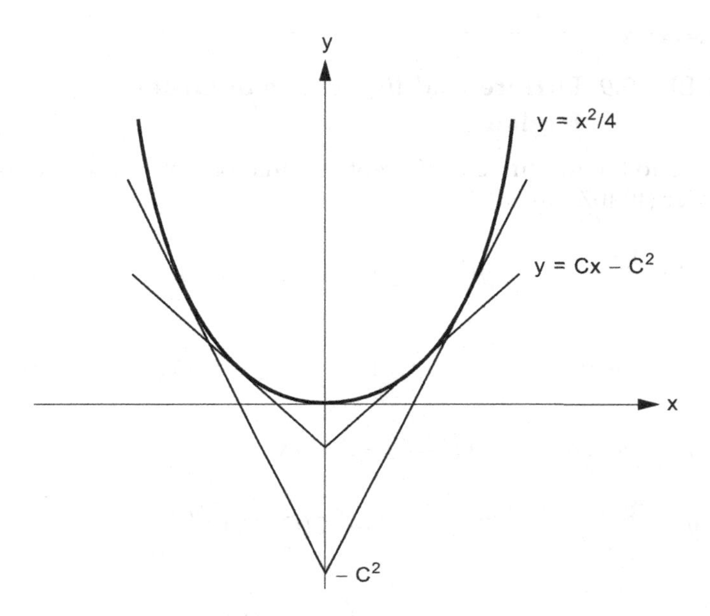

FIGURE 10.4
A family of straight lines distinct from that in Figure 10.3 is the case of ordinate at the origin equal to minus the square of the slope that has a smooth parabola as an envelope.

hence (10.103c) and the general integral is (10.103d) = (10.98b). The C-discriminant (10.104a) leads (10.104b) to the special integral (10.104c) ≡ (10.98c):

$$0 = \frac{\partial y}{\partial C} = x - 2C, \qquad C = \frac{x}{2}, \qquad y(x) = \frac{x^2}{4}. \tag{10.104a–c}$$

The integral curves are *straight lines (10.103d) of slope C and ordinate $-C^2$ at the origin, tangent to the smooth parabola (10.104c), which is their envelope (Figure 10.4).*

E10.8.3 First-Order Equation of Degree Three without Singular Integrals

The ordinary differential equation of first-order third-degree (10.99a) can (standard CIII) be solved (5.62a, b) for y', noting that $y = y'$ is a root, leading to the factorization (10.105):

$$0 = y'^3 - y'^2 y - 4x^2 y' + 4x^2 y = (y' - y)(y'^2 - 4x^2) = (y' - y)(y' - 2x)(y' + 2x); \tag{10.105}$$

there are three solutions (10.106a–c) of (10.105):

$$y_{1-3}(x) = Ce^x, \pm x^2 - C, \quad 0 = [y - y_1(x)][y - y_2(x)][y - y_3(x)], \tag{10.106a–d}$$

so that the product (10.106a–d) ≡ (10.99b) is the general integral. There is no special integral.

EXAMPLE 10.9 Differential Equations of Order Higher than the First

Classify the following fifteen differential equations of the second order or higher order (10.107a–10.122a):

CXI: $y'' = \frac{1}{x}$, $\quad y(x) = C_2 + C_1\,x + x\,\log x - x$, (10.107a, b)

I, CX: $y'' = y' + x$: $\quad y(x) = C_2 + C_1\,e^x - \frac{x^2}{2} - x - 1$, (10.108a, b)

L: $y'' = -y'\tan x$ $\quad y(x) = C_2 + C_1 \sin x$, (10.109a, b)

CVIII: $y'' = \frac{1}{y'}$, $\quad 3y(x) = C_2 + \left[\,2(C_1 + x)\,\right]^{3/2}$, (10.110a, b)

CVIII: $y'' = \frac{3}{2}y^2$, $\quad x(y) = C_2 + \int \left(C_1 + y^3\right)^{-1/2} dy$, (10.111a, b)

CVIII: $y'' = \frac{2y}{3y'}$: $\quad x(y) = C_2 + \int \left(C_1 + y^3\right)^{-1/3} dy$, (10.112a, b)

CVIII: $y'' = -\cosh y$: $\quad x(y) = C_2 + \int \left[\,2\left(C_1 \sinh y\right)\right]^{-1/2} dy$, (10.113a, b)

CVIII: $y'' = \frac{y'}{y}$: $\quad y(x) = C_2 + \int \frac{dy}{C_1 + \log y}$, (10.114a, b)

CXIV: $y''' = \frac{1}{2y''}$: $\quad 15y(x) = C_3 + C_2\,x + 4\,(C_1 + x)^{5/2}$, (10.115a, b)

CXVI: $y''' = -2y''y'$: $\quad x(y) = C_3 + \int \left[C_2 + \log(C_1 + x)\,\right]^{-1/2} dy$, (10.116a, b)

CXIII: $y''' = \frac{y''}{x^2}$: $\quad y(x) = C_3 + C_2\,x + \frac{x^2}{2C_1} - C_1^{-3}\,(1 + C_1 x)\left[\log(1 + C_1 x) - 1\right]$,

(10.117a, b)

CXIII, L: $x\,y^{(N)}(x) = a\,y^{(N-1)}(x)$: $\quad y(x) = \sum_{n=0}^{N-2} C_{n+1}\,x^n + C_N \frac{x^{a+N-1}}{(a+1)\cdots(a+N-1)}$,

(10.118a, b)

CXVII: $y'' + \left(x + \frac{1}{x}\right) y' + 2y = 0$: $y(x) = e^{-x^2/2}\left(C_2 + C_1 \int \frac{e^{x^2/2}}{x} dx\right),$

(10.119a, b)

CXVIII: $xy''y \pm y'y + y'^2 x = 0$: $y_+(x) = \sqrt{C_2 + C_1 \log x},$

$y_-(x) = \sqrt{C_2 x^2 - C_1},$ (10.120a–c)

CXIX: $y''y - y'^2 + 6xy^2 = 0$: $y(x) = C_2 \exp\left[x\left(C_1 - x^2\right)\right],$ (10.121a, b)

CXX: $x^2 y'' + x^2 y'^2 + xy' = 0$: $y(x) = \log\left(C_2 + C_1 \log x\right),$ (10.122a, b)

and obtain the corresponding general integrals (10.107b–10.121b). The roman numerals at left identify the standard in the classification of differential equations in the recollection 10.1.

E10.9.1 Linear Differential Equations with Constant or Variable Coefficients

The linear second-order differential equation (10.107a) involves neither the dependent variable nor its derivative (standard CXI) and is solvable (5.155a, b) by two quadratures: (i) the first integration of (10.107a) leads to (10.123a); (ii) another integration yields the general integral (10.123b) ≡ (10.107b):

$$y'(x) = \log x + C_1, \qquad y(x) = x\left(\log x - 1\right) + C_1 x + C_2. \qquad (10.123\text{a, b})$$

The second-order linear differential equation (10.108a) misses both the independent and dependent variables (standard CX) and is also linear with constant coefficients (1.197a–c) and hence has: (i) characteristic polynomial (10.124a) with (standard I) distinct roots zero and unity corresponding to the general integral in the first two terms on the r.h.s. of (10.124b):

$$0 = P_2(D) = D^2 - D = D(D-1), \qquad y(x) = C_2 + C_1 e^x + \frac{1}{D(D-1)} x;$$

(10.124a, b)

(ii) the last term on the r.h.s. of (10.124b) is (standard XIII) the particular integral (10.124c–e):

$$\frac{1}{D(D-1)} x = \frac{1}{D-1} \frac{x^2}{2} = -\left[1 + D + D^2 + O\left(D^2\right)\right] \frac{x^2}{2} = -\frac{x^2}{2} - x - 1;$$

(10.124c–e)

(iii) sum of (10.124b) and (10.124e) is the complete integral (10.108b). The linear second-order differential equation with variable coefficients (10.109a) ≡ (10.125a) is a separable first-order differential equation (10.125b) in y':

$$\frac{y''}{y'} = -\tan x: \qquad \frac{d}{dx}(\log y') = \frac{d}{dx}\left[\log(\cos x)\right], \tag{10.125a–d}$$

$$y'(x) = C_1 \cos x, \qquad y(x) = C_1 \sin x + C_2, \tag{10.125c, d}$$

and two quadratures (10.125c, d) lead to the general integral (10.125d) = (10.109b).

E10.9.2 Non-Linear Second-Order Differential Equations Omitting the Independent Variable

The second-order differential equation (10.110a) omitting the independent variable (standard CVIII) is equivalent to a first-order differential equation (10.126a) for y', which is solved by two quadratures: (i) the first integration of (10.126a) leads to (10.126b) ≡ (10.126c):

$$y'dy' = dx, \qquad y'^2 = 2(x + C_1), \qquad y' = \left[2(x + C_1)\right]^{1/2}; \tag{10.126a–c}$$

(ii) a further integration of (10.126c) leads to the general integral (10.110b). The second-order differential equation (10.111a) is (standard CVIII) also equivalent (5.138a) to a first-order equation (10.127a) for y':

$$y'dy' = \frac{3}{2}y^2 dy, \qquad y'^2 = y^3 + C_1, \qquad dx = \left(y^3 + C_1\right)^{-1/2} dy, \tag{10.127a–c}$$

leading to (10.127b, c) and hence, to the general integral (10.111b). The non-linear second-order differential equation (10.112a) also (standard CVIII) omits the independent variable and is reducible (5.138a) to a first-order equation (10.128a), the independent variable:

$$3y'^2\,dy' = 2y\,dy: \qquad y'^3 = y^2 + C_1, \qquad dx = \left(y^2 + C_1\right)^{-1/3} dy, \tag{10.128a–c}$$

leading to (10.128b, c) and hence, to the general integral (10.112b). The differential equation (10.113a) is (standard CVIII) reducible to first-order and leads (5.138a) to (10.129a) whose integration yields (10.129b, c):

$$y'dy' = -\cosh y\,dy: \quad y'^2 = 2(C_1 - \sinh y), \quad dx = \left[2(C_1 - \sinh y)\right]^{-1/2} dy, \tag{10.129a–c}$$

and hence to the general integral (10.113b). The non-linear differential equation (10.114a) omits the independent variable (standard CVIII) and leads to a first-order differential equation (10.130a) of degree two:

$$0 = y'\left(\frac{dy'}{dy} - \frac{1}{y}\right): \qquad y' = 0: \qquad y = C_0; \qquad dy' = \frac{dy}{y}, \tag{10.130a–d}$$

which has: (i) a special integral (10.130b) involving only one constant of integration (10.130c); (ii) the second factor (10.130d) in (10.130a) leads (10.131a) to the general integral (10.131b) ≡ (10.114b):

$$y' = C_1 + \log y, \qquad dx = \frac{dy}{C_1 + \log y}. \tag{10.131a, b}$$

The differential equations reducible to the first order may be of the second (higher) order [E10.9.2 (E10.9.3)].

E10.9.3 Higher-Order Differential Equations Reducible to the First Order

The third-order non-linear differential equation (10.115a) is (standard CXIV) of first-order (10.132a) in y'' leading to (10.132b, c):

$$2y''\,dy'' = dx, \qquad (y'')^2 = x + C_1, \qquad y'' = \sqrt{x + C_1}, \tag{10.132a–c}$$

so that double integration of (10.132c) leads to the general integral (10.115b). The third-order non-linear differential equation (10.116a) can (standard CXVI) be factorized (10.133a):

$$y'\left(\frac{dy''}{dy} + 2y''^2\right) = 0: \qquad y' = 0; \qquad y(x) = C_0; \qquad \frac{dy''}{2y''^2} = -dy, \tag{10.133a–d}$$

and hence, has: (i) a special integral (10.133b) involving only one constant of integration (10.133c); (ii) the second factor in (10.133a) leads to (10.133d), which may be integrated as (10.134a) ≡ (10.134b), implying (10.134c) by a second integration:

$$y + C_1 = \frac{1}{2y''}: \qquad 2y'dy' = \frac{dy}{y + C_1}; \qquad y'^2 = C_2 + \log(C_1 + y), \tag{10.134a–c}$$

and yielding the general integral (10.116b) by a third integration. The third-order differential equation (10.117a) is (standard CXVI) non-linear with variable coefficients and: (i) separates (10.135a) to first-order differential equation for y'' leading to (10.135b, c) by a first integration:

$$\frac{dy''}{y''^2} = \frac{dx}{x^2}: \qquad \frac{1}{y''} = C_1 + \frac{1}{x}, \qquad y'' = \frac{x}{1 + C_1 x} = \frac{1}{C_1}\left(1 - \frac{1}{1 + C_1 x}\right); \qquad (10.135\text{a–d})$$

(ii) rewriting the rational function (10.135c) in partial fractions (10.135d) allows (section I.31.8) immediate second integration (10.136):

$$y' = C_2 + \frac{x}{C_1} - C_1^{-2} \log(1 + C_1 x); \qquad (10.136)$$

(iii) a third integration leads to the general integral (10.117b). The differential equation (10.118a) of order N can be solved (standard CXIII) as a linear unforced differential equation with constant coefficients or as a first-order separable (standard L) equation (10.137b) for the derivative (10.137a) of order $N-1$, which may be: (i) integrated once (10.137c, d):

$$z \equiv y^{(N-1)}(x): \quad x z' = a z, \quad \log z = a \log x + \log C_N, \; z = C_N \, x^a = y^{(N-1)}(x); \qquad (10.137\text{a–e})$$

(ii) further $(N-1)$ integrations of (10.137e) lead to the general integral (10.118b).

E10.9.4 Linear Non-Commutative Differential Operators with Variable Coefficients

The linear second-order differential operator (10.119a) results (standard CXVII) from (5.187) the composition of two first-order operators:

$$0 = \left(\frac{d}{dx} + \frac{1}{x}\right)\left(\frac{d}{dx} + x\right) y = \left(\frac{d}{dx} + \frac{1}{x}\right)(y' + xy) = y'' + \left(x + \frac{1}{x}\right) y' + 2y; \qquad (10.138\text{a, b})$$

since the operators have variable coefficients they generally do not commute, that is, (10.138a, b) is distinct from:

$$0 = \left(\frac{d}{dx} + x\right)\left(\frac{d}{dx} + \frac{1}{x}\right) y = \left(\frac{d}{dx} + x\right)\left(y' + \frac{y}{x}\right) = y'' + \left(x + \frac{1}{x}\right) y' + y\left(1 - \frac{1}{x^2}\right), \qquad (10.139\text{a, b})$$

with commutator:

$$\left\{\left(\frac{d}{dx}+\frac{1}{x}\right)\left(\frac{d}{dx}+x\right)-\left(\frac{d}{dx}+x\right)\left(\frac{d}{dx}+\frac{1}{x}\right)\right\}y=\left(1+\frac{1}{x^2}\right)y. \tag{10.140}$$

The second-order ordinary differential equation (10.119a): (i) splits into two first-order equations (10.141a, b):

$$z=y'+xy: \qquad z'+\frac{z}{x}=0; \qquad \frac{dz}{z}+\frac{dx}{x}=0, \qquad z=\frac{C_1}{x}; \tag{10.141a–d}$$

(ii) the equation (10.141b) ≡ (10.141c) has the integral (10.141d); (iii) substitution of (10.141d) in (10.141a) leads to a linear differential equation (10.142a) ≡ (10.142b) ≡ (3.27) with coefficients (10.142c; 10.141e):

$$y'=-xy+\frac{C_1}{x}=Py+Q: \quad P(x)=-x,$$

$$X(x)=\exp\left(-\int^x \xi\,d\xi\right)=\exp\left(-\frac{x^2}{2}\right) \qquad Y(x)=C_1\int^x \frac{e^{\xi^2/2}}{\xi}\,d\xi, \tag{10.142a–f}$$

(iv) from (3.20a; 10.142b)[(3.31a; 10.141e)] follow (10.142d, e)[(10.142f)], which substituted in (3.31b) yield the general integral (10.119b).

E10.9.5 Non-Linear Exact Differential Equation with Variable Coefficients

The differential equation (10.120a) with + (plus) sign is (standard CXVIII) an exact differential (92a):

$$0=xy''y+y'^2x+y'y=\left(xy'y\right)', \qquad C_1=2xy'y=x\left(y^2\right)', \tag{10.143a, b}$$

specifying a first-integral (10.143b); the latter (10.143b) is a first-order differential equation (10.144a):

$$\left(y^2\right)'=\frac{C_1}{x}, \qquad y^2=C_1\log x+C_2, \tag{10.144a, b}$$

whose solution is (10.144b) ≡ (10.120b). The differential equation (10.121a) with – (minus) sign is (standard CXVIII) also an exact differential (10.145a):

$$0 = xy''y + y'^2x + y'y - 2y'y = \left(xy'y - y^2\right)', \quad C_1 = xy'y - y^2 = \frac{x}{2}\left(y^2\right)' - y^2, \tag{10.145a, b}$$

leading to: (i) the first integral (10.145b); (ii) the latter is a non-linear first-order differential equation, which becomes linear (10.145b) ≡ (10.146b) for the variable (10.146a):

$$z \equiv y^2: \quad \frac{x}{2}z' - z = C_1; \quad z' = Pz + Q, \quad \{P, Q\} \equiv \left\{\frac{2}{x}, \frac{2C_1}{x}\right\}. \tag{10.146a–e}$$

(iii) the linear first-order differential equation (3.27) ≡ (10.146b) ≡ (10.146c) with (10.146d, e) leads to (3.20a) ≡ (10.147a, b) and (3.31a) ≡ (10.147c, d):

$$X(x) = \exp\left(\int^x \frac{2}{\xi}d\xi\right) = x^2, \qquad Y(x) = \int^x \frac{2C_1}{\xi^3}d\xi = -\frac{C_1}{x^2}; \tag{10.147a–c}$$

(iv) substitution of (10.147b, d) in (3.31b) leads to (10.147e):

$$z(x) = X(x)\left[C_2 + Y(x)\right] = x^2 C_2 - C_1 = \left[y(x)\right]^2, \tag{10.147e, f}$$

which specifies (10.146a) the general integral (10.147f) ≡ (10.120c).

E10.9.6 Second-Order Homogeneous Differential Equation

The second-order linear differential equation with variable coefficients (10.121a) is (standard CXIX) homogeneous of the first kind (5.200a–d), as follows from (10.148a–d):

$$v \equiv \frac{y'}{y}, \quad \frac{y''}{y} = v' + v^2: \quad 0 = \frac{y''}{y} - \left(\frac{y'}{y}\right)^2 + 6x = v' + 6x; \tag{10.148a–d}$$

hence, (10.121a) is reducible to a first-order equation (10.148d) in the dependent variable (10.148a). The solution of (10.148d) is (10.149a):

$$-3x^2 = v - C_1 = \frac{y'}{y} - C_1, \qquad -x^3 = \log y - C_1 x - \log C_2, \tag{10.149a, b}$$

leading to the general integral (10.149b) ≡ (10.121b). The non-linear differential equation with variable coefficients (10.122a) is (standard CXX) homogeneous of the second kind (5.208) as follows from (5.211a, 5.212b) ≡ (10.150a, b) leading to (10.150c, d):

$$y'x \equiv w, \qquad x^2 y'' = w\left(\frac{dw}{dy} - 1\right): \qquad 0 = x^2 y'' + x^2 y'^2 + y'x = w\left(\frac{dw}{dy} + w\right), \tag{10.150a–d}$$

which is a first-order equation (10.150d) for the dependent variable (10.150a). The special integral solution $w = 0$ of (10.150d) is y = const by (10.150a) and satisfies (10.122a). The general integral solution of (10.150d) is (10.151a):

$$\frac{dw}{dy} = -w: \qquad C_1 e^{-y} = w = x\frac{dy}{dx}, \quad 0 = \frac{C_1}{x}\,dx - e^y dy = C_1 \log x - e^y + C_2, \tag{10.151a–c}$$

leading to (10.151b) and hence (10.150c), to the general integral (10.151d) ≡ (10.122b).

EXAMPLE 10.10 Bending of a Beam under Traction

Consider the linear bending of a uniform beam (6.14f) ≡ (10.152b) under traction (10.152a) in the presence of a shear stress:

$$T > 0: \qquad EI\zeta'''' - T\zeta'' = f(x), \tag{10.152a, b}$$

in the following cases: (a) a clamped beam (10.153a–d) with (Figure 10.5a), a concentrated torque Q in the middle (10.153e); (b) a pinned beam (10.154a–d) with (Figure 10.5b), a concentrated force F in the middle (10.154e); (c) a clamped-pinned beam (10.155a–d) under (Figure 10.5c) its own weight (10.155e); (d) a cantilever beam (10.156a–d) subject (Figure 10.5d) to a shear stress (10.156e) increasing linearly from the clamped end:

$$\zeta(0) = 0 = \zeta'(0); \qquad \zeta(L) = 0 = \zeta'(L): \qquad f(x) = Q\delta'(x - L/2), \tag{10.153a–e}$$

$$\zeta(0) = 0 = \zeta''(0); \qquad \zeta(L) = 0 = \zeta''(L): \qquad f(x) = F\delta(x - L/2), \tag{10.154a–e}$$

$$\zeta(0) = 0 = \zeta'(0); \qquad \zeta(L) = 0 = \zeta''(L): \qquad f(x) = \rho g, \tag{10.155a–e}$$

$$\zeta(0) = 0 = \zeta'(0); \qquad \zeta''(L) = 0 = EI\zeta'''(L) - T\zeta'(L): \qquad f(x) = qx. \tag{10.156a–e}$$

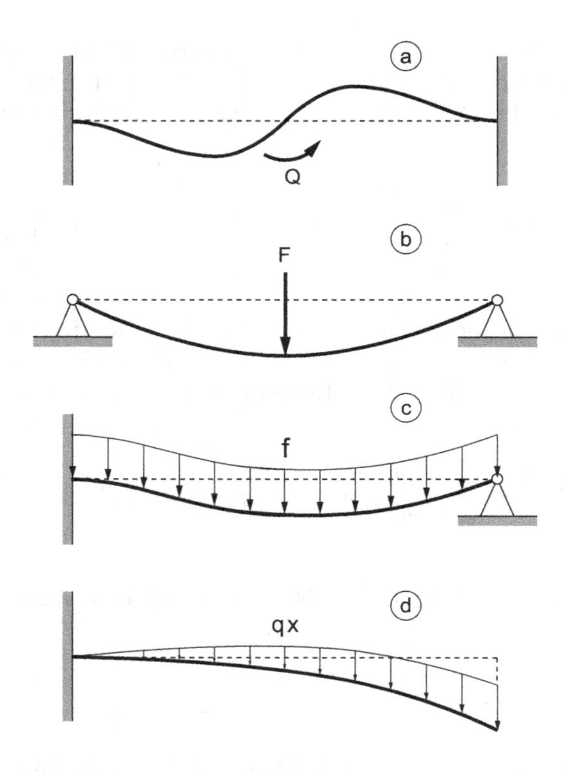

FIGURE 10.5
The linear bending of a beam under traction can be considered for $4 \times 4 = 16$ combinations of support and loads, of which four are illustrated: (i) for a concentrated torque (a) [transverse force (b)] or a constant (c) [linearly increasing (d)] shear stress; (ii) for supports clamped (a) [pinned (b)] at both ends or clamped at one end and pinned (c) [free (d)] at the other end.

The shear stress (10.154e)[(10.153e)] corresponding to a concentrated transverse force F (torque Q) is specified (III.1.34a, b; III.3.11a–c) [(III.1.45a–c; III.3.18a–c)] by a Dirac delta function (its derivative) with singularity [subsection III.1.3 and III.3.1 (III.1.4 and III.3.2)] at the application point.

E10.10.1 Elastica of a Beam under Traction

The problems (10.153a–e; 10.154a–e) may be solved with explicit reference (chapter III.4) to the generalized functions unit jump, unit impulse, and derivatives (chapters III.1 and III.3). It is possible to use only ordinary functions in all four problems (10.153 to 155a–e) as shown next. In the absence of shear stress (10.157a), the differential equation (10.152b) specifying the linear deflection of the elastic becomes (10.157c), involving the parameter (10.157b), which is positive instead of negative for buckling (10.16b):

$$f(x)=0,\ p^2=\frac{T}{EI}>0: \qquad 0=\zeta'''' - p^2\zeta'' = \left\{\frac{d^2}{dx^2}\left(\frac{d}{dx}-p\right)\left(\frac{d}{dx}+p\right)\right\}\zeta(x). \tag{10.157a–d}$$

The characteristic polynomial (10.157d) has a double-zero root and a pair of real symmetric roots $\pm p$, instead of a complex conjugate imaginary pair of roots $\pm ip$; the general integral (10.158) is obtained from (6.18) replacing p by ip:

$$\zeta(x)=A+Bx+C\cosh(px)+D\sinh(px), \tag{10.158}$$

and involves hyperbolic instead of circular functions. The replacement of periodic functions by monotonic functions implies that there is no buckling for a beam under traction; bending is possible only under transverse load. To the general integral (10.158) that specifies the shape of the elastica (10.157c) without shear stress (10.157a) a particular integral of (10.152b) with loads must be added to obtain the complete integral specifying the total deflection in each of (E10.10.2–E10.10.5) the cases (a–d).

E10.10.2 Clamped Beam with a Concentrated Torque

In the case (a) of a beam clamped at both ends (Figure 10.5a) with a concentrated moment Q in the middle, the reaction moment at the support is given by (10.159a) ≡ (III.4.224b):

$$-\frac{Q}{4}=EI\zeta_1''(0); \qquad \zeta_1(0)=0=\zeta_1'(0), \tag{10.159a–c}$$

which specifies the curvature, and the coordinate and slope are zero (10.159b, c). The shape of the beam is skew-symmetric relative to the middle (10.160a)

$$\zeta_1(x)=-\zeta_1(L-x), \qquad \zeta_1\left(\frac{L}{2}\right)=-\zeta_1\left(\frac{L}{2}\right)=0, \tag{10.160a, b}$$

implying that the displacement is zero (10.160b) there. The conditions (10.159b, c) applied to (10.158) lead to (10.161a, b), reducing the number of constants of integration:

$$A+C=0=B+pD: \qquad \zeta_1(x)=A\{1-\cosh(px)\}+D\{\sinh(px)-px\}, \tag{10.161a–c}$$

from four in (10.158) to two in (10.161c). The remaining two constants of integration are determined substituting (10.161c) in (10.159a) [(10.160b)] leading to [(10.162a) [(10.162c)]:

$$Q/4 = EI\,A\,p^2 = AT, \qquad D\{\sinh(pL/2) - pL/2\} = A\{\cosh(pL/2) - 1\}, \tag{10.162a–c}$$

and using (10.157b) in (10.162b). Solving (10.162b, c) for A and D, and substituting into (10.161c) yields:

$$0 \le x \le \frac{L}{2}: \quad \frac{4T}{Q}\zeta_1(x) = 1 - \cosh(px) + \left[\sinh(px) - px\right]\frac{\cosh(pL/2) - 1}{\sinh(pL/2) - pL/2}, \tag{10.163a, b}$$

the shape (10.163b) of the first half (10.163a) of the elastica of the beam under traction (10.157b).

If the traction force is weak in the sense (10.164a), then (III.7.6b) ≡ (10.146b) and (III.7.7b) ≡ (10.146c):

$$(px)^6 \le \left(\frac{pL}{2}\right)^6 = \left(\frac{TL^2}{2EI}\right)^6 << 1: \qquad \cosh(px) - 1 = \frac{p^2x^2}{2} + \frac{p^4x^4}{24} + O(p^6x^6)$$

$$\sinh(px) - px = \frac{p^3x^3}{6} + \frac{p^5x^5}{120} + O(p^7x^7), \tag{10.164a–c}$$

imply (10.164d–f):

$$\frac{\cosh(pL/2) - 1}{\sinh(pL/2) - pL/2} = \frac{3}{px}\left[\left(1 + \frac{p^2x^2}{12}\right)\left(1 + \frac{p^2x^2}{20}\right)^{-1} + O(p^4x^4)\right]$$

$$= \frac{3}{px}\left[1 + p^2x^2\left(\frac{1}{12} - \frac{1}{20}\right) + O(p^4x^4)\right] = \frac{3}{px} + \frac{px}{10} + O(p^3x^3); \tag{10.164d–f}$$

substitution of (10.164b, c, f) and similar expressions with px replaced by $pL/2$ leads from (10.163b) to (10.165c) with the approximation (10.165a):

$$(px)^4 \le \left(\frac{pL}{2}\right)^4 << 1: \qquad \frac{4T}{Q}\zeta_1(x) = -\frac{p^2x^2}{2}\left[1 + \frac{p^2x^2}{12} - \frac{px}{3}\left(\frac{6}{pL} + \frac{pL}{20}\right)\right]; \tag{10.165a–c}$$

the simplication of (10.165b, c) ≡ (10.166a, b):

$$T^2 << \left(\frac{4EI}{L^2}\right)^2: \qquad \zeta_1(x) = -\frac{Qx^2}{8EI}\left[1-\frac{2x}{L}+\frac{Tx}{12EI}\left(x-\frac{L}{5}\right)\right], \qquad (10.166a, b)$$

specifies the shape of the elástica (10.166b) for weak axial traction (10.166a).

The beam equation (10.157c) simplifies to the bar equation (10.167b) in the absence of axial tension (10.167a):

$$T = 0: \qquad \zeta_0'''' = 0; \qquad \zeta_0(x) = \bar{A} + \bar{B}x + \bar{C}x^2 + \bar{D}x^3, \qquad (10.167a\text{–}c)$$

the solution of (10.167b) is a third-degree polynomial (10.167c), which replaces (10.158) for $p = 0$. The four constants of integration in (10.167c) are determined (10.168a–d) from the boundary conditions (10.159a–c; 10.160b):

$$0 = \zeta_{01}(0) = \bar{A}, \quad 0 = \zeta_{01}'(0) = \bar{B}, \quad -\frac{Q}{4EI} = \zeta_{01}''(0) = 2\bar{C},$$
$$0 = \zeta_{01}\left(\frac{L}{2}\right) = \frac{L^2}{4}\left(\bar{C} + \frac{\bar{D}L}{2}\right); \qquad (10.168a\text{–}d)$$

substitution of the non-zero constants (10.168c, d) ≡ (10.169a, b) in (10.167c) leads to the shape of the elástica (10.169c):

$$\bar{C} = -\frac{Q}{8EI}, \qquad \bar{D} = -\frac{2\bar{C}}{L} = \frac{Q}{4EIL}: \qquad \zeta_{10}(x) = -\frac{Qx^2}{8EI}\left(1-\frac{2x}{L}\right), \qquad (10.169a\text{–}c)$$

which coincides with (10.166b) ≡ (III.4.220b) for zero tension (10.167a). *Thus, the (problem 222) linear bending (10.152b) of a uniform beam (6.10a, b) subject to a traction (10.152a) clamped at both ends (10.153a–d) under a concentrated torque (10.153e) leads to: (i) the transverse displacement of the first (10.163a, b) [second(10.170a, b)] half of the elastica, which is skew-symmetric (10.160a):*

$$\frac{L}{2} \le x \le L: \qquad \frac{4T}{Q}\zeta_1(x) = \cosh\left[p(L-x)\right] - 1$$
$$-\left[\sinh\left[p(L-x)\right] - p(L-x)\right]\frac{\cosh(pL/2)-1}{\sinh(pL/2)-pL/2}, \qquad (10.170a, b)$$

confirming that the displacement is zero at the clamped ends (10.153a, c) and in the middle (10.160b); (ii) the slope (10.171b) is symmetric (10.171a):

$$\zeta_1'(L-x)=\zeta_1'(x)=\frac{Qp}{4T}\left\{-\sinh(px)+\left[\cosh(px)-1\right]\frac{\cosh(pL/2)-1}{\sinh(pL/2)-pL/2}\right\}, \tag{10.171a, b}$$

confirming it vanishes at the clamped end (10.153b, d); (iii) the curvature (10.172c) is skew-symmetric (10.172b) and specifies the bending moment (10.172a) and implies that $M_1(0)=-Q/4$ in agreement (10.159a) with the bending moment at the support:

$$\begin{aligned} M_1(x) &= -EI\zeta_1''(L-x)=EI\zeta_1''(x) \\ &= \frac{Q}{4}\left\{-\cosh(px)+\sinh(px)\frac{\cosh(pL/2)-1}{\sinh(pL/2)-pL/2}\right\}, \end{aligned} \tag{10.172a–c}$$

(iv) the slope (10.171b) becomes (10.172d) at the mid-position:

$$\zeta_1'\left(\frac{L}{2}\right)=\frac{Qp}{4T}\,\frac{2-2\cosh(pL/2)+(pL/2)\sinh(pL/2)}{\sinh(pL/2)-pL/2}. \tag{10.172d}$$

The shape of the elastica simplifies to (10.169c) for a bar in the absence of axial tension (10.167a); the lowest-order correction for a beam in the case of weak axial traction (10.166a) is (10.166b).

E10.10.3 Pinned Beam with a Concentrated Force

In the case (b) of a transverse force P concentrated at the middle of the beam, the traction at the support (10.159a) is replaced by the transverse force (10.173a):

$$-\frac{P}{2}=EI\zeta_2'''(0)-T\zeta'(0), \qquad \zeta_2'\left(\frac{L}{2}\right)=0, \tag{10.173a, b}$$

and (10.160b) is replaced by a condition of zero slope at the middle (10.173b). The latter arises because the shape of the beam is symmetric relative to the middle (10.174a):

$$\zeta_2(x)=\zeta_2(L-x), \qquad \zeta_2'(x)=-\zeta_2'(L-x), \qquad \zeta_2'(L/2)=-\zeta_2'(L/2)=0, \tag{10.174a–d}$$

and hence, the slope (10.174b) is skew-symmetric (10.174c) leading to (10.174d) ≡ (10.173b). Considering the case (Figure 10.5b) of a beam pin-joined at both ends, by symmetry (10.175a) it is sufficient to consider in (10.158) only one end where the boundary conditions (10.154a, b) ≡ (10.175a, b):

$$\zeta(0) = 0 = \zeta_2''(0): \qquad A = 0 = C, \quad \zeta_2(x) = Bx + D\sinh(px), \tag{10.175a–e}$$

specify the constants (10.175c, d) and lead to (10.175e). Substitution of (10.175e) in (10.173a, b) specifies:

$$-\frac{P}{2} = -TB, \qquad 0 = B + pD\cosh\left(\frac{pL}{2}\right), \tag{10.176a, b}$$

the two remaining constants of integration, and hence:

$$0 \le x \le \frac{L}{2}: \qquad \frac{2T}{P}\zeta_2(x) = x - \frac{1}{p}\sinh(px)\operatorname{sech}\left(\frac{pL}{2}\right), \tag{10.177a, b}$$

the shape (10.177a, b) of the elastica of the beam.

In the case of weak traction force (10.178a) the inverse of (10.164b) is (10.178b) to third order in (10.178c, d):

$$\begin{aligned}(px)^6 \le \left(\frac{pL}{2}\right)^6 \ll 1: \quad \operatorname{sech}(px) &= \left(1 + \frac{p^2x^2}{2} + \frac{p^4x^4}{24}\right)^{-1} \\ &= 1 - \frac{p^2x^2}{2} - \frac{p^4x^4}{24} + \left(\frac{p^2x^2}{2}\right)^2 = 1 - \frac{p^2x^2}{2} + \frac{5p^4x^4}{24};\end{aligned} \tag{10.178a–d}$$

substitution of (10.164c; 10.178d) in (10.177b) leads to (10.179a):

$$\begin{aligned}\frac{2T}{Px}\zeta_2(x) &= 1 - \left(1 + \frac{p^2x^2}{6}\right)\left(1 - \frac{p^2L^2}{8} + \frac{5p^4L^4}{384}\right) \\ &= -\frac{p^2x^2}{6} + \frac{p^2L^2}{8} - \frac{5p^4L^4}{384} + \frac{p^4L^2x^2}{48},\end{aligned} \tag{10.179a}$$

which simplifies to the shape of the elastica (10.179c):

$$T^2 \ll \left(\frac{4EI}{L^2}\right)^2: \qquad \zeta_{02}(x) = -\frac{Px}{12EI}\left[x^2 - \frac{3L^2}{4} - \frac{TL^2}{8EI}\left(x^2 - \frac{5L^2}{8}\right)\right], \tag{10.179b, c}$$

under weak traction (10.179b). In the absence of axial tension (10.167a) the beam (10.157c) becomes a bar (10.167b) and the constants in the shape (10.167c) of the elastica are determined by the boundary conditions (10.175a, b; 10.173a, b) ≡ (10.180a–d):

$$0 = \zeta_{02}(0) = \bar{A}, \quad 0 = \zeta_{02}''(0) = 2\bar{C}, \quad -\frac{P}{2EI} = \zeta_{02}'''(0) = 6\bar{D}, \qquad 0 = \zeta_{02}'\left(\frac{L}{2}\right) = \bar{B} + \frac{3\bar{D}L^2}{4}; \tag{10.180a–d}$$

the non-zero constants (10.180c, d) ≡ (10.181a, b) in (10.167c) specify the shape of the elástica (10.181c) of the bar:

$$\bar{D} = -\frac{P}{12EI}, \quad \bar{B} = -\frac{3\bar{D}L^2}{4} = \frac{PL^2}{16EI}: \qquad \zeta_{20}(x) = -\frac{P}{12EI}\left(x^2 - \frac{3L^2}{4}\right), \tag{10.181a–c}$$

which coincides with (10.179c) ≡ (III.4.114b) for zero axial tension (10.167a).

In conclusion, (problem 223) *the linear bending (10.152b) of a uniform beam (6.10a, b) pinned at both ends (10.154a–d) under traction (10.152a) with a concentrated force (10.154e) at the middle (Figure 10.5b) leads to: (i) the transverse displacement of the first (10.177a, b) [second (10.182a, b)] half of the elastica, which is symmetric (10.175a):*

$$\frac{L}{2} \le x \le L: \qquad \frac{2T}{P}\zeta_2(x) = L - x - \frac{1}{p}\sinh\left[p(L-x)\right]\operatorname{sech}\left(\frac{pL}{2}\right), \tag{10.182a, b}$$

confirming that it vanishes at both ends (10.154a, c); (ii) the slope (10.183b):

$$\zeta_2'(x) = -\zeta_2'(L-x) = \frac{P}{2T}\left[1 - \cosh(px)\operatorname{sech}\left(\frac{pL}{2}\right)\right], \tag{10.183a, b}$$

which is skew-symmetric (10.183a), confirming it vanishes in the middle (10.173b); (iii) the curvature (10.184c), which is symmetric (10.184b) and specifies the bending moment (10.184a):

$$M_2(x) = -EI\zeta_2''(x) = -EI\zeta_2''(L-x) = -T\sinh(px)\operatorname{sech}\left(\frac{pL}{2}\right), \tag{10.184a–c}$$

which vanishes at the pinned ends; (iv) the maximum deflection (slope in modulus) is:

$$\zeta_{2\max} = \zeta_2\left(\frac{L}{2}\right) = \frac{PL}{4T}\left[1 - \frac{2}{pL}\tanh\left(\frac{pL}{2}\right)\right], \tag{10.185}$$

$$\zeta'_{2\max} = \zeta'_2(0) = \frac{P}{2T}\left[1 - \operatorname{sech}\left(\frac{pL}{2}\right)\right] = -\zeta'_2(L), \tag{10.186a, b}$$

at the middle (10.185) [at the supports (10.186a, b)]. In the absence of tension (10.167a) the shape of the elastica of the bar is (10.181a–c) and the lowest-order correction for a beam under weak traction (10.179b) is (10.179c).

E10.10.4 Heavy Clamped-Pinned Beam

Continuous loads instead of concentrated loads are considered next. The simplest case is a uniform shear stress (10.155e), such as a beam with mass density per unit length ρ in a gravity field with uniform acceleration g:

$$EI\zeta_3'''' - T\zeta_3'' = \rho g; \tag{10.187}$$

a particular integral of the forced linear differential equation with constant coefficients (10.187) is given by the method (§3.17) of inverse polynomial of derivatives:

$$D \equiv \frac{d}{dx}: \qquad \zeta_{3*}(x) = \left(EID^4 - TD^2\right)^{-1}\rho g = -\frac{\rho g}{T}D^{-2}(1) = -\frac{\rho g x^2}{2T}. \tag{10.188a–d}$$

Adding (10.189a) to (10.158) the general integral (10.158) of the unforced equation (10.157c) specifies the complete integral (10.189b):

$$\bar{\zeta}_3(x) = \zeta(x) + \zeta_{3*}(x) = A + Bx - \frac{\rho g x^2}{2T} + C\cosh(px) + D\sinh(px). \tag{10.189a, b}$$

In the case (c) of a beam (Figure 10.5c) clamped (10.155a, b) ≡ (10.190a, b) at one end substitution of (10.189b) yields (10.161a, b), so that only two constants of integration remain in (10.190c):

$$\bar{\zeta}_3(0) = 0 = \bar{\zeta}'_3(0): \qquad \zeta_3(x) = A\{1 - \cosh(px)\} + D\{\sinh(px) - px\} - \frac{\rho g x^2}{2T}. \tag{10.190a–c}$$

The other end is pin-joined (10.155c, d) ≡ (10.191a, b) leading to the linear inhomogeneous system of equations (10.191c):

$$\bar{\zeta}_3(L) = 0 = \bar{\zeta}_3''(L): \quad \begin{bmatrix} 1-\cosh(pL) & \sinh(pL)-pL \\ -\cosh(pL) & \sinh(pL) \end{bmatrix} \begin{bmatrix} A \\ D \end{bmatrix} = \begin{bmatrix} \rho g L^2/2T \\ \rho g/p^2 T \end{bmatrix}; \tag{10.191a–c}$$

the determinant (10.192b):

$$pL > 0: \qquad \Delta \equiv \sinh(pL) - pL\cosh(pL) = \cosh(pL)\{\tanh(pL) - pL\} \neq 0, \tag{10.192a–c}$$

is non-zero (10.192c) for (10.192a), showing that there is no buckling under traction, in contrast with the case of compression. Since $\Delta \neq 0$, the system can be solved uniquely for A, D:

$$\begin{bmatrix} A \\ D \end{bmatrix} = \begin{bmatrix} \sinh(pL) & pL-\sinh(pL) \\ \cosh(pL) & 1-\cosh(pL) \end{bmatrix} \begin{bmatrix} \rho g L^2/2T\Delta \\ \rho g/p^2 T\Delta \end{bmatrix}; \tag{10.193}$$

substitution of (10.193) in (10.190c) specifies the shape of the beam under traction.

In the absence of traction (10.194a), the shape of a bar under its own weight is (10.187) given by (10.194b):

$$T = 0: \qquad \zeta_{03}'''' = \frac{\rho g}{EI}, \quad \bar{\zeta}_{03}(0) = \frac{\rho g x^4}{24EI} + \bar{A} + \bar{B}x + \bar{C}x^2 + \bar{D}x^3, \tag{10.194a–c}$$

whose complete integral (10.194c) consists of the sum of: (i) a particular integral of the unforced equation (10.194b), which is the first term; (ii) the general integral (10.167c) of the unforced equation (10.167b). The boundary conditions for clamping (10.190a, b) at one end, and pin-joint (10.191a, b) at the other end determine the constants of integration in (10.194c), namely (10.195a–c):

$$\bar{A} = 0 = \bar{B}, \qquad \begin{bmatrix} 1 & L \\ 2 & 6L \end{bmatrix} \begin{bmatrix} \bar{C} \\ \bar{D} \end{bmatrix} = -\frac{\rho g L^2}{24EI} \begin{bmatrix} 1 \\ 12 \end{bmatrix}, \tag{10.195a–c}$$

leading to (10.196a, b):

$$\bar{C} = \frac{\rho g L^2}{16EI}, \qquad \bar{D} = -\frac{5\rho g L}{48EI}; \qquad \bar{\zeta}_{03}(x) = \frac{\rho g x^2}{8EI}\left(\frac{x^2}{3} - \frac{5xL}{6} + \frac{L^2}{2}\right), \tag{10.196a–c}$$

the shape of the bar is given by (10.194c) with (10.195a, b; 10.196a, b) leading to (10.196c) ≡ (III.4.64).

In conclusion, (problem 224) *the linear bending (10.152b) of a heavy (10.155e) uniform (6.10a, b) beam under traction (10.152a) clamped (10.155a, b) at one end and pinned (10.155c, d) at the other end leads to: (i) the transverse displacement of the elastica (10.190c) with (10.193) confirming that the displacement is zero at the supports (10.190a; 10.191a); (ii) the slope (10.197):*

$$\bar{\zeta}_3'(x) = p\left\{-A\sinh(px) + D\left[\cosh(px) - 1\right]\right\} - \frac{\rho g x}{T}; \tag{10.197}$$

(iii) the curvature (10.198b) specifying the bending moment (10.198a):

$$M_3(x) = -EI\bar{\zeta}_3''(x) = T\left[A\cosh(px) - D\sinh(px)\right] + \frac{\rho g EI}{T}; \tag{10.198a, b}$$

(iv) the transverse force (10.199a, b):

$$F_3(x) = EI\bar{\zeta}_3'''(x) - T\bar{\zeta}_3'(x) = \rho g x + pTD, \qquad f_3(x) = F_3'(x) = \rho g, \tag{10.199a–d}$$

leading to the shear stress (10.199c), in agreement with (10.199d) ≡ (10.155e). The bending momenta at the clamped support is (10.200a):

$$M_3(0) = TA + \frac{\rho g EI}{T}; \qquad F_3(0) = pTD, \qquad F_3(L) = F_3(0) + \rho g L, \tag{10.200a–c}$$

and the transverse force at the two supports (10.200b, c) differs by the weight of the beam.

E10.10.5 Cantilever Beam with a Linearly Increasing Shear Stress

The case (d) of a linearly increasing shear stress (10.156e) leads (10.152b) to (10.201):

$$EI\zeta_4'''' - T\zeta_4'' = qx, \tag{10.201}$$

which is a forced linear differential equation with constant coefficients, whose particular integral can be obtained, as in the case (10.188a–d) of uniform shear stress:

$$D \equiv \frac{d}{dx}: \qquad \zeta_{4*}(x) = \left(EID^4 - TD^2\right)^{-1} qx = -\frac{q}{T} D^{-2}(x) = -\frac{qx^3}{6T}. \qquad \text{(10.202a–d)}$$

Adding (10.202d) to the general integral (10.158) of the unforced case (10.157c) leads (10.202e) to (10.202f):

$$\bar{\zeta}_4(x) = \zeta(x) + \zeta_{4*}(x) = A + Bx - \frac{qx^3}{6T} + C\cosh(px) + D\sinh(px), \qquad \text{(10.202e, f)}$$

for the complete integral.

In the case (Figure 10.5d) of a beam clamped at one end (10.156a, b) ≡ (10.203a, b), substitution of (10.202b) yields (10.161a, b) implying (10.203c):

$$\zeta(0) = 0 = \zeta'(0): \qquad \bar{\zeta}_4(x) = A\left\{1 - \cosh(px)\right\} + D\left\{\sinh(px) - px\right\} - \frac{qx^3}{6T}.$$

(10.203a–c)

The boundary conditions (10.156c) ≡ (10.204a) [(10.156d) ≡ (10.205a)] at the free end:

$$\bar{\zeta}_4'''(L) - p^2\,\bar{\zeta}_4'(L) = 0: \qquad 0 = -\frac{q}{T} + p^3 D + \frac{qp^2L^2}{2T}, \qquad \text{(10.204a, b)}$$

$$\bar{\zeta}_4'(L) = 0: \qquad A\sinh(pL) - D\left[\cosh(pL) - 1\right] = -\frac{qL^2}{2Tp}, \qquad \text{(10.205a, b)}$$

determine the remaining two constants of integration (10.206a) [(10.206b)]:

$$p^3 D = \frac{q}{T} - \frac{qL^2}{2EI}, \quad A = D\left[\tanh(pL) - \operatorname{csch}(pL)\right] - \frac{qL^2}{2Tp}\operatorname{csch}(pL);$$

(10.206a, b)

substitution of (10.206a, b) into (10.203c), specifies the shape of the beam under traction.

In the case of a bar in the absence of traction (10.207a), the equation (10.201) is replaced by (10.207b):

$$T = 0: \qquad \zeta_{04}'''' = \frac{q\,x}{E\,I}, \quad \bar{\zeta}_{04}(x) = \frac{q\,x^5}{120E\,I} + \bar{A} + \bar{B}\,x + \bar{C}\,x^2 + \bar{D}\,x^3, \qquad \text{(10.207a–c)}$$

whose complete integral is (10.207c) the sum of (10.158) with the particular integral of (10.207b). The constants of integration are determined by the boundary conditions at the: (i) clamped end (10.156a, b) leading to (10.195a, b); (ii) at the free end (10.156c, d) leading to (10.208a, b):

$$0 = \zeta_{04}'''(L) = 6\bar{D} + \frac{q\,L^2}{2E\,I}, \quad 0 = \bar{\zeta}_{04}''(L) = 2\bar{C} + 6\bar{D}L + \frac{q\,L^3}{6E\,I} = 2\bar{C} - \frac{q\,L^3}{3E\,I}; \qquad \text{(10.208a–c)}$$

substitution of (10.208a) in (10.208b) specifies the remaining constant of integration (10.208c); substitution of (10.195a, b; 10.208a, c) in (10.207c) yields:

$$\bar{\zeta}_{04}(x) = \frac{q\,x^2}{120E\,I}\left\{x^3 - 10\,x\,L^2 + 20\,L^3\right\}, \qquad \text{(10.209)}$$

for the shape of the bar.

In conclusion, (problem 225) *the linear bending (10.152b) of a uniform (6.10a, b) cantilever (10.156a–d) beam under compression (10.152a) subject to a shear stress (10.156e) increasing linearly along its length (10.201) leads to: (i) the transverse displacement of the elastica (10.203c) with (10.206a, b) confirming the zero displacement at the clamped end (10.156a); (ii) the slope (10.210):*

$$\zeta_4'(x) = p\left[D\cosh(px) - 1 - A\sinh(px)\right] - \frac{q\,x^2}{2T}, \qquad \text{(10.210)}$$

confirming that it vanishes at the clamped end (10.156b); (iii) the curvature (10.211b), which specifies the bending moment (10.211a):

$$M_4(x) = -E\,I\,\zeta_4''(x) = T\left[A\cosh(p\,x) - D\sinh(p\,x)\right] + \frac{q\,x\,E\,I}{T}; \qquad \text{(10.211a, b)}$$

(iv) the transverse force (10.212a, b):

$$F_4(x) = E\,I\,\bar{\zeta}'''(x) - T\bar{\zeta}'(x) = p\,T\,D - \frac{q\,E\,I}{T} + \frac{q\,x^2}{2}, \quad f_4(x) = F_4'(x) = q\,x, \qquad \text{(10.212a–d)}$$

leading to the shear stress (10.212c) in agreement with (10.212d) ≡ (10.156e). The displacement (slope) at the free end is given by (10.203c) [(10.210)] with $x = L$, and the bending moment (transverse force) at the clamped end by (10.213a) [(10.213b)]:

$$M_4(0) = T\,A, \qquad F_4(0) = p\,T\,D - \frac{q\,E\,I}{T}. \tag{10.213a, b}$$

with D given by (10.206a; 10.157b).

Thus, the shape of a beam (bar) under (under no) traction (10.152a) [(10.167a, b)] has been obtained in the following four cases: (E10.10.2) clamped at both ends (Figure 10.5a) with a concentrated moment Q at the middle (10.163a, b; 10.170a, b)[(10.166a, b)]; (E10.10.3) pin-joined at both ends (Figure 10.5b) with a concentrated force P in the middle (10.177a, b; 10.182a, b) [(10.181c)]; (E10.10.4) under its own weight (Figure 10.5c) with one end clamped and the other pinned (10.190c; 10.192b, c; 10.193) [(10.196c)]; (E10.10.5) under a linearly increasing load (Figure 10.5d) with one end clamped and the other free (10.203c; 10.206a, b) [(10.209)]. The first-order correction to the linear approximation was obtained (10.165a–c) [(10.179b, c)] in the cases (i) [(ii)]. The preceding four cases (E10.10.2–E10.10.5) are a cross sample of the 16 combinations of four loads (10.153e–10.156e) and four supports (10.153a–d to 10.156a–d).

EXAMPLE 10.11 Linear Bending of a Circular Heavy Plate with a Circular Hole

Consider the problem for all combinations of clamped, supported, or free edges at the inner and outer boundary, with a vertical offset.

The shape of the neutral surface or directrix of a heavy plate with polar symmetry is specified by (6.502e) ≡ (10.214b):

$$D = \frac{Eh^3}{12\left(1-\sigma^2\right)}: \quad \zeta(r) = \frac{\rho g r^4}{64D} + C_1 + C_2 \log r + (C_3 - C_4) r^2 + C_4 r^2 \log r, \tag{10.214a, b}$$

where C_{1-4} are arbitrary constants to be determined by four boundary conditions. The shape of the neutral surface or directrix (10.214b) implies the slope (10.215a, b), the curvature (10.216a, b):

$$\zeta'(r) \equiv \frac{d\zeta}{dr} = \frac{\rho g r^3}{16D} + \frac{C_2}{r} + 2C_3 r - C_4 r + 2C_4 r \log r, \tag{10.215a, b}$$

$$\zeta''(r) \equiv \frac{d^2\zeta}{dr^2} = \frac{3\rho g r^2}{16D} - \frac{C_2}{r^2} + 2C_3 + C_4 + 2C_4 \log r, \tag{10.216a, b}$$

$$\begin{aligned} M_r(r) = -D\left(\zeta'' + \frac{\sigma}{r}\zeta'\right) = -\frac{\rho g r^2}{16}(3+\sigma) \\ +D(1-\sigma)\left(\frac{C_2}{r^2} - C_4\right) - D(1+\sigma)\left[C_3 + C_4 \log r\right], \end{aligned} \tag{10.217a, b}$$

$$N_r(r) = -\left[\frac{D}{r}\left(r\zeta'\right)'\right]' = -\frac{\rho g r}{2} - \frac{4C_4 D}{r}, \tag{10.218a, b}$$

the stress couple (10.217a, b), and the turning moment (10.218a, b).

The linear bending of a heavy circular plate with a concentric (10.219a) circular hole (Figure 10.6) leads (Table 10.2) to (problem 272) eight cases (Table 10.1):

$$b \le r \le a; \tag{10.219a–e}$$

$$\text{I:} \quad \zeta(a) = 0 = \zeta'(a), \qquad \zeta(b) = -d, \qquad \zeta'(b) = 0,$$

$$\text{II:} \quad \zeta(a) = 0 = \zeta'(a), \qquad \zeta(b) = -d, \qquad M_r(b) = 0, \tag{10.220a–d}$$

$$\text{III:} \quad \zeta(a) = 0 = \zeta'(a), \qquad M_r(b) = 0 = N_r(b), \tag{10.221a–d}$$

$$\text{IV:} \quad \zeta(a) = 0 = M_r(a), \qquad M_r(b) = 0 = N_r(b), \tag{10.222a–d}$$

$$\text{V:} \quad \zeta(a) = 0 = M_r(a), \qquad \zeta(b) = -d, \qquad M_r(b) = 0, \tag{10.223a–d}$$

TABLE 10.1

Combinations of Boundary Conditions for a Circular Plate with a Circular Hole

Boundary		**Outer**		
	Support	**Clamped**	**Supported**	**Free**
Inner	Clamped	case I, Figure 10.6a	VI ≡ reverse case II	VII ≡ reverse case III
	Supported	case II, Figure 10.6b	case V, Figure 10.6e	VIII ≡ reverse case IV
	Free	case III, Figure 10.6c	case IV, Figure 10.6d	statically unstable

Note: There are $3 \times 3 = 9$ combinations of clamped/pinned/free boundaries for the weak bending of a circular elastic plate with a circular hole; of these eight are static cases, consisting of five distinct cases (Table 10.2 and Figures 10.5a–c) and three interchanges.

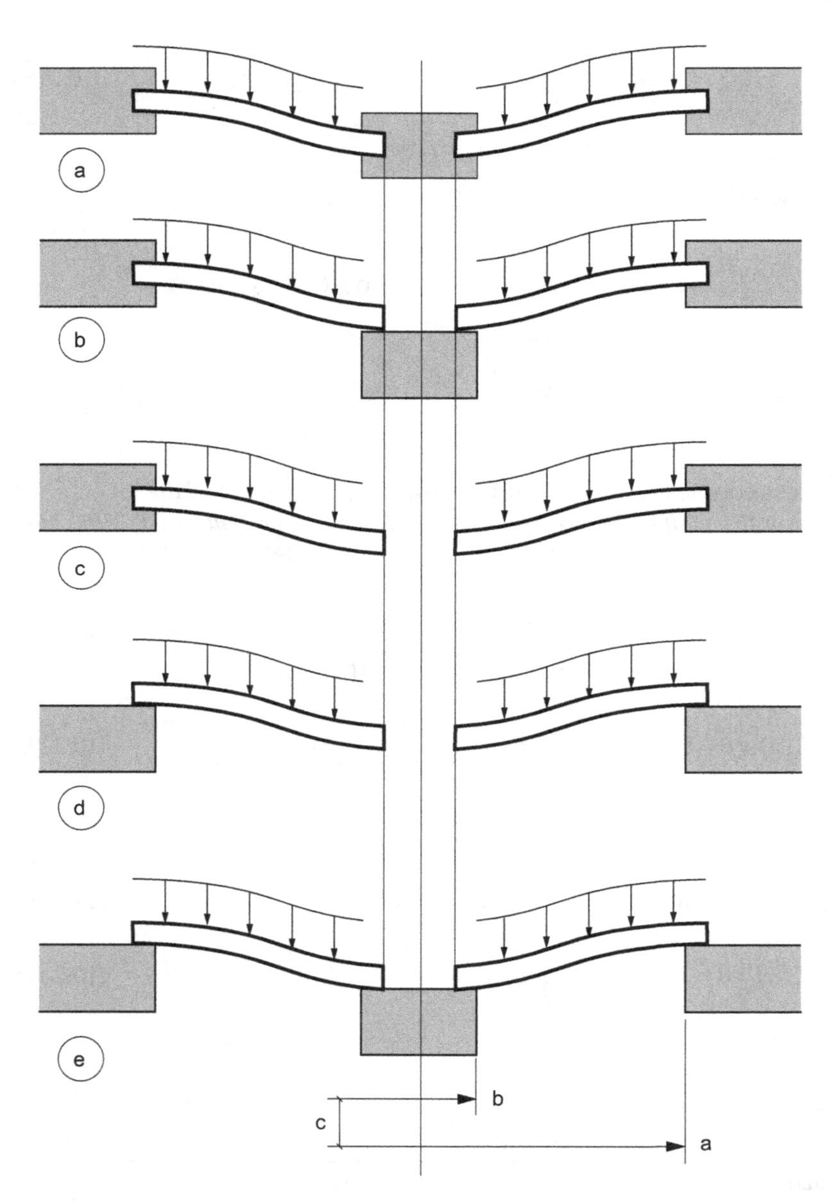

FIGURE 10.6
The linear bending of a circular elastic plate with a concerntric circular hole (Table 10.1) leads to five distinct cases (Table 10.2), namely: (a) the case I: clamped at both boundaries; (b) the case II: clamped at the outer boundary and supported at the inner boundary (and vice-versa for the case VI); (c) the case III: clamped at the outer boundary and free at the inner boundary (and vice-versa for the case VII); (d) the case IV: supported at the outer boundary and free at the inner boundary (and vice-versa for the case VIII): (e) the case V supported at both the outer and inner boundaries. The case IX free at both boundaries is not static and is omitted.

TABLE 10.2

Constants in the Shape of Neutral Surface of Heavy Circular Plate with a Circular Hole

Case	I	II	III	IV	V
Figure	10.6a	10.6b	10.6c	10.6d	10.6e
Outer Boundary	Clamped	Clamped	Clamped	Supported	Supported
	$\zeta(a)=0$	$\zeta(a)=0$	$\zeta(a)=0$	$\zeta(a)=0$	$\zeta(a)=0$
	$\zeta'(a)=0$	$\zeta'(a)=0$	$\zeta'(a)=0$	$M_r(a)=0$	$M_r(a)=0$
Inner Boundary	Clamped	Supported	Free	Free	Supported
	$\zeta(b)=-d$	$\zeta(b)=-d$	$N_r(b)=0$	$N_r(b)=0$	$\zeta(a)=-d$
	$\zeta'(b)=0$	$M_r(b)=0$	$M_r(b)=0$	$M_r(b)=0$	$M_r(b)=0$

Note: For the distinct cases (Figures 10.5a–e) of a circular heavy elastic plate with a concentric circular hole (Table 10.1) the boundary conditions are indicated.

namely: (I) clamped at both boundaries (Figure 10.6a) with (10.219b–e) a height difference d; (II) clamped at the outer boundary (10.220a, b) and supported at the inner boundary (10.220c, d) (Figure 10.6b): (III) clamped at the outer boundary (10.221a, b) and free at the inner boundary (10.221c, d) (Figure 10.6c); (IV) supported at the outer boundary (10.222a, b) and free at the inner boundary (10.222c, d) (Figure 10.6d); (V) supported both at the outer boundary (10.223a, b) and the inner boundary (10.223c, d) (Figure 10.6e); (VI, VII, VIII) the cases II, III, IV of unequal boundaries can be reversed, respectively, for (VI) supported outside and clamped inside, (VII) clamped inside and free outside and (VIII) supported inside and free outside. The remaining combination IX of $3\times 3=9$ is free both at the inner boundary and the outer boundary, which is not statically stable because there is no support.

EXAMPLE 10.12 Vibrations of a Membrane under Uniform or Non-Uniform Tension

Consider a homogeneous elastic membrane held at two parallel sides by a normal uniform tension (Figure 10.7) or non-uniform tension (Figure 10.8). The tension parallel to the sides is constant and there is no shear stress.

The linear transverse displacement of an elastic membrane is specified by (10.224b), which balances the stresses (6.369a) against minus the inertia force (6.754b):

$$T_{xy}=0: \qquad T_{xx}\frac{\partial^2\zeta}{\partial x^2}+T_{yy}(x)\frac{\partial^2\zeta}{\partial y^2}=\rho\frac{\partial^2\zeta}{\partial t^2}, \qquad (10.224a, b)$$

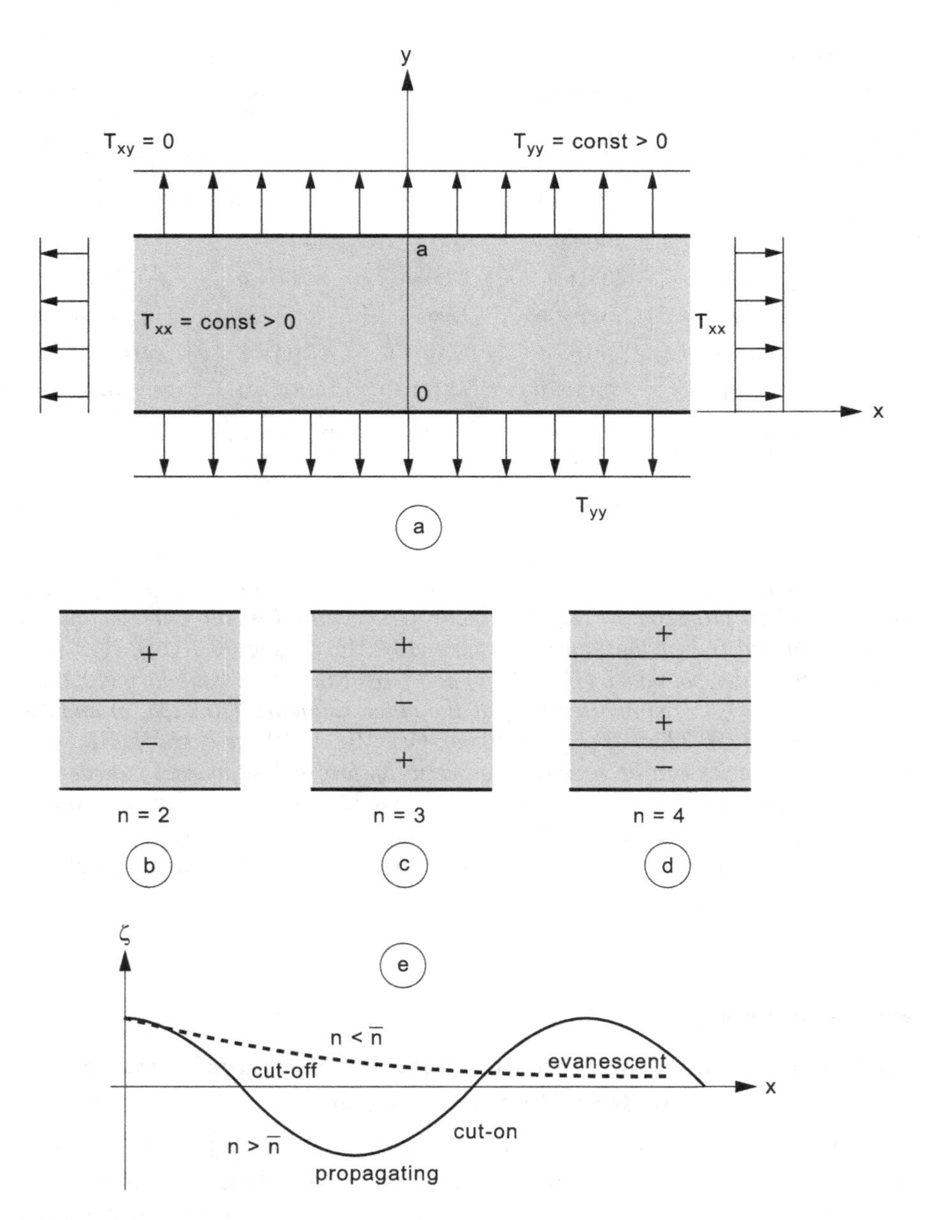

FIGURE 10.7
A homogeneous elastic membrane held at two parallel boundaries and (a) like an infinite strip in the orthogonal direction, subject to constant normal tractions and no shear stress, has transverse modes of oscillation of all orders, for example, (b) two, (c) three, and (d) four. The modes below (above) a transition value $\bar{n}$ are (e) cut-on (cut-off) or propagating (evanescent).

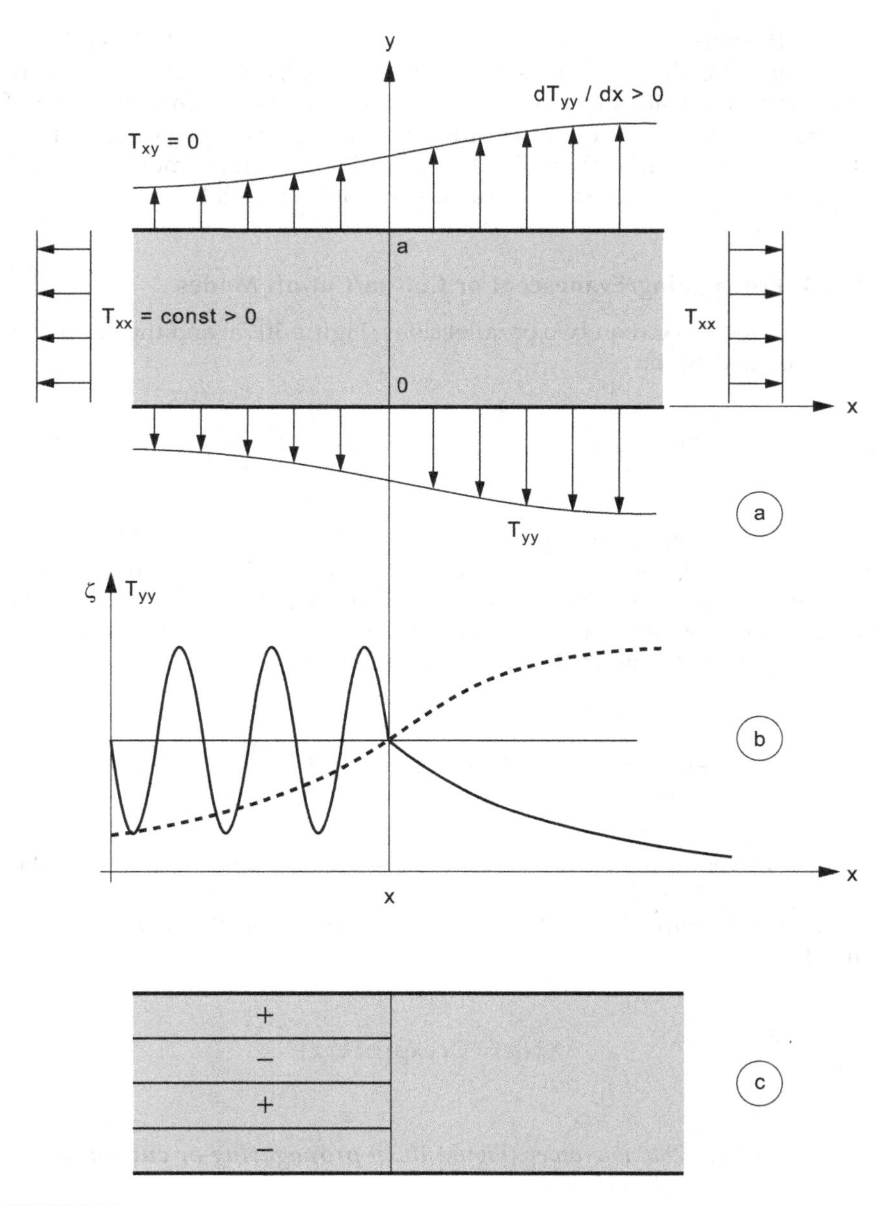

FIGURE 10.8
In Figure 10.6[a], the stress normal to the boundary (a) increases monotonically with distance along the boundary, each transverse mode has a turning point, such that before (after) (b) the modes are oscillating (decaying), corresponding to (c) propagating (evanescent) waves.

where: (i) the mass density per unit area ρ is constant because the membrane is homogeneous; (ii) there is no shear stress (10.224a); (iii)(iv) the stress parallel (normal) to the sides is constant (non-uniform or constant). The case of constant tension is considered first (E10.12.1) leading to propagating (evanescent) that is cut-on (cut-off) modes. The case of non-uniform motion leads to turning points (E10.12.2), as in the ray theory (notes 5.10–5.19).

E10.12.1 Propagating/Evanescent or Cut-on/Cut-off Modes

The membrane is fixed on two parallel sides (Figure 10.7a) and the boundary conditions (10.225a, b):

$$\zeta(x,y=0,t)=0=\zeta(x,y=a,t): \quad \zeta_n(x,y,t)=e^{i\omega t}\sin\left(\frac{n\pi y}{a}\right)X(x), \qquad (10.225\text{a–c})$$

are met by the y-dependence in the transverse displacement (10.225c), corresponding to transverse modes of order n, of which $n = 2, 3, 4$ are represented in Figure 10.7b, c, d. Considering a vibration of frequency ω in (10.225c), the dependence of the transverse displacement on the longitudinal coordinate is specified by substitution in (10.224b), leading to (10.226a):

$$d^2X_n/dx^2 + k_n^2 X_n = 0, \qquad \sqrt{T_{xx}}\,k_n = \left|\rho\omega^2 - T_{yy}\left(\frac{\pi n}{a}\right)^2\right|^{1/2}, \qquad (10.226\text{a, b})$$

where the wavenumbers k_n are is specified by (10.226b). The traction parallel to the supports T_{xx} is always constant. *Consider the case in when the traction at the supports is uniform (Figure 10.7a). A real wavenumber in (10.226b) corresponds to (10.227a):*

$$n < \frac{\omega a}{\pi}\sqrt{\frac{\rho}{T_{yy}}} \equiv \bar{n}: \qquad X_n^{\pm}(x) = C_{\pm}\exp(\pm i k_n x), \qquad (10.227\text{a, b})$$

to (10.227a) ≡ (10.228b) low-order (Figure 10.7e) ***propagating or cut-on modes*** *(10.227b; 10.225c) ≡ (10.228b):*

$$n < \bar{n}: \qquad \zeta_n^{\pm}(x,y,t) = C_{\pm}\sin\left(\frac{n\pi y}{a}\right)\exp\left[i(\omega t \pm k_n x)\right], \qquad (10.228\text{a, b})$$

$$= C_{\pm}\sin\left(\frac{n\pi y}{a}\right)\exp\left[i k_n (u_n t \pm x)\right], \qquad (10.228\text{c})$$

propagating in the negative (positive) direction corresponding to the + (–) sign in (10.228b) ≡ (10.228c) with phase speed (10.229c):

$$u_0 = \sqrt{\frac{T_{xx}}{\rho}}: \qquad u_n = \frac{\omega}{k_n} = u_0 \left| 1 - \frac{T_{yy}}{\rho}\left(\frac{\pi n}{\omega a}\right)^2 \right|^{-1/2}, \tag{10.229a–c}$$

where (10.229a) is the speed (10.229b) of the zero-order mode. The modes of order higher (10.230a) than (10.227a) are (Figure 10.7e) ***cut-off or evanescent modes*** *(10.230b; 10.225c) ≡ (10.230c):*

$$n > \bar{n}: \quad X_n^{\pm}(x) = C_{\pm}\exp(\pm k_n x), \quad \zeta_n^{\pm}(x, y, t) = C_{\pm}\sin\left(\frac{n\pi y}{a}\right)\exp(\pm k_n x)\cos(\omega t), \tag{10.230a–c}$$

whose amplitude decays as $x \to +\infty\ (x \to -\infty)$ *choosing the lower – sign (upper +) sign in (10.230c).*

E10.12.2 Turning Point Due to Non-Uniform Tension

Consider next a fixed mode n and let the transverse traction at the supports be non-uniform, for example, steadily increasing with x in Figure 10.8a. There is a turning point $\bar{x}$ *for which the wavenumber (10.226b) vanishes (10.231a):*

$$k_n(\bar{x}) = 0: \qquad T_{yy}(\bar{x}) = \rho\left(\frac{a\omega}{n\pi}\right)^2: \qquad \begin{cases} x > \bar{x}: & \text{propagation,} \\ x < \bar{x}: & \text{evanescence,} \end{cases} \tag{10.231a–d}$$

and the traction takes the value (10.131b). Before the turning point (10.231c), there are vibrations like (10.228a–c; 10.229a, b) cut-on or propagating modes (Figure 10.8b, c); beyond the turning point, the modes decay like cut-off or evanescent modes (10.230a–c). In a strict sense, the wavenumber k only exists (10.226b) when it is constant, that is for uniform traction (Figure 10.7a–e), corresponding to sinusoidal vibrations; in the case of non-uniform tension the wavenumber (10.226b) is not constant:

$$k_n(x) = \left| \frac{\rho\omega^2}{T_{xx}} - \frac{T_{yy}(x)}{T_{xx}}\left(\frac{n\pi}{a}\right)^2 \right|^{1/2}, \tag{10.232}$$

and the cut-on (cut-off) or propagating (evanescent) wavefields are given by (10.233a, b) [(10.234a, b)] in the ray approximation (5.274a, b):

$$x > \bar{x}: \qquad \zeta_n(x,y,t) = C_\pm \left[k_n(x)\right]^{-1/2} \sin\left(\frac{n\pi y}{a}\right) \exp\left\{i\left[\omega t \pm \int^x k_n(\xi)\right] d\xi\right\}, \tag{10.233a, b}$$

$$x < \bar{x}: \qquad \zeta_n(x,y,t) = C_\pm \left[k_n(x)\right]^{-1/2} \sin\left(\frac{n\pi y}{a}\right) \cos(\omega t) \exp\left\{\pm \int^x k_n(\xi) d\xi\right\}, \tag{10.234a, b}$$

when (7.431a–g) the local wavelength is much smaller than the lengthscale of variation of the stress:

$$\left[\lambda_n(x)\right]^2 = \left[\frac{2\pi}{k_n(x)}\right]^2 \le L^2 = T_{yy}^2 \left(\partial T_{yy}/dx\right)^{-2}. \tag{10.235}$$

If the ray approximation (notes 5.16–5.17, 7.35–7.27) does not hold, then the notion of wavenumber or wavelength loses its meaning, even locally, and exact global solutions must be sought to describe accurately vibrations or waves. The vibrations of a membrane held are similar to quasi-one-dimensional waves in non-uniform medium (notes 7.28–7.45), so analogous methods apply.

EXAMPLE 10.13 Curve as the Tangent to a Vector Field or as of the Intersection Surfaces

Obtain the curves defined as: (i) tangent to the vector field (10.236a):

$$\{X,Y,Z\} = \left\{y^2 - z^2, z^2 - x^2, x^2 - y^2\right\};$$

$$x^2(dx)^2 - y^2(dy)^2 + (dz)^2 - 2x\,dx\,dz = 0. \tag{10.236a, b}$$

(ii) specified by the differential of degree two in three variables (10.236b).

From (10.236a), follow the identities (10.237a, b):

$$X + Y + Z = 0 = x^2X + y^2Y + z^2Z; \qquad \frac{dx}{X} = \frac{dy}{Y} = \frac{dz}{Z}; \tag{10.237a–c}$$

the curve tangent to the vector field (10.236a) satisfies (7.12a–c) ≡ (10.237c) leading to (10.238a, b):

$$dx + dy + dz = 0 = x^2\, dx + y^2 dy + z^2 dz: \qquad x + y + z = C_1, \quad x^3 + y^3 + z^3 = C_2, \tag{10.238a–d}$$

the corresponding primitives (10.238c, d) show that *the two-parameter family of curves to which the vector field (10.236a) is tangent are the intersection of the cubic surface (10.238d) with the plane (10.238c).*

The differential (10.236b) ≡ (10.239) of second-degree has coefficients (10.240a–f):

$$0 = A(dx)^2 + B(dy)^2 + C(dz)^2 + 2D\,dx\,dy + 2E\,dx\,dz + 2F\,dy\,dz; \tag{10.239}$$

$$\{A, B, C, D, E, F\} = \{x^2, -y^2, 1, 0, -x, 0\}. \tag{10.240a–f}$$

which satisfy the condition (3.365b) ≡ (10.240g):

$$ABC + 2DEF - AF^2 - BE^2 - CD^2 = -x^2 y^2 + x^2 y^2 = 0; \tag{10.240g}$$

this leads to the factorization (3.366) ≡ (10.241a–c):

$$\begin{aligned} 0 &= (C\,dz + E\,dx + F\,dy)^2 - \left(\sqrt{E^2 - CA}\, dx + \sqrt{F^2 - CB}\, dy\right)^2 \\ &= (dz - x\,dx)^2 - (y\,dy)^2 = (dz - x\,dx - y\,dy)(dz - x\,dx + y\,dy). \end{aligned} \tag{10.241a–c}$$

The solutions (10.242a, b) of (10.241c) show that:

$$x^2 + y^2 = 2z + C_1, \qquad x^2 - y^2 = 2z + C_2, \tag{10.242a, b}$$

the differential (10.236b) of second degree in three variables determines a two-parameter family of curves specified by the in tersection of circular (10.242a) and hyperbolic (10.242b) paraboloids with a common axis.

EXAMPLE 10.14 Differentials of First Degree in Three/Four Variables

Solve the following first-degree differentials in three variables:

LXXIV: $$y^2\,dx+\left(2xy+z^2\right)dy+2yz\,dz=0;\quad xy^2+yz^2=C; \qquad (10.243a, b)$$

LXXV: $$yz\,dx+2xz\,dy+3xy\,dz=0;\qquad xy^2z^3=C; \qquad (10.244a, b)$$

LXXVI: $$2y\,dx-x\,dy+z\,dz=0,\quad y=C_1x:\quad C_1x^2+z^2=C_2; \qquad (10.245a–c)$$

and in four variables:

LXXXII: $$y^2dx+\left(2xy+z^2\right)dy+\left(2yz+u^2\right)dz+2zu\,du=0:\quad xy^2+yz^2+zu^2=C; \qquad (10.246a, b)$$

$$yzu\,du+2xzu\,dy+3xyu+4xyz\,du=0:\qquad xy^2z^3u^4=C; \qquad (10.247a, b)$$

$$y\,dx+x\,dy+z\,dz-z\,du=0,\qquad y=C_1x,\qquad u=C_2z:\qquad 2C_1x^2-C_2z^2=-z^2. \qquad (10.248a–d)$$

In the cases where a first-degree differential in three (four) variables is not exact one (two) subsidiary conditions is (are) used. The Roman numerals at left indicate the standard in the recollection 10.1.

E10.14.1 Exact, Inexact, and Non-Integrable Differentials

The differential (10.243a) ≡ (10.241a) has vector (10.249b) with zero curl (7.27e) ≡ (10.249c):

$$0=\vec{X}.d\vec{x},\qquad \vec{X}=\left\{y^2,2xy+z^2,2yz\right\};\qquad \nabla\wedge\vec{X}=0, \qquad (10.249a–c)$$

$$0=\vec{X}.d\vec{x}=y^2dx+2xy\,dy+z^2\,dy+2yz\,dz=d\left(y^2x+z^2y\right), \qquad (10.249d)$$

and hence, is (7.27 a–e) immediately integrable (10.249d) ≡ (10.243a); thus, *the family of surfaces (10.243b) is orthogonal to the vector field (10.249b).* The differential (10.244a) ≡ (10.243a, b) is (7.28a–d) inexact (10.250c) but integrable (7.28d) ≡ (10.250d):

$$0=\vec{X}.d\vec{x},\quad \vec{X}=\left\{yz,2xz,3xy\right\};\quad \nabla\wedge\vec{X}=\left\{x,-2y,z\right\},\quad \vec{X}.\left(\nabla\wedge\vec{X}\right)=0; \qquad (10.250a–d)$$

$$\lambda = y z^2: \quad 0 = \lambda \vec{X}.d\vec{x} = y^2 z^3 dx + 2xyz^3 dy + 3xy^2 z^2 dz = d\left(xy^2 z^3\right), \qquad (10.250e, f)$$

the integrating factor (10.250e) leads to the solution (10.250f) ≡ (10.244b). Thus, *the family of surfaces (10.244b) is orthogonal to the vector field (10.250b).* The differential (10.245a) ≡ (10.251a, b) is (7.29 a–d) inexact (10.251c) and non-integrable (10.251d):

$$0 = \vec{X}.d\vec{x}, \qquad \vec{X} = \{2y, -x, z\}; \qquad \nabla \wedge \vec{X} = \{0, 0-3\}, \qquad \vec{X}.\left(\nabla \wedge \vec{X}\right) = -3z; \qquad (10.251a–d)$$

$$y = C_1 x: \qquad 0 = 2y\,dx - x\,dy + z\,dz = C_1\,x\,dx + z\,dz = \frac{1}{2}\,d\left(C_1\,x^2 + z^2\right), \qquad (10.251e, f)$$

the subsidiary condition (10.251e) ≡ (10.245b) leads to the solution (10.251f) ≡ (10.245c). Thus, *on the family of planes (10.251e) ≡ (10.245b) lie the family of curves (10.245c) orthogonal to the vector field (10.251b).*

E10.14.2 Immediate and Complete Integrability and Subsidiary Conditions

The first-degree differential in four variables (10.246a) corresponds (10.252a) to the vector field (10.252b); the differential is exact because the vector field satisfies (3.278d). Hence, it is immediately (10.252c) integrable (10.252d) ≡ (10.246b):

$$0 = \vec{X}.d\vec{x}: \qquad \vec{X} = \left\{y^2, 2xy + z^2, 2yz + u^2, 2zu\right\}, \qquad (10.252a, b)$$

$$0 = \left(y^2 dx + 2xy\,dy\right) + \left(z^2 dy + 2yz\,dz\right) + \left(u^2\,dz + 2zu\,du\right) = d\left(y^2 x + z^2 y + u^2\,z\right). \qquad (10.252c, d)$$

Thus, *the family of hypersurfaces (10.246b) is orthogonal to the four-dimensional vector field (10.252b).* The differential (10.247a) corresponds (10.253a) to the vector field (10.253b). It is inexact but integrable because the vector field does not satisfy (3.278d) but does satisfy (3.282). It has the integrating factor (10.253c):

$$0 = \vec{X}.d\vec{x}: \qquad \vec{X} = \{yzu, 2xzu, 3xyu, 4xyz\}, \qquad (10.253a, b)$$

$$\lambda = yz^2u^3: \qquad \lambda\left(yzu\,dx + 2xzu\,dy + 3xyu\,dz + 4xy\,z\,du\right)$$

$$= y^2 z^3 u^4 dx + 2xyz^3u^4 dy + 3xy^2z^2u^4 dz + 4xy^2z^3u^3\,du = d\left(xy^2z^3u^4\right), \qquad (10.253c–e)$$

leading (10.253d) to (10.253e) ≡ (10.247b). Thus, *the family of hypersurfaces (10.247b) is orthogonal to the four-dimensional vector field (10.253b).* The differential (10.248a) corresponds (10.254a) to the vector field (10.254b); the differential (10.248a) is inexact and non-integrable, since the vector field does not satisfy (3.282). The subsidiary conditions (10.248b, c) lead to (10.254c, d):

$$0=\vec{X}.d\vec{x}: \qquad \vec{X}=\{y,x,z,-z\}, \tag{10.254a, b}$$

$$\begin{aligned}0&=C_1x\,dx+x\,d(C_1x)+z\,dz-z\,d(C_2z)=2C_1x\,dx+(1-C_2)z\,dz\\&=d\left[C_1\,x^2+(1-C_2)\frac{z^2}{2}\right],\end{aligned} \tag{10.254c–e}$$

which coincides with (10.254c) ≡ (10.258d). Thus, *the hyperplanes (10.248b, c) intersect on a plane where lies the family of curves (10.248d) orthogonal to the four-dimensional vector field (10.254b).*

EXAMPLE 10.15 General Boundary Conditions for the Bending of a Plate

Obtain the general boundary condition (6.609a) for an isotropic (6.453b) [pseudo-isotropic orthotropic (6.608b)] plate including the explicit stress couple (6.609b) and turning moment (6.609c).

The method starts with the boundary integral in (6.453b) for an isotropic plate (E10.15.1) extended to a pseudo-isotropic orthotropic plate using (6.808b). An integration by parts along the boundary (E10.15.2) leads to the expression (6.609a) determining (E10.15.3) the stress couple and turning moment, which is simplified if the plate has a fixed boundary (E10.15.4). Thus, the general boundary conditions are obtained for the weak bending of a pseudo-isotropic orthotropic plates (E10.15.5) including the particular case of an isotropic plate. The boundary conditions apply to a plate whose boundary is an arbitrary closed regular curve (E10.15) including, in particular, circular and rectangular shapes (subsections 6.7.12–6.7.14). The boundary conditions are given in the three most important cases of (i) clamped E10.15.6); (ii) supported or pinned (E10.15.7) and (iii) with a free boundary (E10.15.8) and are summarized (E10.15.9) in Table 10.3.

TABLE 10.3

Boundary Conditions for the Bending of a Plate

Shape of Boundary	Arbitrary Regular Curve	Circular	Rectangular
Figure	6.24a	6.24b	6.24c
Equation	(6.467e)	(6.467c)	(6.467a)
Slope	(6.464a)	(6.464c)	(6.464e)
Stress Couple*	(10.261)/(10.280)	(10.283b)/(6.471d)	(10.283d)/(6.471b)
Turning Moment*	(10.262)/(10.281)	(6.467d)/(6.467d)	(6.467b)/(6.467b)
Clamped* (10.271a–e) Figure 6.23a	(6.474a, b, d; 10.263b) (6.474a–d)	(6.473a, b, d; 10.284)/ (6.473a–d)	(6.472a–d)/(6.472a–d)
Supported or Pinned* (10.273a–e) Figure 6.23b, c	(6.477a, b, d; 10.285)/ (6.477a–d)	(6.476a, b, d; 10.276)/ (6.476a–d)	(6.475a–d)/(6.475a–d)
Free Boundary* (10.277a–e) Figure 6.23d	(6.480a, b; 10.278; 10.279)/ (6.480a–d)	(6.479a, b, d; 10.276)/ (6.479a–d)	(6.478a, b, d; 10.282)/ (6.478a–d)

* for a plate made of a pseudo-isotropic orthotropic (isotropic) material before (after) the dash:
* first bending stiffness (6.413c, d) [(6.579a; 6.581a)];
* second bending stiffness (10.255a) [(10.255b)];
* stiffness ratio parameter (10.274a) [(10.275a)]

Note: The boundary conditions for the linear bending of an elastic plate lead to $3 \times 3 \times 2 = 18$ cases combining: (i) three types of boundary: clamped, pinned, and free; (ii) three shapes: arbitrary closed regular curve, circular, and straight; (iii) two types of elastic material: isotropic and pseudo-isotropic orthotropic.

E10.15.1 Elastic Energy along the Boundary of a Plate

The boundary condition is (problem 301) the vanishing (10.255c) of the elastic energy along the boundary on the r.h.s. of (6.453b):

$$\bar{C}_{44} = \frac{h^3}{12} C_{44} \to D(1-\sigma) = \text{const}:$$

$$\hat{E}_d = \int_{\partial C} \left\{ D\left(\nabla^2 \zeta\right) \partial_n (\delta\zeta) - \partial_n \left[D\left(\nabla^2 \zeta\right)\right] \delta\zeta + \bar{C}_{44}\, I_n \right\} ds, \tag{10.255a–c}$$

where the first bending stiffness (6.593a; 6.595a) [(6.413c, d)] for a pseudo-isotropic orthotropic (isotropic) plate need not be constant, and the second stiffness (10.255b) [(10.255a)] is constant (6.454a). The coefficient of the first (second) term of (10.255c) is in agreement with (6.609b) [(6.609c)] the turning moment (6.430a) [the stress couple (6.422a–c; 6.423a–c)] with additional contributions coming from the third term on the r.h.s. of (10.255c). The latter involves the deformation vector $\vec{I}$ given by (6.448d) whose normal component (6.451e) appears in (10.255c). Designating by θ the angle of the normal with the x-axis (Figure 6.24a) leads to the unit normal (6.462a) [tangent (6.462c)] vectors and associated derivatives (6.462b) [(6.462d)]. Using (6.462a), the normal component of the deformation vector (6.448d) is given by:

$$I_n = \vec{I}.\vec{n} = \cos\theta\left[\left(\partial_{xy}\zeta\right)\partial_y(\delta\zeta) - \left(\partial_{yy}\zeta\right)\partial_x(\delta\zeta)\right] + \sin\theta\left[\left(\partial_{xy}\zeta\right)\partial_x(\delta\zeta) - \left(\partial_{xx}\zeta\right)\partial_y(\delta\zeta)\right], \quad (10.256)$$

for substitution in the last term of the r.h.s. of (10.255c), leading to an integration by parts along the boundary (E10.15.2).

E10.15.2 Integration by Parts along a Closed Regular Boundary

Substituting (10.256) in the integral along the boundary in the third term on the r.h.s. of (10.255c) leads to (10.257):

$$\int_{\partial c}\bar{C}_{44}I_n ds = \int_{\partial c}\bar{C}_{44}\left\{\left[2\sin\theta\cos\theta\left(\partial_{xy}\zeta\right) - \sin^2\theta\left(\partial_{xx}\zeta\right) - \cos^2\theta\left(\partial_{yy}\zeta\right)\right]\delta\left(\partial_n\zeta\right) + \left[\cos\theta\sin\theta\left(\partial_{yy}\zeta - \partial_{xx}\zeta\right) + \left(\cos^2\theta - \sin^2\theta\right)\partial_{xy}\zeta\right]\partial_s(\delta\zeta)\right\}ds, \quad (10.257)$$

where (6.463b, c) was used to transform the gradient of $\delta\zeta$ in Cartesian coordinates $\{\partial_x, \partial_y\}$ to local normal ∂_n and tangential ∂_s derivatives. The integrand in the second term in square brackets on the r.h.s. of (10.257) is (10.258):

$$X \equiv \frac{\sin(2\theta)}{2}\left(\partial_{yy}\zeta - \partial_{xx}\zeta\right) + \cos(2\theta)\partial_{xy}\zeta, \quad (10.258)$$

leading to an integration by parts along the closed regular boundary (10.259a):

$$\int_{\partial c}\bar{C}_{44}\, X\, \partial_s(\delta\zeta)ds + \int_{\partial c}\delta\zeta\partial_s\left(\bar{C}_{44}\, X\right)ds = \int_{\partial c}\partial_s\left(\bar{C}_{44}\, X\,\delta\zeta\right)ds = \left[\bar{C}_{44}\, X\,\delta\zeta\right] = 0, \quad (10.259\text{a–d})$$

where (10.259b) is the difference of the expression in square brackets at the right-hand side (r.h.s.) and left-hand side (l.h.s) of the same point (10.259c) and hence, is zero by continuity (10.259d). Substituting (10.259d) in (10.252) and then in (10.255c) leads to (6.609a) ≡ (10.260), the elastic energy per unit length of the boundary:

$$\tilde{E}_d = \frac{d\hat{E}_d}{ds} = \left\{ -\left[\partial_n\left(D\nabla^2\zeta\right)\right] + \bar{C}_{44}\,\partial_s\left[\sin\theta\cos\theta\left(\partial_{xx}\zeta - \partial_{yy}\zeta\right) - \cos(2\theta)\partial_{xy}\zeta\right]\right\}\delta\zeta,$$
$$+\left\{D\nabla^2\zeta + \bar{C}_{44}\left[\sin(2\theta)\partial_{xy}\zeta - \sin^2\theta\,\partial_{xx}\zeta - \cos^2\theta\,\partial_{yy}\zeta\right]\right\}\delta(\partial_n\zeta), \tag{10.260}$$

where (E10.15.3) minus the coefficient of $\delta\zeta\left[\partial_n\left(\delta\zeta\right)\right]$ is the normal component of the stress couple (6.609b) [turning moment (6.609c)].

E10.15.3 Stress Couple and Turning Moment

Thus, *(problem 302) in the weak linear bending of a thin plate whose boundary is an arbitrary closed regular curve (Figure 6.24a) the stress couple (turning moment) normal to the boundary (10.260) ≡ (6.609a) is given by (10.261) ≡ (6.609b) [(10.262) ≡ (6.609c)], which has the dimensions of force (moment) per unit length:*

$$M_n = -\,D\nabla^2\zeta - \bar{C}_{44}\left[\sin(2\theta)\partial_{xy}\zeta - \sin^2\theta\,\partial_{xx}\zeta - \cos^2\theta\,\partial_{yy}\zeta\right] \tag{10.261}$$

$$N_n = \partial_n\left(D\nabla^2\zeta\right) - \bar{C}_{44}\,\partial_s\left[\sin\theta\cos\theta\left(\partial_{xx}\zeta - \partial_{yy}\zeta\right) - \cos(2\theta)\partial_{xy}\zeta\right]. \tag{10.262}$$

In the case of the nonlinear strong bending of a plate with in-plane stresses, the augmented turning moment is given by (6.682a–c). If the bending moment D is constant: (i) it can be taken out of the derivative in the first term on the r.h.s. of (10.262); (ii) from (10.255b) the Poisson ratio is also constant. If (problem 303) the plate is supported (Figure 6.23b) or pinned (Figure 6.23c) the vanishing of the displacement on the boundary (10.263a) simplifies the stress couple (10.261) [turning moment (10.262)] to (10.263b) [(10.263c, d)]:

$$\zeta = 0: \qquad M_n = -D\left(\partial_{nm}\zeta + \frac{d\theta}{ds}\partial_n\zeta\right) + \bar{C}_{44}\frac{d\theta}{ds}\partial_n\zeta. \tag{10.263a, b}$$

$$D = const: \qquad \frac{N_n}{D} = \partial_n\left(\nabla^2\zeta\right) = \partial_{nnn}\zeta + \frac{d\theta}{ds}\partial_{nn}\zeta. \tag{10.263c, d}$$

If (problem 304) the plate is clamped (Figure 6.23a) the conditions (10.264a, b) simplify the stress couple to (10.264c) and leaves the turning moment unchanged (10.263d) ≡ (10.264d):

$$\zeta = 0 = \partial_n: \qquad M_n = -D\partial_{nn}\zeta, \qquad \frac{N_n}{D} = \partial_{nnn}\zeta + \frac{d\theta}{ds}\partial_{nn}\zeta. \tag{10.264a–d}$$

The relations (10.261, 10.262; 10.263a–d; 10.264a–d) hold for a plate with any shape (Figure 6.24a) provided that the boundary is a closed regular curve. The proof of (10.263a–d) is made next (E10.15.4) before considering the three main types of boundary conditions (E10.15.6–E.10.15.8) for pseudo-isotropic orthotropic and isotropic plates (E10.15.5).

E10.15.4 Plate with Arbitrary Closed Regular Boundary

The condition (10.263a) ≡ (10.265a) applies to clamped (Figure 6.23a), supported (Figure 6.23b), and pinned (Figure 6.23c) plates, and implies that: (i) the derivatives of all orders along the boundary vanish (10.265b, c); (ii) the gradient in Cartesian coordinates (6.463b, c) simplifies to (10.265d, e):

$$\zeta = 0: \qquad \partial_s \zeta = 0 = \partial_{ss} \zeta, \qquad \{\partial_x \zeta, \partial_y \zeta\} = \{\cos\theta, \sin\theta\} \partial_n \zeta. \qquad (10.265\text{a–e})$$

The second-order derivatives of the transverse displacement in Cartesian coordinates are given (6.463b, c; 10.265d, e) by (10.266a–c):

$$\partial_{xy} \zeta = (\cos\theta\, \partial_n - \sin\theta\, \partial_s) \sin\theta\, \partial_n \zeta = \cos\theta \sin\theta \left(\partial_{nn} \zeta - \frac{d\theta}{ds} \partial_n \zeta \right), \qquad (10.266\text{a})$$

$$\partial_{yy} \zeta = (\sin\theta\, \partial_n + \cos\theta\, \partial_s) \sin\theta\, \partial_n \zeta = \sin^2\theta\, \partial_{nn} \zeta + \cos^2\theta \frac{d\theta}{ds} \partial_n \zeta, \qquad (10.266\text{b})$$

$$\partial_{xx} \zeta = (\cos\theta\, \partial_n - \sin\theta\, \partial_s) \cos\theta\, \partial_n \zeta = \cos^2\theta\, \partial_{nn} \zeta + \sin^2\theta \frac{d\theta}{ds} \partial_n \zeta, \qquad (10.266\text{c})$$

where (10.267a) was used since θ is the direction of the normal, hence, does not vary along it, implying (10.267b), which is the inverse (10.267c) of the radius of curvature (6.461c):

$$\partial_n \theta = 0, \qquad \partial_s \theta \equiv \frac{d\theta}{ds} = \frac{1}{R}; \qquad \zeta = 0: \qquad \nabla^2 \zeta = \partial_{xx} \zeta + \partial_{yy} \zeta = \partial_{nn} \zeta + \frac{d\theta}{ds} \partial_n \zeta, \qquad (10.267\text{a–f})$$

from (10.266b, c) follows that the Laplacian (10.267e) along the boundary (10.267d) is given by (10.267f) in terms of normal derivatives in agreement with the term in curved brackets in (6.474d). These results apply to pseudo-isotropic orthotropic plates, which include as the particular case the isotropic plate (E10.15.5).

E10.15.5 Isotropic and Pseudo-Isotropic Orthotropic Plates

Substituting (10.266a–c) in (10.262) the term in square brackets cancels and the turning moment simplifies to (10.268a) leading to (10.268b) using the Lapacian (10.267f):

$$N_n = \partial_n\left(D\nabla^2\zeta\right) = \partial_n\left[D\left(\partial_{nn}\zeta + \frac{d\theta}{ds}\partial_n\zeta\right)\right]; \tag{10.268a, b}$$

from (10.268b) follows (10.263d) for constant bending stiffness (10.263c). Substitution of (10.266a–c) in the term in square brackets in (10.261) cancels the coefficient of $\partial_{nn}\zeta$ and leaves only the coefficient of $\partial_n\zeta$:

$$\begin{aligned} &2\sin\theta\cos\theta\,\partial_{xy}\zeta - \sin^2\theta\,\partial_{xx}\zeta - \cos^2\theta\,\partial_{yy}\zeta \\ &= -\left(2\sin^2\theta\cos^2\theta + \sin^4\theta + \cos^4\theta\right)\frac{d\theta}{ds}\partial_n\zeta \\ &= -\left(\sin^2\theta + \cos^2\theta\right)^2\frac{d\theta}{ds}\partial_n\zeta = -\frac{d\theta}{ds}\partial_n\zeta. \end{aligned} \tag{10.269}$$

Substitution of (10.269) in (10.261) proves (10.263b) for a pseudo-isotropic orthotropic plate. Thus, *(problem 305) a clamped plate (Figure 6.23b) or a pinned plate (Figure 6.23c) has a turning moment (10.268a, b), that simplifies to (10.263d) ≡ (10.264d) for constant bending stiffness (10.263c); the turning moment is the same for isotropic (pseudo-isotropic orthotropic) plates with bending stiffness specified by (6.413c, d) [(6.593a; 6.595a)]. The same applies for the stress couple (10.264c) of clamped (Figure 6.23a) plate (10.129a, b). For a supported plate (Figure 6.23b) or pinned plate (Figure 6.23c) the stress couple (10.263b) for a pseudo-isotropic orthotropic plate simplifies for an isotropic plate (10.255b) to (10.270a):*

$$-\frac{M_n}{D} = \nabla^2\zeta - (1-\sigma)\frac{d\theta}{ds}\partial_n\zeta = \partial_{nn}\zeta + \sigma\frac{d\theta}{ds}\partial_n\zeta, \tag{10.270a, b}$$

where the Lapacian (10.267f) was used in (10.270b). The boundary conditions are considered next for the three main cases of (i) clamped plate (E10.15.6), (ii) supported or pinned plate (E10.15.7), and (iii) free boundary (E10.15.8).

E10.15.6 General or Rectangular Clamped Plate

For the weak linear bending of plate whose boundary is an arbitrary closed regular curve (10.271a) the clamping (Figure 6.23a) is specified by zero displacement (10.271b) and slope (10.271c), and it implies non-zero stress couple (10.271d) [turning moment (10.271e)]:

$$s(\theta) \in C^1(\partial C): \qquad \zeta = 0 = \partial_n\zeta, \qquad M_n \neq 0 \neq N_n, \tag{10.271a–e}$$

given by (10.263b) [(10.263d)] for a pseudo-isotropic orthotropic plate that simplify to (6.474a–d) for an isotropic plate. For a clamped circular plate, the boundary conditions in the isotropic case (6.473a–d) hold also for pseudo-isotropic orthotropic plates replacing (6.473c) by (10.272a, b):

$$M_r = -D\left(\partial_{rr}\zeta + \frac{1}{r}\partial_r\zeta\right) - \bar{C}_{44}\frac{1}{r}\partial_r\zeta = -D\,\partial_{rr}\zeta - \left(D + \bar{C}_{44}\right)\frac{1}{r}\partial_r\zeta. \qquad (10.272\text{a, b})$$

For the straight $y = 0$ side of a rectangular plate, the boundary conditions (6.472a, d) for the isotropic case apply also to the pseudo-isotropic orthotropic case.

E10.15.7 Boundary Conditions for Supported or Pinned Plates

The boundary conditions for general shape (10.271a) ≡ (10.273a) for support plates (Figure 6.23b) or pinning plates (Figure 6.23c) are zero displacement (10.273b) implying the non-zero turning moment (10.273e) and the non-zero slope (10.273c) implying the zero stress couple (10.273d):

$$s(\theta)\in C^1(\partial C): \qquad \zeta = 0 \neq \partial_n\zeta, \qquad M_n = 0 \neq N_n. \qquad (10.273\text{a–e})$$

The non-zero normal component of the turning moment is given by (10.263d) both for isotropic and pseudo-isotropic orthotropic plates; the vanishing of the normal component of the stress couple (10.263b) leads to the second boundary condition (10.274b) involving the stiffness ratio parameter (6.606a–c) ≡ (10.274a):

$$\chi \equiv \frac{\bar{C}_{44}}{D}: \qquad \partial_{nn}\zeta + \frac{d\theta}{ds}\partial_n\zeta = \chi\frac{d\theta}{ds}\partial_n\zeta; \qquad (10.274\text{a, b})$$

in the case of an isotropic plate (6.607a–c) ≡ (10.275a), the boundary condition (10.274b) simplifies to (10.275b) in agreement with (6.477c) ≡ (10.275b):

$$\chi = 1 - \sigma: \qquad \partial_{nn}\zeta + \sigma\frac{d\theta}{ds}\partial_n\zeta = 0. \qquad (10.275\text{a, b})$$

In the case of a supported or pinned circular plate, made of an isotropic material, the boundary conditions are (6.476a–d), where only (6.476c) is changed for a pseudo-isotropic orthotropic material to (10.276):

$$\partial_{rr}\zeta + \frac{1}{r}\partial_r\zeta = \frac{\chi}{r}\partial_r\zeta. \qquad (10.276)$$

For a supported or pinned rectangular plate, the boundary conditions (6.475a–d) are the same in the isotropic and pseudo-isotropic orthotropic cases.

E10.15.8 General, Circular, or Rectangular Plate with Free Boundary

At the free boundary of a plate with arbitrary shape (10.271a) ≡ (10.273a) ≡ (10.277a) neither the displacement (10.277b) [nor the slope (10.277c)] are zero and thus, the turning moment (10.277e) [and stress (couple (10.277d)] must be zero:

$$s(\theta)\in C^1(\partial C): \qquad \zeta\neq 0\neq\partial_n\zeta: \qquad M_n=0=N_n. \tag{10.277a–e}$$

The vanishing of the stress couple (10.261) [turning moment (10.262)] at the free boundary lead to the first (10.278) [second (10.279)] boundary conditions for a pseudo-isotropic orthotropic plate involving the parameter (6.606a–c):

$$-\chi^{-1}\nabla^2\zeta=\sin(2\theta)\,\partial_{xy}\zeta-\cos^2\theta\,\partial_{xx}\zeta-\sin^2\theta\,\partial_{yy}\zeta. \tag{10.278}$$

$$\chi^{-1}\,\partial_n\left(\nabla^2\zeta\right)=\partial_s\left[\,\sin\theta\cos\theta\left(\partial_{xx}\zeta-\partial_{yy}\zeta\right)-\cos(2\theta)\partial_{xy}\zeta\right]. \tag{10.279}$$

In the case (10.275a) of an isotropic plate, the general stress couple (10.261) [turning moment (10.262)] simplifies to (10.280) [(10.281)]:

$$M_n=-D\left\{\nabla^2\zeta-(1-\sigma)\left[\sin(2\theta)\partial_{yy}\zeta-\sin^2\theta\,\partial_{yy}\zeta-\cos^2\theta\,\partial_{yy}\zeta\right]\right\}, \tag{10.280}$$

$$N_n=\partial_n\left(D\nabla^2\zeta\right)-D(1-\sigma)\partial_s\left[\sin\theta\cos\theta\left(\partial_{xx}\zeta-\partial_{yy}\zeta\right)-\cos(2\theta)\partial_{yy}\zeta\right]. \tag{10.281}$$

The vanishing of (10.261; 10.262) [(10.280; 10.281)] at the free boundary of a pseudo-isotropic orthotropic (isotropic) plate leads to the same boundary conditions (10.278; 10.279) with different stiffness ratio parameter (6.606a–c) [(6.607a–c)]. At the free boundary of a circular (rectangular) plate, the boundary conditions (6.479a–d) [(6.478a–c)] in the isotropic case also apply in the pseudo-isotropic orthotropic case, replacing (6.479c) [(6.478c)] by (10.276) [(10.282)]:

$$\partial_{yy}\zeta+(1-\chi)\partial_{xx}\zeta=0. \tag{10.282}$$

The $2\times3\times3=18$ sets of boundary conditions combining different materials ($\times2$), shapes ($\times3$) and support ($\times3$) are summarized next (E10.15.9).

E10.15.9 Sets of Boundary Conditions for the Bending of a Plate

The 18 sets of boundary conditions (problem 306) for the linear bending of a thin plate are summarized in Table 10.3 according to three criteria: (i) the boundary is an arbitrary closed regular curve (Figure 6.24a) and, in particular, [Figure 6.24b(c)] circular (straight); (ii) the elastic plate is made of a pseudo-isotropic orthotropic material, in particular isotropic; (iii) the three main boundary conditions are clamped (Figure 6.23a), supported (Figure 6.23b), or pinned (Figure 6.23c) or free boundary (Figure 6.23d). The boundary conditions (6.480a–d) involve the displacement, the slope, and the normal components of the stress couple and the turning moment. Normal component means radial for a circular plate and along the y-axis for the straight side along the x-axis of a rectangular plate. For arbitrary/circular/rectangular plate the boundary is given, respectively, by (6.467e, c, a) and the slope by (6.464a, c, e). The normal component of the stress couple (turning moment) is given by (10.261) [(10.262)] for a pseudo-isotropic orthotropic plate and by (10.280) [(10.281)] for an isotropic plate. The stress couple for a pseudo-isotropic orthotropic (isotropic) plate simplifies to (10.283b) [(6.471d)] for a circular plate (10.283a) and to (10.283d) [(6.471b)] for a straight boundary (10.273c):

$$r = const: \quad -\frac{M_r}{D} = \partial_{rr}\zeta + \frac{1-\chi}{r}; \qquad y = 0: \quad -\frac{M_y}{D} = \partial_{yy}\zeta + (1-\chi)\partial_{xx}\zeta. \tag{10.283a–d}$$

The turning moment for a circular (6.467d) [rectangular (6.467b)] plate is the same for the isotropic and the pseudo-isotropic orthotropic plate.

The general form of the stress general couple (10.261) [turning moment (10.262)] simplifies: (i) to (10.263b)-[(10.263d)] for supported or pinned boundary (10.263a, c); (ii) to (10.264c) [(10.264d)] for clamped boundary (10.264a, b). Thus, the boundary conditions for arbitrary/circular/straight boundaries, respectively, of a pseudo-isotropic orthotropic (isotropic) plate are: (i) for clamped (6.474a, b, d; 10.263b)/(6.473a, b, d; 10.284)/(6.472a–d) [(6.474a–d)/(6.473a–d)/(6.472a–d)]:

$$M_r = -D\left(\partial_{rr}\zeta + \frac{1}{r}\partial_r\zeta\right) - \bar{C}_{44}\frac{1}{r}\partial_r\zeta; \tag{10.284}$$

(ii) for supported or pinned boundary (6.477a, b, d; 10.285)/(6.476a, b, d; 10.276)/(6.475a–d) [(6.477a–d)/(6.476a–d)/(6.475a–d)]:

$$\partial_{rr}\zeta + \frac{1-\chi}{r}\partial_r\zeta = 0; \tag{10.285}$$

(iii) for a free boundary (6.480a, b; 10.278, 10.279)/(6.479a, b, d; 10.276)/(6.478a, b, d; 10.282) [(6.480a–d)/(6.479a–d)/(6.478a–d)].

EXAMPLE 10.16 Strong Bending of a Pseudo-Isotropic Orthotropic Plate

Generalize the equations of strong bending of a thick elastic plate from an isotropic material (Foppl, 1907) to a pseudo-isotropic orthotropic material.

The balance equation (6.656) remains (problem 317) valid (10.286):

$$\frac{f}{h} = \frac{D}{h}\nabla^2\zeta - (\partial_{yy}\Theta)(\partial_{xx}\zeta) - (\partial_{xx}\Theta)(\partial_{yy}\zeta) + 2(\partial_{xy}\Theta)(\partial_{xy}\zeta), \tag{10.286}$$

replacing the first bending stiffness for an isotropic plate (6.413d) ≡ (10.287a) by that for a pseudo-isotropic orthotropic plate (6.593a; 6.595a) ≡ (10.287b):

$$\frac{E h^3}{12(1-\sigma^2)} \leftarrow D \rightarrow \frac{h^3}{12}\left(C_{11} - C_{13}\frac{C_{13}}{C_{23}}\right). \tag{10.287a, b}$$

Concerning the second complementary equation (6.657) of the pair: (i) the derivation from (6.659a, b) to the first equality in (6.666a–c) is independent of the type of material; (ii) the elimination of the in-plane displacements is made (10.288), as in (6.667a), retaining the strains from the first equality in (6.666a–c) leading to:

$$\frac{1}{2}\left[\partial_{yy}(\partial_x\zeta)^2 + \partial_{xx}(\partial_x\zeta)^2 - 2\partial_{xy}(\partial_x\zeta)(\partial_y\zeta)\right] = \partial_{yy}S_{xx} + \partial_{xx}S_{yy} + 2\partial_{xy}S_{xy}; \tag{10.288}$$

(iii) the l.h.s. of (10.288) is simplified as in (6.667b):

$$\begin{aligned}(\partial_{xy}\zeta)^2 - (\partial_{xx}\zeta)(\partial_{yy}\zeta) = {} & \partial_{yy}(A_{11}T_{xx} + A_{12}T_{yy}) + \partial_{xx}(A_{12}T_{xx} + A_{22}T_{yy}) \\ & + 2\partial_{xy}(A_{44}T_{xy}),\end{aligned} \tag{10.289}$$

and on the r.h.s. the compliance matrix (6.583) is used for an orthotropic material, bearing in mind that there are only in-plane stresses (6.312c–e); (iv) substituting (6.655e) in (10.289) it follows that (problem 318) *the complementary equation relating the transverse displacement to the stress function for the strong bending of an orthotropic plate (10.290b):*

$$A_{ab} = const: \quad \begin{aligned}&(\partial_{xy}\zeta)^2 - (\partial_{xx}\zeta)(\partial_{yy}\zeta) \\ &= A_{22}\,\partial_{xxxx}\Theta + A_{11}\,\partial_{yyyy}\Theta - 2(A_{12} + A_{44})\partial_{xxyy}\Theta,\end{aligned} \tag{10.290a, b}$$

assuming that the components of the compliance matrix are constant (10.290a).

The first (10.286) [second (10.290a, b)] equation of the coupled pair is valid for a pseudo-isotropic (general) orthotropic plate. In the complementary equation (10.290b), there are three coefficients (10.291a–c) specified by the compliance matrix (6.583):

$$\left\{ A_{22}, A_{11}, 2(A_{12}+A_{44}) \right\} = \left\{ \frac{1}{E_y}, \frac{1}{E_x}, -2\frac{\sigma_{yx}}{E_x} + \frac{1}{G_{yz}} \right\}. \tag{10.291a–c}$$

Several coefficients (10.292a–g) of the stiffness matrix (6.586):

$$\begin{aligned} &\left\{ C_{11}, C_{22}, C_{33}, C_{44}, C_{12}, C_{13}, C_{23} \right\} \\ &= \left\{ \frac{1-\sigma_{yz}\sigma_{zy}}{C_0 E_y E_z}, \frac{1-\sigma_{xz}\sigma_{zx}}{C_0 E_x E_z}, \frac{1-\sigma_{xy}\sigma_{yx}}{C_0 E_x E_y}, 2G_{yz}, \right. \\ &\qquad \left. \frac{\sigma_{yx}+\sigma_{yz}\,\sigma_{zx}}{C_0 E_y E_z}, \frac{\sigma_{zx}+\sigma_{zy}\,\sigma_{yx}}{C_0 E_y E_z}, \frac{\sigma_{zy}+\sigma_{zx}\,\sigma_{xy}}{C_0 E_x E_z} \right\}, \end{aligned} \tag{10.292a–g}$$

are needed, namely: (i)(ii) three (one) in the first (10.287b) ≡ (10.293b) [second (6.595b) ≡ (10.293a)] bending stiffness:

$$\bar{C}_{44} = \frac{h^3 G_{yz}}{6}, \; D = \frac{h^3}{12 C_0 E_y E_z}\left[1-\sigma_{yz}\,\sigma_{zy} - \frac{E_x}{E_y}\frac{\left(\sigma_{zx}+\sigma_{zy}\,\sigma_{yx}\right)^2}{\sigma_{zy}+\sigma_{zx}\,\sigma_{xy}} \right]; \tag{10.293a, b}$$

(iii)(iv) five (six) in the first (6.596a) ≡ (10.294a) [second (6.596b) ≡ (10.294b)] conditions for a pseudo-isotropic orthotropic material:

$$\begin{aligned} &E_z\left(1-\sigma_{xy}\sigma_{yx}\right)\left[E_y\left(1-\sigma_{xz}\sigma_{zx}\right)-E_x\left(1-\sigma_{yz}\sigma_{zy}\right)\right] \\ &\qquad = \left[E_y\left(\sigma_{zy}+\sigma_{zx}\,\sigma_{xy}\right)\right]^2 - \left[E_x\left(\sigma_{zx}+\sigma_{zy}\sigma_{yx}\right)\right]^2, \end{aligned} \tag{10.294a}$$

$$\begin{aligned} &E_z\left(1-\sigma_{xy}\,\sigma_{yx}\right)\left[1-\sigma_{xz}\,\sigma_{zx} - \frac{E_x}{E_y}\left(\sigma_{yx}+\sigma_{yz}\,\sigma_{zx}\right) \right] \\ &= \left(\sigma_{xy}+\sigma_{xz}\,\sigma_{zy}\right)\left[E_y\left(\sigma_{zy}+\sigma_{zx}\,\sigma_{xy}\right)-E_x\left(\sigma_{yz}+\sigma_{yz}\,\sigma_{zx}\right)\right]. \end{aligned} \tag{10.294b}$$

In conclusion, (problem 319) *the transverse displacement and stress function in the strong non-linear deflection of an elastic plate, made of a pseudo-isotropic orthotropic material, satisfy the coupled non-linear fourth-order partial differential equations (10.286; 10.290a, b) where: (i) the first bending stiffness (10.287b) is given by (10.293b); (ii) the second bending stiffness that appears in the boundary conditions (10.261; 10.262) is given by (10.293a). Four (seven) terms of the compliance (6.583) [stiffness (6.586)] matrix appear (10.291a–c) [(10.292a–g)] in the balance* *equations (i-ii) and the boundary conditions (ii-iii). The three Young moduli E_i, six Poisson ratio σ_{ij}, and three shear moduli G_{ij} satisfy (6.584b) [(6.587a–c)] in the compliance (stiffness) matrix for an orthotropic material. In addition, (problem 320) a pseudo-isotropic orthotropic material satisfies two additional relations (6.596a, b) ≡ (10.294a, b).*

EXAMPLE 10.17 Non-Linear and Linear Coupled Systems of Differential Equations

The simultaneous systems of differential equations are illustrated in the simplest case of two coupled differential equations, either non-linear (E10.17.1) or linear (E10.17.2).

E10.17.1 Simultaneous System of Non-Linear Ordinary Differential Equations

Eliminate the system of two simultaneous non-linear second-order ordinary differential equations:

$$y''z + y z' = 0, \qquad z'' + zy = 0, \qquad (10.295\text{a, b})$$

in two possible ways and conclude that it is of order four.

The system (10.295a, b) is equivalent to the system of four first-order equations:

$$\frac{dy}{dx} = y' \equiv u, \quad \frac{dz}{dx} = z' \equiv v, \quad u' = y'' = -\frac{yv}{z}, \quad v' = z'' = -zy. \qquad (10.296\text{a–d})$$

Thus, the order of the system cannot exceed four, but could be less. Eliminating for y leads to:

$$y'''y = -y\left(\frac{yv}{z}\right)' = -\frac{y'yv}{z} - \frac{y^2v'}{z} + \frac{y^2vz'}{z^2} = y'y'' + y^3 + \left(\frac{yv}{z}\right)^2 = y'y'' + y^3 + y''^2,$$
$$(10.297\text{a–d})$$

which is of the third-order. Thus, the system could be of order three or order four. To find out which is the case, the system is eliminated for z:

$$z''' = -(zy)' = -z'y - y'z = \frac{z'z''}{z} - y'z, \qquad (10.298\text{a–c})$$

$$z^2 z'''' = z^2 \left(\frac{z'z''}{z}\right)' - z^2 z'y' - z^3 y'' = z''' z'z + z''^2 z - z''z'^2 + z^2 z'\left(\frac{z''}{z}\right)' + z^2 z'y,$$

$$= 2z'''z'z + z''^2 z - 2z''z'^2 - z''z'z,$$

(10.299a–c)

proving that it is of the fourth order.

E10.17.2 Linear Differential System with a Given Characteristic Polynomial

Consider the coupled system of linear differential equations (10.300a, b):

$$y'' + cz'' + \alpha y + \beta z = 0 = y' + z' + \gamma y + \delta z, \qquad (10.300\text{a, b})$$

and determine the constant coefficients $(\alpha, \beta, \gamma, \delta)$ so that (10.301a) [(10.302a)]:

$$c = 0: \qquad P_3(D) = (D-1)(D+1)(D+2), \qquad (10.301\text{a, b})$$

$$c = 1: \qquad P_2(D) = \lambda(D-\mu)^2, \qquad (10.302\text{a, b})$$

the characteristic polynomial (10.301b) [(10.302b)]: (i) is of the third (second) degree; (ii) has three distinct roots $\pm 1, -2$ (a double root μ); and (iii) the coefficient of the leading power is $1(\lambda)$.

The coupled system of linear differential equations with constant coefficients (10.300a, b) ≡ (10.303):

$$\begin{bmatrix} D^2 + \alpha & cD^2 + \beta \\ D + \gamma & D + \delta \end{bmatrix} \begin{bmatrix} y(x) \\ z(x) \end{bmatrix} = 0, \qquad (10.303)$$

has the characteristic polynomial:

$$P_3(D) = \left(D^2 + \alpha\right)(D + \delta) - \left(cD^2 + \beta\right)(D + \gamma)$$

$$= (1-c)D^3 + (\delta - c\gamma)D^2 + (\alpha - \beta)D + \alpha\delta - \beta\gamma, \qquad (10.304\text{a, b})$$

which simplifies to (10.305b) [(10.306b)]:

$$c = 0: \qquad P_3(D) = D^3 + \delta D^2 + (\alpha - \beta)D + \alpha\delta - \beta\gamma, \qquad (10.305\text{a, b})$$

$$c = 1: \qquad P_2(D) = (\delta - \gamma)D^2 + (\alpha - \beta)D + \alpha\delta - \beta\gamma, \qquad (10.306\text{a, b})$$

for (10.301a) ≡ (10.305a) [(10.302a) ≡ (10.306a)].

In the case (10.301a) ≡ (10.305a) ≡ (10.307a), the characteristic polynomial (10.301b) ≡ (10.307b) ≡ (10.307c):

$$c = 0: \qquad P_3(D) = (D^3 - 1)(D + 2) = D^3 + 2D^2 - D - 2, \tag{10.307a–c}$$

coincides with (10.305b) if (10.308a–c) hold:

$$\delta = 2: \qquad \beta - \alpha = 1, \qquad \beta\gamma - \alpha\delta = 2: \qquad \beta = 1 + \alpha, \quad \gamma = 2, \tag{10.308a–e}$$

leading to (10.308d, e). Substituting (10.308a, d, e) in (10.300a, b; 10.301a) specifies the differential system (10.309a, b):

$$y'' + \alpha y + (1 + \alpha) z = 0 = y' + z' + 2(y + z). \tag{10.309a, b}$$

The roots (10.310a) of the characteristic polynomial (10.301b) lead to the general integral (10.310b):

$$a_{1-3} = \pm 1, -2: \qquad y(x) = C_1 e^{-2x} + C_2 \cosh x + C_3 \sinh x, \tag{10.310a, b}$$

where C_{1-3} are arbitrary constants.

In the case (10.302a) ≡ 10.306a) ≡ (10.311a), the characteristic polynomial (10.302b) ≡ (10.311b):

$$c = 1: \qquad P_2(D) = \lambda D^2 - 2\lambda\mu D + \mu^2\lambda, \tag{10.311a, b}$$

coincides with (10.306b) if (10.312a–c) hold:

$$\delta - \gamma = \lambda, \qquad \beta - \alpha = 2\lambda\mu, \qquad \alpha\delta - \beta\gamma = \mu^2\lambda, \tag{10.312a–c}$$

the compatibility of (10.312a–c) requires:

$$\alpha\delta - \beta\gamma = \mu^2\lambda = \frac{(2\mu\lambda)^2}{4\lambda} = \frac{(\beta - \alpha)^2}{4(\delta - \gamma)}, \tag{10.313a–d}$$

that the constants $(\alpha, \beta, \gamma, \delta)$ be related by (10.313d) ≡ (10.314a):

$$(\beta - \alpha)^2 = 4(\delta - \gamma)(\alpha\delta - \beta\gamma): \qquad \lambda = \delta - \gamma, \qquad 2\mu = \frac{\beta - \alpha}{\delta - \gamma}, \tag{10.314a–c}$$

in which case the parameters (λ,μ) are given by (10.312a, b) ≡ (10.314b, c). The differential system (10.300a, b; 10.302a) ≡ (10.315a, b):

$$y'' + z'' + \alpha y + \beta z = 0 = y' + z' + \gamma y + \delta z, \qquad y(x) = e^{\mu x}\left(D_1 + D_2\, x\right). \tag{10.315a–c}$$

has the general integral (10.315c) where D_{1-2} are arbitrary constants.

In the case (10.309a, b) substitution of (10.310b) in (10.309a) ≡ (10.316a) leads to the second general integral (10.316b):

$$(1+\alpha)z(x) = -y''(x) - \alpha y(x) = -(\alpha+4)C_1 e^{-2x} - (1+\alpha)\left(C_2 \cosh x + C_3 \sinh x\right). \tag{10.316a, b}$$

In the case (10.315a, b) substitution of (10.315c; 10.317a) in (10.315b) leads to (10.317b, c):

$$z(x) = e^{\mu x}\left(E_1 + E_2 x\right): \qquad D_2(\mu+\gamma) + E_2(\mu+\delta) = 0,$$

$$D_1(\mu+\gamma) + D_2 + E_1(\mu+\delta) + E_2 = 0. \tag{10.317a–c}$$

Solving (10.317b, c) for $E_{1,2}$ leads to (10.318a, b):

$$E_2 = -D_2 \frac{\mu+\gamma}{\mu+\delta}, \quad E_1 = -D_1 \frac{\mu+\gamma}{\mu+\delta} + D_2 \frac{\gamma-\delta}{(\mu+\delta)^2}, \tag{10.318a, b}$$

and hence (10.317a) to the general integral (10.319):

$$\frac{\mu+\delta}{\mu+\gamma} z(x) = -e^{\mu x}\left[D_1 + D_2\, x - D_2 \frac{\gamma-\delta}{(\mu+\gamma)(\mu+\delta)}\right]. \tag{10.319}$$

In conclusion, *the coupled system of linear differential equations with constant coefficients (10.300a, b) for (10.301a) [(10.302a)]: (i) simplifies to (10.309a, b) [(10.315a, b)]; (ii) has the cubic (10.301b) [quadratic (10.302b)] characteristic polynomial if the four constants satisfy (10.308a, d, e)[(10.314a–c)]; (iii) has the general integral (10.310b; 10.316b) [(10.315c; 10.319)] where* $C_{1,2,3}\left(D_{1,2}\right)$ *are arbitrary constants.*

EXAMPLE 10.18 Three Coupled Systems with a Matrix of Characteristic Polynomials

The simultaneous systems with matrix of characteristic polynomials are illustrated in the simplest case of two coupled forced equations of three types; (i)(ii) linear differential equations with constant (homogeneous) coefficients

[E10.18.1 (E10.18.2)]; (iii) linear finite difference equations with constant coefficients (E10.18.3–E10.18.6).

E10.18.1 Forced Coupled Linear Differential System with Constant Coefficients

Consider the system (10.320a, b):

$$y' + z' - y = e^{2x} + x, \qquad y'' + z' - y + z = e^{x} + x^2, \tag{10.320a, b}$$

and obtain the complete integral.

The forced coupled system of linear differential equations with constant coefficients (10.320a, b) ≡ (10.321a, b):

$$D \equiv \frac{d}{dx}: \qquad \begin{bmatrix} D-1 & D \\ D^2-1 & D+1 \end{bmatrix}\begin{bmatrix} y(x) \\ z(x) \end{bmatrix} = e^{2x}\begin{bmatrix} 1 \\ 0 \end{bmatrix} + e^{x}\begin{bmatrix} 0 \\ 1 \end{bmatrix} + \begin{bmatrix} x \\ x^2 \end{bmatrix}, \tag{10.321a, b}$$

has the characteristic polynomial (10.322a–c):

$$P_3(D) = \begin{vmatrix} D-1 & D \\ D^2-1 & D+1 \end{vmatrix} = (D^2-1)(1-D) = -(D-1)^2(D+1) = -D^3 + D^2 + D - 1, \tag{10.322a–d}$$

with double (single) root 1(–1) leading to the general integral (10.323a) for $y(x)$, where (A, B, C) are arbitrary constants:

$$y(x) = (A + Bx)e^{x} + Ce^{-x}; \qquad z'(x) = y(x) - y'(x), \tag{10.323a, b}$$

the general integral (10.323b) for z follows from (10.320a) without forcing and substitution of (10.323a) leads to (10.323c):

$$z'(x) = -Be^{x} + 2Ce^{-x}, \qquad z(x) = -Be^{x} - 2Ce^{-x}, \tag{10.323c, d}$$

and hence by integration to (10.323d).

The forcing by the first term on the r.h.s. of (10.321b), which is a non-resonant exponential (7.121a, b) uses the inverse matrix of (10.321b) and leads to the particular integrals (10.324a–d):

$$\begin{bmatrix} y(x) \\ z(x) \end{bmatrix} = \lim_{b\to 2} \frac{e^{bx}}{P_3(b)}\begin{bmatrix} b+1 & -b \\ 1-b^2 & b-1 \end{bmatrix}\begin{bmatrix} 1 \\ 0 \end{bmatrix} = \frac{e^{2x}}{P_3(2)}\lim_{b\to 2}\begin{bmatrix} b+1 \\ 1-b^2 \end{bmatrix} = -\frac{e^{2x}}{3}\begin{bmatrix} 3 \\ -3 \end{bmatrix} = e^{2x}\begin{bmatrix} -1 \\ 1 \end{bmatrix}. \tag{10.324a–d}$$

The forcing by the second term on the r.h.s. of (10.321b), which is a doubly resonant exponential (7.122a, b) is given by (10.325a–d):

$$\begin{bmatrix} y(x) \\ z(x) \end{bmatrix} = \lim_{b\to 1} \frac{1}{P_3''(b)} \frac{\partial^2}{\partial b^2} \left\{ e^{bx} \begin{bmatrix} b+1 & -b \\ 1-b^2 & b-1 \end{bmatrix} \begin{bmatrix} 0 \\ 1 \end{bmatrix} \right\}$$

$$= \lim_{b\to 1} \frac{1}{2-6b} \frac{\partial^2}{\partial b^2} \left\{ e^{bx} \begin{bmatrix} -b \\ b-1 \end{bmatrix} \right\}$$

$$= -\frac{1}{4} \lim_{b\to 1} e^{bx} \left\{ x^2 \begin{bmatrix} -b \\ b-1 \end{bmatrix} + 2x \begin{bmatrix} -1 \\ 1 \end{bmatrix} \right\} \tag{10.325a–d}$$

$$= \frac{e^x}{4} \begin{bmatrix} x(x+2) \\ -2x \end{bmatrix}.$$

The forcing by the last term on the r.h.s. of (10.321b) leads to particular integrals (10.326a–d) using the inverse matrix of polynomials of derivatives:

$$\begin{bmatrix} y(x) \\ z(x) \end{bmatrix} = \frac{1}{P_3(D)} \begin{bmatrix} D+1 & -D \\ 1-D^2 & D-1 \end{bmatrix} \begin{bmatrix} x \\ x^2 \end{bmatrix} = -\frac{1}{1-D-D^2+O(D^3)} \begin{bmatrix} 1-x \\ 3x-x^2 \end{bmatrix}$$

$$= -\left[1+D+2D^2+O(D^3)\right] \begin{bmatrix} 1-x \\ 3x-x^2 \end{bmatrix} = \begin{bmatrix} x \\ x^2-x+1 \end{bmatrix}. \tag{10.326a–d}$$

Adding the general integral (10.323a, d) of the unforced system on the l.h.s. of (10.320a, b) ≡ (10.321a, b) to the particular integrals (10.324d; 10.325d; 10.326d) corresponding to the three forcing terms on the r.h.s. leads to:

$$y(x) = (A+Bx)e^x + Ce^{-x} - e^{2x} + \frac{x(x+2)}{4}e^x + x, \tag{10.327a}$$

$$z(x) = -Be^x - 2Ce^{-x} + e^{2x} - \frac{xe^x}{2} + x^2 - x + 1, \tag{10.327b}$$

as the complete integral (10.327a, b) of the coupled forced system of linear differential equations with constant coefficients (10.320a, b) ≡ (10.321a, b).

E10.18.2 Forced Coupled Linear Differential System with Homogeneous Coefficients

Consider the system (10.328a, b):

$$xy' + xz' - y = x^2 + \log x, \quad x^2 y'' + xy' + xz' - y + z = x + 2\log x, \quad (10.328\text{a, b})$$

and obtain the general integral.

The forced coupled linear system of differential equations with homogeneous coefficients (10.328a, b) ≡ (10.329a, b):

$$\delta \equiv x\frac{d}{dx}: \qquad \begin{bmatrix} \delta - 1 & \delta \\ \delta(\delta-1)+\delta-1 & \delta+1 \end{bmatrix} \begin{bmatrix} y(x) \\ z(x) \end{bmatrix} = x^2 \begin{bmatrix} 1 \\ 0 \end{bmatrix} + x \begin{bmatrix} 0 \\ 1 \end{bmatrix} + \begin{bmatrix} 1 \\ 2 \end{bmatrix} \log x, \quad (10.329\text{a, b})$$

has the same matrix (10.321b) ≡ (10.329b) replacing homogeneous (10.329a) by ordinary (10.321a) derivatives. Hence, the changes of variables (10.10a, b) lead from (10.327a, b) to:

$$y(x) = (A + B\log x)x + \frac{C}{x} - x^2 + \frac{x}{4}\log x(2 + \log x) + \log x, \quad (10.330\text{a})$$

$$z(x) = -Bx - \frac{2C}{x} + x^2 - \frac{x}{2}\log x + \log^2 x - \log x + 1, \quad (10.330\text{b})$$

as the complete integral (10.330a, b) of the forced coupled linear system of differential equations with homogeneous coefficients (10.328a, b) ≡ (10.329a, b).

E10.18.3 Forced Coupled System of Finite Difference Equations

Consider the system (10.331a, b):

$$y_{n+1} + z_{n+1} - y_n = 0, \qquad y_{n+2} + z_{n+1} - y_n + z_n = 0, \quad (10.331\text{a, b})$$

and obtain the complete solution.

The unforced coupled linear system of finite difference equations with homogeneous coefficients (10.331a, b) ≡ (10.332a, b):

$$\Delta\{y_n, z_n\} \equiv \{y_{n+1}, z_{n+1}\}: \qquad \begin{bmatrix} \Delta - 1 & \Delta \\ \Delta^2 - 1 & \Delta + 1 \end{bmatrix} \begin{bmatrix} y_n \\ z_n \end{bmatrix} = 0, \quad (10.332\text{a, b})$$

coincides with the unforced part of (10.321b) [(10.329b)] replacing ordinary (10.321a) [homogeneous (10.329a)] derivatives by forward finite differences

(10.332a). The changes of variable (1.445c, 1.446c, 1.447c) ≡ (10.33a, b) and (1.448b–d) ≡ (10.333c, d):

$$e^{ax} \quad \leftrightarrow \quad x^a \quad \leftrightarrow \quad a^n, \qquad x^n \quad \leftrightarrow \quad \log^n x \quad \leftrightarrow \quad n, \qquad \text{(10.333a–d)}$$

lead from the first three (two) terms of (10.327a) ≡ (10.330a) [(10.327b) ≡ (10.330b)] to (10.334a) [(10.334b)]:

$$y_n = A + Bn + C(-)^n, \qquad z_n = -B - 2C(-)^n, \qquad \text{(10.334a, b)}$$

as the general solution (10.334a, b) of the coupled unforced system of linear finite difference equations with constant coefficients (10.331a, b).

E10.18.4 System of Finite Difference Equations with Oscillatory Forcing

Consider the forcing of a coupled linear system of finite difference equations with constant coefficients by products consisting of (i) power with integral exponent and (ii) an hyperbolic [and/or (iii) circular] cosine or sine of multiple angles; in particular, determine a particular solution of the system:

$$y_{\ell+1} - y_\ell - z_\ell = b^\ell \cos(2\ell\phi), \qquad y_{\ell+1} + z_{\ell+1} + y_\ell = b^\ell \cos(2\ell\phi), \qquad \text{(10.335a, b)}$$

for all values of (b, ϕ). The solution of (10.335a, b) includes oscillatory (non-oscillatory) general (particular) cases [E10.18.5 (E10.18.6)].

E10.18.5 Forcing by Power Multiplied by a Cosine

Consider the coupled linear system of finite difference equations with constant coefficients forced (10.335a, b) ≡ (10.336a, b) product of (i) a power with integral exponent by (ii) an circular cosine of the double of the same multiple of an angle:

$$\begin{bmatrix} \Delta - 1 & -1 \\ \Delta + 1 & \Delta \end{bmatrix} \begin{bmatrix} y_\ell \\ z_\ell \end{bmatrix} = \begin{bmatrix} 1 \\ 1 \end{bmatrix} b^\ell \cos(2\ell\phi) = \operatorname{Re}\left(b^\ell e^{i2\ell\phi}\right). \qquad \text{(10.336a, b)}$$

The matrix of polynomials of finite differences (10.336a) ≡ (10.337a) has the matrix of co-factors (10.337b):

$$R_{m,r}(\Delta) = \begin{bmatrix} \Delta - 1 & -1 \\ \Delta + 1 & \Delta \end{bmatrix}, \qquad \overline{R}_{m,r}(\Delta) = \begin{bmatrix} \Delta & 1 \\ -\Delta - 1 & \Delta - 1 \end{bmatrix}, \qquad \text{(10.337a, b)}$$

and the determinant specifying (10.338a–c) the characteristic polynomial:

$$R_2(\Delta) = Det\left[R_{m,r}(\Delta)\right] = \Delta(\Delta - 1) + \Delta + 1 = \Delta^2 + 1; \qquad \text{(10.338a–c)}$$

in the solution (7.299b) appear (10.339a, b):

$$\bar{R}_{r,m}(\Delta)G_m = \begin{bmatrix} \Delta & 1 \\ -\Delta-1 & \Delta-1 \end{bmatrix}\begin{bmatrix} 1 \\ 1 \end{bmatrix} = \begin{bmatrix} 1+\Delta \\ -2 \end{bmatrix}. \tag{10.339a, b}$$

Substitution of (10.337b; 10.338c) in (7.299b) leads to the particular solution (10.340):

$$\begin{bmatrix} y_\ell \\ z_\ell \end{bmatrix} = \left\{ \lim_{\Delta \to b e^{i2\phi}} \frac{\Delta^\ell}{1+\Delta^2}\begin{bmatrix} 1+\Delta \\ -2 \end{bmatrix} \right\}, \tag{10.340}$$

of (10.335a, b) ≡ (10.336a, b).

The characteristic polynomial (10.338c) ≡ (10.341) appears in (10.340):

$$R_2\left(b e^{i2\phi}\right) = b^2 e^{4i\phi} + 1 = b^2 \cos(4\phi) + 1 + i b^2 \sin(4\phi), \tag{10.341}$$

in the inverse form (10.342b, c):

$$b^2 e^{i4\phi} \neq -1: \quad \frac{1}{R_2\left(b e^{i2\phi}\right)} = \frac{b^2\cos(4\phi)+1-ib^2\sin(4\phi)}{\left[b^2\cos(4\phi)+1\right]^2 + b^4\sin^2(4\phi)} = \frac{b^2 e^{-i4\phi}+1}{1+b^4+2b^2\cos(4\phi)}, \tag{10.342a–c}$$

excluding the special case (10.342a), which is considered separately (E10.18.5). Substituting (10.342c) in (10.340) leads to (10.343a–c):

$$\begin{aligned} b e^{i2\phi} \neq \pm i: \quad \begin{bmatrix} y_\ell \\ z_\ell \end{bmatrix} &= \operatorname{Re}\left\{ \frac{\left(b e^{i2\phi}\right)^\ell \left(1+b^2 e^{-i4\phi}\right)}{1+b^4+2b^2\cos(4\phi)} \begin{bmatrix} 1+b e^{i2\phi} \\ -2 \end{bmatrix} \right\} \\ &= \frac{b^\ell}{1+b^4+2b^2\cos(4\phi)} \times \operatorname{Re}\begin{bmatrix} e^{i2\ell\phi} + b e^{i2(\ell+1)\phi} + b^2 e^{i2(\ell-2)\phi} + b^3 e^{i2(\ell-1)\phi} \\ -2e^{i2\ell\phi} - 2b^2 e^{i2(\ell-2)\phi} \end{bmatrix}, \end{aligned} \tag{10.343a–c}$$

which specifies the particular solution (10.344b, c) of (10.335a, b) ≡ (10.336a, b):

$$(b,\phi) \neq \left(1, \pm\frac{\pi}{4}\right): \qquad z_\ell = -\,2b^\ell \frac{\cos(2\ell\phi) + b^2\cos\left[2(\ell-2)\phi\right]}{1+b^4+2b^2\cos(4\phi)}, \tag{10.344a, b}$$

$$y_\ell = b^\ell \frac{\cos(2\ell\phi) + b\cos\left[2(\ell+1)\phi\right] + b^2\cos\left[2(\ell-2)\phi\right] + b^3\cos\left[2(\ell-1)\phi\right]}{1+b^4+2b^2\cos(4\phi)}, \tag{10.344c}$$

except in the special case (10.344a), which is considered next (E10.18.5).

E10.18.6 Special Case of Constant Forcing

The case (10.344a), which is excluded from (10.344b, c), corresponds to (10.343a) ≡ (10.345a) in (10.335a, b) ≡ (10.345b, c):

$$c \equiv b e^{i2\phi} = \pm i: \qquad y_{\ell+1} - y_\ell - z_\ell = \operatorname{Re}\left(c^\ell\right) = y_{\ell+1} + z_{\ell+1} + y_\ell, \tag{10.345a–c}$$

which is equivalent to (10.345a–c) ≡ (10.346a–c):

$$\operatorname{Re}\left(c^\ell\right) = \operatorname{Re}\left(e^{\pm i\pi\ell/2}\right): \qquad y_{\ell+1} - y_\ell - z_\ell = \cos\left(\frac{\pi\ell}{2}\right) = y_{\ell+1} + z_{\ell+1} + y_\ell. \tag{10.346a–c}$$

The system (10.345b, c) ≡ (10.347):

$$\begin{bmatrix} \Delta - 1 & -1 \\ \Delta + 1 & \Delta \end{bmatrix} \begin{bmatrix} y_\ell \\ z_\ell \end{bmatrix} = c^\ell \begin{bmatrix} 1 \\ 1 \end{bmatrix}, \tag{10.347a}$$

has for (10.347b) the solutions (10.347c, d), where (10.337b; 10.338c) were used:

$$c \neq \pm i: \qquad \begin{bmatrix} y_\ell \\ z_\ell \end{bmatrix} = \frac{c^\ell}{R_2(c)} \begin{bmatrix} c & 1 \\ -c-1 & c-1 \end{bmatrix} \begin{bmatrix} 1 \\ 1 \end{bmatrix} = \frac{c^\ell}{1+c^2} \begin{bmatrix} 1+c \\ -2 \end{bmatrix}. \tag{10.347b–d}$$

The resonant case (10.347e) leads (7.300b) to (10.347f–i):

$$\begin{aligned} c \neq \pm i: \qquad \begin{bmatrix} y_\ell \\ z_\ell \end{bmatrix} &= \operatorname{Re}\left\{ \lim_{c \to \pm i} \left[\frac{1}{R_2'(c)} \frac{\partial}{\partial c} \left(c^\ell \begin{bmatrix} 1+c \\ -2 \end{bmatrix} \right) \right] \right\} \\ &= \operatorname{Re}\left\{ \lim_{c \to \pm i} \left[\frac{\log c}{2c} \right] \begin{pmatrix} c^\ell + c^{\ell+1} \\ -2 \end{pmatrix} \right\} = \frac{\pi}{4} \operatorname{Re}\left\{ c^{\pm i\pi\ell/2} \begin{bmatrix} 1 \pm i \\ -2 \end{bmatrix} \right\} \\ &= \frac{\pi}{4} \begin{bmatrix} \cos(\pi\ell/2) - \sin(\pi\ell/2) \\ -2\cos(\pi\ell/2) \end{bmatrix}. \end{aligned} \tag{10.347e–i}$$

Thus, *the system (10.345b, c) [(10.346b, c)] has particular solution (10.347c, d) ≡ (10.348a–c) [(10.347e, c) ≡ (10.349a–c):*

$$c \neq \pm i: \qquad y_\ell = c^\ell \frac{1+c}{1+c^2}, \qquad z_\ell = -\frac{2c^\ell}{1+c^2}; \tag{10.348a–c}$$

$$c = \pm i: \qquad y_\ell = \frac{\pi}{4}\left[\cos\left(\frac{\pi\ell}{2}\right) - \sin\left(\frac{\pi\ell}{2}\right)\right], \qquad z_\ell = -\frac{\pi}{2}\cos\left(\frac{\pi\ell}{2}\right). \tag{10.349a–c}$$

In conclusion, *the particular solution of (10.335a, b) ≡ (10.336a, b) is (10.344b, c) except (10.344a) ≡ (10.343a) ≡ (10.342a) for the special case (10.346a, c; 10.349b, c).*

E10.18.7 General and Complete Solutions

In both cases, the general solution is (10.350a, b):

$$y_\ell = A\cos\left(\frac{\ell\pi}{2}\right) + B\sin\left(\frac{\ell\pi}{2}\right), \tag{10.350a}$$

$$z_\ell = (B - A)\cos\left(\frac{\ell\pi}{2}\right) - (A + B)\sin\left(\frac{\ell\pi}{2}\right), \tag{10.350b}$$

whose value is indicated in Table 10.4, where (A,B) are arbitrary constants determined by initial values. The complete solution adds to the general solution (10.350a, b), the particular solutions (10.344a–c), simplifying to (10.348a–c) for (10.345a–c) and (10.349a–c) for (10.349a, b). The general solution (10.350a, b) is obtained as follows: (i) the characteristic polynomial (10.338c) has roots (10.351a, b) leading to the solutions (10.351c, d):

$$\Delta = \pm i = e^{\pm i\pi/2}: \qquad \left(e^{\pm i\,\pi/2}\right)^\ell = e^{\pm i\ell\pi/2} = \cos\left(\frac{\ell\pi}{2}\right) \pm i\,\sin\left(\frac{\ell\pi}{2}\right), \tag{10.351a–d}$$

TABLE 10.4

General Solution (10.350a, b) of Coupled System of Finite Difference Equations (10.346a, b)

$\ell =$	$4n$	$4n+1$	$4n+2$	$4n+3$
$\cos\left(\frac{\ell\pi}{2}\right)$	1	0	–1	0
$\sin\left(\frac{\ell\pi}{2}\right)$	0	1	0	–1
y_ℓ	A	B	$-A$	$-B$
z_ℓ	$B - A$	$A - B$	$A - B$	$A + B$

Note: The general integral (10.350a, b) of the coupled system of linear finite difference equations with constant coefficients (10.334a, b) leads to four cases, for ℓ, a multiple of 4, or adding 1, 2, or 3.

of which a real linear combination with arbitrary constants *(A, B)* was chosen in the r.h.s. (10.350a); (ii) substituting (10.350a) in the l.h.s. of (10.335a) leads to (10.351e, f):

$$z_\ell = y_{\ell+1} - y_\ell = A\left[\cos\left(\frac{\ell\pi}{2}+\frac{\pi}{2}\right) - \cos\left(\frac{\ell\pi}{2}\right)\right] + B\left[\sin\left(\frac{\ell\pi}{2}+\frac{\pi}{2}\right) - \sin\left(\frac{\ell\pi}{2}\right)\right]$$
$$= A\left[-\sin\left(\frac{\ell\pi}{2}\right) - \cos\left(\frac{\ell\pi}{2}\right)\right] + B\left[\cos\left(\frac{\ell\pi}{2}\right) - \sin\left(\frac{\ell\pi}{2}\right)\right], \tag{10.351e–g}$$

which coincides with (10.351g) ≡ (10.350b).

EXAMPLE 10.19 Asymptotic Stability of a Damped Non-Linear Oscillator

Prove that the damped oscillator with parameters depending on position (9.109a) ≡ (9.111b) is asymptotically stable in all cases, including $v = 0$ when the total energy (9.112c) as stability function is inconclusive because $\dot{H} = 0$ in (9.113e).

The stability function is chosen (10.352b) as total energy (9.112a) plus an extra term (10.352c):

$$f(x) = k(x)x: \qquad H = E + \alpha m v f = \frac{m}{2}v^2 + \int_0^x f(\xi)d\xi + \alpha v m f, \tag{10.352a–c}$$

where (10.352a) is the restoring force, and α is a constant to be chosen at will. To prove the asymptotic stability, in all cases, it is sufficient to show that there is a value of α for which: (i) the stability function (10.352c) is positive-definite (10.353a):

$$H > 0 > \dot{H} = \frac{\partial H}{\partial x}\frac{dx}{dt} + \frac{\partial H}{\partial v}\frac{dv}{dt} = v\frac{\partial H}{\partial x} - \frac{\mu v + f}{m}\frac{\partial H}{\partial v}; \tag{10.353a–d}$$

(ii) its time derivative (10.353c, d) following the differential system is negative-definite (10.353b). In order to prove the inequalities (10.353a, b), use will be made of the identity (10.354a, b):

$$\beta > 0: \qquad \left(\frac{a}{\sqrt{\beta}} + b\sqrt{\beta}\right)^2 > 0 \quad \rightarrow \; -2ab < \frac{a^2}{\beta} + b^2\beta, \tag{10.354a–c}$$

in the form (10.354c).

E10.19.1 Positive-Definite Stability Function

The inequality (10.354c) with (10.355a) is applied to the last term of the stability function (10.352b) leading to (10.355b, c):

$$\beta = 1: \qquad H \geq E - \frac{m\alpha}{2}\left(v^2 + f^2\right) = \frac{m}{2}(1-\alpha)v^2 + \int_0^x f(\xi)\, d\xi - \frac{m}{2} f^2 \alpha. \tag{10.355a–c}$$

The middle term is compared with the last term on the r.h.s. of (10.355c) using L'Hôpital rule (I.19.35):

$$\lim_{x\to 0} \frac{\left[f(x)\right]^2}{\int_0^x f(\xi) d\xi} = \lim_{x\to 0} \frac{2f' f}{f} = 2 f'(0) = 2 \lim_{x\to 0}\left[x k(x)\right]' = 2k(0) > 0, \tag{10.356a–d}$$

where $k(0)$ is the resilience of the spring at zero displacement, as for a linear restoring force. It follows that there exists a constant (10.357a) such that (10.357b) holds:

$$c > 0: \qquad \left[f(x)\right]^2 \leq c \int_0^x f(\xi) d\xi; \quad H \geq \frac{m}{2}(1-\alpha)v^2 + \left(1 - \frac{m\alpha c}{2}\right)\int_0^x f(\xi) d\xi, \tag{10.357a–c}$$

substitution of (10.357b) in (10.355c) leads to (10.357c), showing that the Lyapounov or the stability function can be made positive-definite (10.358c) by choosing α to satisfy (10.358a, b):

$$\alpha < \left\{1, \frac{2}{mc}\right\}: \qquad H > 0; \qquad f(x) > 0 < \int_0^x f(\xi) d\xi. \tag{10.358a–e}$$

In (10.357a), as in (10.358d, e), the restoring force is positive; otherwise there would no stable of equilibrium and the system would not be an oscillator. Having proved the condition (10.353a) it remains to prove (10.353b).

E10.19.2 Negative-Definite Time Derivative of the Stability Function

Denoting by prime (10.359b)[dot (10.359a)], the spatial (time) derivative implies (10.359c):

$$\dot{g} \equiv \frac{dg}{dt}, \qquad g' = \frac{dg}{dx}: \qquad \dot{g} = \frac{dg}{dx}\frac{dx}{dt} = g' v, \tag{10.359a–d}$$

which is used in the time derivative (10.353d) of the stability function (10.352c), specified by (10.360a–c):

$$\dot{H} = m\dot{v}\left(v+\alpha f\right)+f v+\alpha m\, f' v^2 = -\left(\mu v+f\right)\left(v+\alpha f\right)+v\left(f+\alpha m f' v\right)$$
$$= -\mu v^2 + \alpha m\, f' v^2 - \alpha f^2 - \alpha\mu f v. \tag{10.360a–c}$$

The inequality (10.354c) is applied to the last term on the r.h.s. of (10.359c) leading to (10.360d):

$$\dot{H} \le -\mu v^2 + \alpha m\, v^2 f' - \alpha f^2 + \frac{\mu\alpha}{2}\left(v^2\beta + \frac{f^2}{\beta}\right). \tag{10.360d}$$

Introducing the upper bound (10.361a) for $f'(x)$, which must be finite, leads to (10.361b, c):

$$B = \max\left|f'(x)\right|: \qquad \dot{H} \le -\mu v^2\left(1-\frac{\alpha m B}{\mu}-\frac{\alpha\beta}{2}\right)-\alpha f^2\left[\left(1-\frac{\mu}{2\beta}\right)\right]<0. \tag{10.361a–c}$$

The derivative of the stability function (10.361b) can be made negative-definite (10.361c) by choosing: (i) a large enough β so that (10.362a), the last term on the r.h.s. of (10.361b), is negative:

$$\beta > \frac{2}{\mu}; \qquad \alpha < \frac{1}{\dfrac{mB}{\mu}+\dfrac{\beta}{2}} < \frac{\mu}{1+mB}, \tag{10.362a–c}$$

(ii) a small enough α so that (10.362b), the first term on the r.h.s. of (10.361b), is also negative; (iii) the value (10.362c) of α is compatible with (10.358a) since it suffices to comply with the smallest of the two upper bounds. Thus, α meeting (10.358a; 10.361c) is sufficient to ensure the conditions (10.353a, b) of asymptotic stability, quod erat demonstrandum (QED).

EXAMPLE 10.20 Solutions of the Generalized Circular and Hyperbolic Differential Equation

Obtain the solution of the generalized circular (10.363b)[hyperbolic (10.363c)] differential equations for negative integer values of the parameter (10.363a):

$$-m \in |N: \qquad y'' \pm x^m\, y = 0, \tag{10.363a–c}$$

which is in the cases when the generalized circular and hyperbolic cosine and sine (subsections 9.4.12–9.4.20) do not apply directly.

The analysis is distinct for: (i)(ii) a simple $m=-1$ (double $m=-2$) pole [E10.20.1(E10.20.2)], for which the origin is a regular singularity leading to regular integrals (elementary power solutions); (iii)(iv) a pole of third $m=-3$ (higher $m=-4-5....$) order [E10.20.3(E10.20.4–E10.20.5)], for which the origin is an irregular singularity and irregular integrals are needed.

E10.20.1 Simple Pole and Regular Integrals

The case of a simple pole (10.364a) leads to the differential equations (10.364b, c):

$$m=-1: \qquad xy'' \pm y = 0, \qquad y(x) = \sum_{k=0}^{\infty} x^{k+a} c_k(a), \tag{10.364a–d}$$

which have regular integrals (10.364d) leading to:

$$\begin{aligned} k=n+1: \qquad 0 &= \sum_{k=0}^{\infty}(k+a)(k+a-1)x^{k+a-1}c_k(x) \pm \sum_{n=0}^{\infty} x^{a+n} c_n(a) \\ &= x^a \sum_{n=0}^{\infty} x^n \left[(n+a)(n+a+1)\, c_{n+1}(a) \pm c_n(a)\right]. \end{aligned} \tag{10.365a–c}$$

From (10.365c) follows the recurrence formula for the coefficients (10.366a):

$$(n+a)(n+a-1)\, c_n(a) = \mp c_{n-1}(a), \quad n=0: \qquad a_{\pm} = 0, 1, \tag{10.366a–d}$$

and for (10.366b) the indices (3.366c, d). The higher index (10.366d) leads (10.366a) to the coefficients (10.367a–c):

$$c_n(1) = \mp \frac{c_{n-1}(1)}{(n+1)n} = (\mp)^n \frac{c_0(1)}{(n+1)n^2(n-1)^2 \dots 2^2} = (\mp)^n \frac{c_0(1)}{(n+1)!n!}. \tag{10.367a, b}$$

Setting (10.368a) one particular integral of the differential equation (10.364b, c) is (10.368b):

$$c_0(1) = 1: \qquad y_1^{\pm}(x) = \sum_{n=0}^{\infty} \frac{(\mp)^n}{n!} \frac{x^{n+1}}{(n+1)!}, \tag{10.368a, b}$$

which is (subsection 9.5.9) a regular integral of the first kind.

Since the indices (10.366c, d) differ by an integer the second particular integral linearly independent from (10.368b) is a regular integral of the second kind, second type (9.412) specified by:

$$y_0^{\pm}(x) = \lim_{a\to 0} \frac{\partial}{\partial a}\left[a \sum_{n=0}^{\infty} x^{a+n}\, c_n(a)\right], \tag{10.369}$$

with the coefficients specified by recurrence (10.370) from (10.366a):

$$c_n(a) = \frac{(\mp)^n\, c_0(a)}{(n+a)(n+a-1)^2 \ldots (a+1)^2\, a}. \tag{10.370}$$

Substituting (10.370) in (10.369) the vanishing factor $a \to 0$ cancels in the numerator and denominator and setting (10.371a) the differentiation in (10.371b):

$$c_0(a) = 1: \qquad y_0^{\pm}(x) = \lim_{a\to 0} \frac{\partial}{\partial a}\left\{x^a\left[a + \sum_{n=1}^{\infty} \frac{(\mp x)^n}{(n+a)(n+a-1)^2 \ldots (a+1)^2}\right]\right\}, \tag{10.371a, b}$$

leads to:

$$\begin{aligned}
y_0^{\pm}(x) &= \lim_{a\to 0}\left\{x^a\left[1 + a\log x + \sum_{n=1}^{\infty} \frac{(\mp x)^n}{(n+a)(n+a-1)^2 \ldots (a+1)^2}\right.\right.\\
&\qquad \left.\left.\left(\log x - \frac{1}{n+a} - \frac{2}{n+a-1} \ldots - \frac{2}{a+1}\right)\right]\right\}\\
&= 1 + \sum_{n=1}^{\infty} \frac{(\mp x)^n}{n!\,(n-1)!}\left(\log x - \frac{1}{n} - \frac{2}{n-1} \ldots - 2\right)\\
&= 1 + \sum_{n=1}^{\infty} \frac{(\mp x)^n}{n!(n-1)!}\left[\log x - \psi(1+n) - \psi(n) + 2\psi(1)\right]\\
&= 1 + \log x\, y_1^{\pm}(x) - \sum_{m=0}^{\infty} \frac{(\mp x)^n}{m!(m+1)!}\left[\psi(2+m) + \psi(1+m) - 2\psi(1)\right],
\end{aligned} \tag{10.372a–d}$$

consisting of the sum of three terms: (i) a constant preliminary function equation equal to unity; (ii) a logarithmic factor multiplying the function of the first kind (10.368b); (iii) a complementary function involving digamma functions (9.466a).

The constant factor $-2\psi(1)$ in the square brackets is a constant multiple of (10.368b) and can be incorporated in the arbitrary constant c_0 in the general integral (10.373b) of (10.363a, b):

$$|x| < \infty: \qquad y^{\pm}(x) = C_1\, y_1^{\pm}(x) + C_0\, y_0^{\pm}(x). \qquad (10.373\text{a, b})$$

Thus, the general integral (10.373b) of the generalized hyperbolic (circular) differential equation (10.364b)[(10.364c)] with parameter (10.364a) in (10.363a–c) is (standard CCLXXXV) a linear combination (10.373b) with arbitrary constants (C_0, C_1), *valid in the finite complex x-plane (10.373a) of: (i) a regular integral of the first kind (10.368b); (ii) a regular integral of the second kind type two (10.372d) consisting (10.374a) of the sum of: (ii-1) a preliminary function equal to unity; (ii-2) a logarithm multiplying a function of the first kind:*

$$y_0^{\pm}(x) = \log x\, y_1^{\pm}(x) + y_0^{\pm}(x): \qquad y_0^{\pm}(x) = 1 - \sum_{n=1}^{\infty} \frac{(\mp x)^n}{n!(n+1)!}\left[\psi(1+n) + \psi(n)\right], \qquad (10.374\text{a, b})$$

(ii-3) a complementary function (9.374b) of order $O(1)$. The case $m = -2$ of (10.363b, c) is the simpler because it leads to exact integrals in finite terms (E10.20.2).

E10.20.2 Double Pole and Elementary Integrals

The generalized hyperbolic (10.36b)[circular (10.363c)] differential equation with a double pole in the coefficient:

$$m = -2: \qquad x^2 y'' \mp y = 0, \qquad (10.375\text{a–c})$$

is linear with homogeneous derivatives (10.375b)[(10.375c)] and has simple power solutions (10.376a) with exponents (10.376c) that are the roots of the characteristic polynomial (10.376b):

$$y(x) = x^a: \qquad 0 = a(a-1) \mp 1 = P_2^{\pm}(a), \qquad 2a_{\pm} = 1 \pm \sqrt{1 \pm 4}. \qquad (10.376\text{a–c})$$

The upper sign leads to the roots (10.377a) and the general integral (10.377b):

$$2a_{\pm} = 1 \pm \sqrt{5}: \qquad y(x) = x^{1/2}\left[C_0 \cosh\left(\frac{\sqrt{5}}{2}\log x\right) + C_1 \sinh\left(\frac{\sqrt{5}}{2}\log x\right)\right], \qquad (10.377\text{a, b})$$

$$2a_{\pm} = 1 \pm i\sqrt{3}: \qquad y(x) = x^{1/2}\left[C_0 \cos\left(\frac{\sqrt{3}}{2}\log x\right) + C_1 \sin\left(\frac{\sqrt{3}}{2}\log x\right)\right], \qquad (10.378\text{a, b})$$

and the lower sign leads to the roots (10.378a) and the general integral (10.378b). *Thus, the generalized hyperbolic (circular) differential equation (10.375b) [(10.375c)] with a double pole (10.375a) in (10.363b) [(10.363c)] has (standard CCLXXXVI) general integral (9.377b) [(9.378b)] where* (C_0, C_1) *are arbitrary constants.* The cases of (10.363a–c) remaining are poles of order higher than the second leading to an irregular singularity at the origin and irregular integrals (E10.20.3).

E10.20.3 Triple Pole and Asymptotic Integrals

The generalized circular (10.363b) [hyperbolic (10.363c)] differential equation with a pole of order higher than two (10.379a, b) in the coefficient:

$$p \in |N_0; \qquad m = -3 - p: \qquad y'' \pm x^{-3-p} y = 0, \tag{10.379a–d}$$

has an irregular singularity at the origin (10.379c) [(10.379d)] and hence, the solution has an essential singularity, which is involving unending descending powers x^{-n}. This suggests as change of variable the inversion relative to the origin (9.553a, b) ≡ (10.380a, b) leading (9.555c–e) the differential equation (10.380c):

$$\xi = \frac{1}{x}, \qquad w(\xi) = y(x): \qquad 0 = \xi w'' + 2w' \pm \xi^p w. \tag{10.380a–d}$$

In the case of a triple pole (10.381a, b), the differential equation (10.381c, d) has a regular singular at infinity:

$$m = -3; \qquad p = 0: \qquad \xi w'' + 2w' \pm w = 0, \tag{10.381a–d}$$

and the solution is specified by regular (10.382a) [irregular (10.382b)] integrals in the inverse (10.380a) [direct x] variable:

$$\sum_{n=0}^{\infty} \xi^{n+a} e_n(a) = w(\xi) = y(x) = \sum_{n=0}^{\infty} x^{-n-a} e_n(a), \tag{10.382a, b}$$

with the index and the coefficients to be determined.

Substitution of (10.382a) in (10.381c, d) leads to (10.383b):

$$k = n+1: \qquad 0 = \sum_{k=0}^{\infty} (k+a)(k+a+1) \xi^{k+a-1} e_k(a) \pm \sum_{n=0}^{\infty} \xi^{n+a} e_n(a)$$

$$= \xi^a \sum_{n=0}^{\infty} \xi^n \left[(n+a+1)(n+a+2)\, e_{n+1}(a) \pm e_n(a) \right], \tag{10.383a–c}$$

which is equivalent to (10.383c) with the change of summation variable (10.383a). The vanishing of the coefficients of all powers in (10.383c) leads to the recurrence formula (10.384a) for the coefficients:

$$(n+a)(n+a+1)\,e_n(a) = \mp\, e_{n-1}(a); \qquad n=0: \qquad a_\pm = 0,-1, \tag{10.384a–d}$$

setting (10.384b) leads to the índices (10.384c, d). The recurrence formula (10.384a) may be applied iteratively (10.385b, c) up to the zero order coefficient to which may be given the value unity (10.385a):

$$e_1(a)=1: \qquad e_n(a) = \mp\frac{e_{n-1}(a)}{(n+a)(n+a+1)} = \frac{(\mp)^n}{(n+a+1)(n+a)^2\dots(2+a)^2(1+a)}. \tag{10.385a–c}$$

The higher índex (10.384c) together with (10.385a, c) substituted in (10.382b) lead to:

$$y_0^\pm(x) = \sum_{n=0}^{\infty} x^{-n} e_n(0) = \sum_{n=0}^{\infty} \frac{(\mp x)^{-n}}{n!(n+1)!}, \tag{10.386a, b}$$

which is a regular asymptotic integral of the first kind.

Since the indices (10.384c, d) differ by an integer, a linearly independent solution is (9.412) a regular integral of the second kind, second type:

$$\begin{aligned}
w_{-1}^\pm(\xi) &= \lim_{a\to-1}\frac{\partial}{\partial a}\left[(a+1)\,\xi^a\sum_{n=0}^{\infty}\xi^n\,e_n(a)\right] \\
&= \lim_{a\to-1}\frac{\partial}{\partial a}\left\{\xi^a\left[a+1+\sum_{m=1}^{\infty}\frac{(\mp\xi)^m}{(m+a+1)(m+a)^2\dots(a+2)^2}\right]\right\} \\
&= \lim_{a\to-1}\xi^a\left[1+(a+1)\log\xi+\sum_{m=1}^{\infty}\frac{(\mp\xi)^m}{(m+a+1)(m+a)^2\dots(a+2)^2}\right. \\
&\qquad\left.\left(\log x-\frac{1}{m+a+1}-\frac{2}{m+2}-\dots-\frac{2}{a+2}\right)\right] \\
&= \xi^{-1}+\xi^{-1}\sum_{m=1}^{\infty}\frac{(\mp\xi)^m}{m!(m-1)!}\left(\log\xi-\frac{1}{m}-\frac{2}{m-1}-\dots-2\right) \\
&= \xi^{-1}+\sum_{n=0}^{\infty}\frac{(\mp\xi)^n}{n!(n+1)!}\left[\log\xi-\psi(2+n)-\psi(1+n)+2\psi(1)\right],
\end{aligned} \tag{10.387a–e}$$

consisting of a preliminary function, plus the function of the first kind (10.386b) multiplied by a logarithm plus a complementary function.

Bearing in mind (10.380a, b) it follows that *the generalized circular (10.379c) [hyperbolic (10.379b)] differential equation with a triple pole (10.388a):*

$$m=-3: \qquad x^3 y'' \pm y = 0, \qquad (10.388a–c)$$

has the general integral (standard CCLXXXVII) valid outside the origin (9.389a), specified by a linear combination (9.389b) with arbitrary constants (C_0, C_1):

$$x \neq 0: \qquad y(x) = C_0\, y_0^{\pm}(x) + C_1\, y_{-1}^{\pm}(x), \qquad (10.389a, b)$$

of asymptotic regular integrals of the first kind (10.386b) and the second kind (10.387e) ≡ (10.390a):

$$y_{-1}^{\pm}(x) = x - \log x\, y_0^{\pm}(x) - y_2^{\pm}(x); \quad y_2^{\pm}(x) = \sum_{n=0}^{\infty} \frac{(\mp x)^{-n}}{n!(n+1)!}\left[\psi(2+n)+\psi(1+n)\right],$$

(10.390a, b)

the asymptotic regular integral of the second kind (10.390a) is of the second type and consists of: (i) a preliminary function x; (ii) the integral of the first kind (10.386b) multiplied by a logarithm; (iii) the complementary function (10.390b). The only remaining case of solution of the generalized circular (hyperbolic differential equation (10.363b) [(10.363c)] is the case of a pole of order more than three that is solvable in terms of the generalized circular (hyperbolic) functions of the inverse variable (E10.20.4).

E10.20.4 High-Order Poles and Asymptotic Analytic Integrals

The general circular (10.363b) [hyperbolic (10.363c)] differential equation with a pole of order higher than three (10.391a):

$$m = -4, -5, \ldots: \qquad y'' \pm x^m y = 0, \qquad (10.391a–c)$$

leads for the inverse variable (10.379b; 10.380a–d) to the differential equation (10.392a):

$$0 = \xi w'' + 2w' \pm \xi^{-m-3} w = (\xi w)'' \pm \xi^{-m-4}\, \xi w, \qquad (10.392a, b)$$

which may be written (10.392b); comparing (10.392b) with (9.313a) [(9.295a)] it follows that it is a generalized circular (hyperbolic) differential equation with a non-negative integer parameter (10.393a):

$$-m-4 = 0, 1, 2, \ldots \in |N_0: \qquad \xi w(\xi) = \frac{1}{x} y(x), \qquad (10.393a, b)$$

whose solutions are given (10.378b) [(10.377b)] by a linear combination of generalized circular (10.394) [hyperbolic (10.395)] cosines and sines:

$$\xi w_+(\xi) = B_0 \cos(\xi; -m-4) + B_1 \sin(\xi; -m-4), \tag{10.394}$$

$$\xi w_-(\xi) = E_0 \cosh(\xi; -m-4) + E_1 \sinh(\xi; -m-4), \tag{10.395}$$

with arbitrary constants (B_0, B_1) $[(E_0, E_1)]$. Substituting (10.393b) in (10.394) [(10.395)] it follows that the general integral of *the generalized circular (10.391b) [hyperbolic (10.391c)] differential equation with a pole of order higher than three (10.391a) is (standard CCLXXXVIII) a linear combination (10.396)[(10.397)] with arbitrary constants* $(B_0, B_1)[(E_0, E_1)]$ *of generalized circular (hyperbolic) cosines and sines of the inverse variable 1/x, with parameter* $-m-4$, *multiplied by x:*

$$y_+(x) = x\left[B_0 \cos\left(\frac{1}{x}; -m-4\right) + B_1 \sin\left(\frac{1}{x}; -m-4\right)\right], \tag{10.396}$$

$$y_-(x) = x\left[E_0 \cosh\left(\frac{1}{x}; -m-4\right) + E_1 \sinh\left(\frac{1}{x}; -m-4\right)\right]. \tag{10.397}$$

In the case of a pole of order four $m = -4(-5)$ these solutions involve (E10.20.5) the original circular and hyperbolic cosine and sine (Airy functions).

E10.20.5 Circular, Hyperbolic, and Airy Functions of the Inverse Variable

Setting $m = -4$ in (10.396)[(10.397)] it follows that *the generalized circular (10.398a) [hyperbolic (10.399a)] differential equation with a pole of order four has the (standard CCLXXXIX) general integral specified by (10.398b)[(10.399b)] a linear combination with arbitrary constants* $(B_0, B_1)[(E_0, E_1)]$ *of circular (hyperbolic) functions of the inverse variable 1/x multiplied by the variable x:*

$$x^4 y'' + y = 0: \qquad y(x) = x\left[B_0 \cos\left(\frac{1}{x}\right) + B_1 \sin\left(\frac{1}{x}\right)\right], \tag{10.398a, b}$$

$$x^4 y'' - y = 0: \qquad y(x) = x\left[E_0 \cosh\left(\frac{1}{x}\right) + E_1 \sinh\left(\frac{1}{x}\right)\right]. \tag{10.399a, b}$$

Setting $m = -5$ in (10.396) and using (9.311a–d; 9.312a–d), it follows that *the generalized hyperbolic differential equation with a pole of order five (9.400a) has (standard CCLXXXIX) general integral specified (10.400b) by a linear combination with arbitrary constants* (C_0, C_1) *of the two Airy functions of the inverse variable 1/x multiplied by the variable x:*

$$x^5 y'' + y = 0: \qquad y(x) = x\left[C_0\, Ai\left(\frac{1}{x}\right) + C_1\, Bi\left(\frac{1}{x}\right)\right]. \qquad (10.400a, b)$$

The general integral of the generalized hyperbolic (9.295a)[circular (9.313a)] differential equation that is (10.363c)[(10.363b)] with the lower – (upper +) sign has been obtained for (standard CCXC) all values of the parameter m, namely: (i) for all complex values, excluding negative integers as a linear combination (9.295b) [(9.313b)] of generalized hyperbolic (9.305; 9.306) ≡ (9.307a–c; 9.308a–c) [circular (9.315; 9.316) ≡ (9.317a–c; 9.318a–c)] cosines and sines including as particular cases the original functions for zero parameter (9.296a–d) [(9.314a–d)] and also the Airy functions for parameter unity (9.310a–c; 9.311a–d; 9.312a–d); (ii) simple power solutions with complex exponents (10.377a, b) [(10.378a, b) for double pole (10.375a–c); (iii) (iv) regular (regular asymptotic) integrals of the first kind (10.368b)[(10.386b)] and second kind, second type (10.374a, b) [(10.390a, b)] for (10.373a, b) [(10.389a, b)] a simple (10.364a–c) [triple (10.388a–c)] pole; (v) for poles of order higher than three to generalized hyperbolic (10.397) [circular (10.396)] functions of the inverse variable, including the original functions (10.398a, b;10.399a, b) [Airy functions (10.400a, b)] for poles of order four (five).

Conclusion 10

Two examples of integral curves or streamlines of a flow: (Figure 10.1) all passing through the origin; (Figure 10.2) not passing through the origin, except for the six asymptotes. The cusped (smooth) parabola is the envelope of a one-parameter family of straight lines [Figure 10.3 (10.4)]. A beam, which is a bar under axial tension, can be subject to 16 possible combinations of loads and supports, of which four are illustrated (Figures 10.5a–d), using four types of (i) support: clamped, pinned, clamped-pinned or cantilever; (ii) loads: concentrated torque or force or uniform or linearly increasing shear stress. The linear bending of a circular plate with a circular hole allows for eight combinations (Table 10.1), of which five are distinct (Table 10.2), namely: (Figure 10.6a/e): clamped/supported at both boundaries; (Figure 10.6b/c) clamped at the outer boundary and supported/free at the inner boundary; (Figure 10.6d) supported at the outer boundary and free at the inner boundary. For an elastic membrane without shear stress and under uniform tension parallel to the supports and with uniform (non-uniform) traction at the supports [Figure 10.7a (10.8a)], there are modes of all orders $n = 1, 2, ...,$ for example orders 2, 3, 4, respectively, in Figures 10.7b, c, d. The low– (high–) order modes (Figure 10.7e) are cut-on (cut-off) or propagating (evanescent). For a given mode or fixed n, a non-uniform traction (Figure 10.8a) causes a turning point (Figure 10.8b) beyond which propagating modes become evanescent, that is, the cut-on mode becomes the cut-off mode (Figure 10.8c). The values of the arbitrary constant (Table 10.4) include 16 cases of the general integral of the linear coupled system of finite difference equations (10.350a, b). The boundary conditions for the weak bending of an elastic plate depend (Table 10.3) on the shape, type of support, and material.

Classification 10.1

500 Standards (I to M) of Single and Simultaneous Systems of Ordinary Differential Equations

Classification 10.1 on the mathematical classes of ordinary differential equations consists of 500 standards with roman numerals I to M to distinguish from the arabic numerals 1 to 500 in Classification 10.2 on typical applications to physics and engineering problems. The 500 standards consist of: (i) 256 distinct differential equations written explicitly as a look-up table; (ii) 244 related properties of the solutions that are referred to in the text. Classification 10.1 serves at least two purposes: (a) as a summary of types of differential equations and methods to solve them, often with one or more examples of their integrals; (b) in case there is a specific differential equation to be solved, it may fall into one of the standards, thus indicating a suitable method of solution. The 500 standards with roman numerals I to M, are divided into 26 sections with capital letters A to Z, and subsections with a lowercase letter, such as A.a, A.b, . . . There are six groups. The first group, consisting of the sections A to H and standards I to XLIX, consists mostly of differential and finite difference equations having a characteristic polynomial for which the: (i) general integral can always be determined from the roots of the characteristic polynomial; (ii) the latter also specifies the complete integral for a variety of forcing functions. The second group, consisting of the sections I to L and standards L to CXX, includes a variety of linear and non-linear differential equations of the first and higher orders, whose general and special integrals can be determined in finite terms. The third group, consisting of the sections M to P and standards CXXI to CLXXVIII, concerns simultaneous systems of ordinary differential equations, which can be solved by extensions of the methods that apply to the first two groups, for example, matrices of characteristic polynomials.

If an ordinary differential equation or a simultaneous system cannot be solved explicitly by the preceding methods, then a numerical or approximate solution may be sought. In this case, the theorems of existence and unicity of solution, ensuring other properties may be useful, form the fifth group, consisting of the sections R to T and the standards CCII to CCLIV. The numerical and approximate methods may fail for singular differential equations, in which case it is critical to know in what form the solution exists. The linear differential equations with variable coefficients are considered in the sections U to Z and standards CCII to M, which form the sixth group; they relate to the special or higher transcendental functions that appear in many situations. A typical case is the solution of the partial differential equations of mathematical physics by separation of variables, which appears as the fourth group, consisting of the section Q and the standards CLXXIX to CCI. The fifth group relating to the special functions is too extensive to cover in a single volume; the methods of solution of linear differential equations with variable coefficients are presented in detail and are illustrated with generalized Bessel and other special functions. Classification 10.1 with 500 standards on the methods of solution of differential equations is complemented by Classification 10.2, with detailed application to 500 physical and engineering problems.

A. Linear Differential Equation with Constant Coefficients –ℓ.o.d.e.c. (sections 1.3–1.5):

$$\sum_{n=0}^{N} A_n \frac{d^n y}{dx^n} = B(x). \tag{10.401}$$

A. a. Unforced (section 1.3): $B(x)=0$; roots of the characteristic polynomial:

$$0 = P_N(a) = \sum_{n=0}^{N} A_n\, a^n. \tag{10.402}$$

*standard I. Single root (subsections 1.3.1–1.3.2);
*standard II. Two distinct real roots (subsection 1.3.3);
*standard III. Pair of complex conjugate roots (subsection 1.3.4);
*standard IV. Multiple root (subsections 1.3.6–1.3.9);
*standard V. Multiple pairs of real roots (subsection 1.3.10);
*standard VI. Multiple pairs of complex conjugate roots (subsection 1.3.10).

A. b. Forced (section 1.4): **Direct Method** $B(x) \neq 0$:

*standard VII. Forcing by an exponential (subsections 1.4.1–1.4.3):

$$B(a) = B e^{x}. \tag{10.403}$$

*standard VIII. Forcing by hyperbolic cosine or sine (subsection 1.4.4):

$$B(x) = B \cosh, \sinh(c\,x); \tag{10.404}$$

*standard IX. Forcing by circular cosine or sine (subsection 1.4.5):

$$B(x) = B \cos, \sin(a\,x); \tag{10.405}$$

*standard X. Forcing by the product of an exponential and hyperbolic cosine or sine (subsection 1.4.6):

$$B(x) = B e^{bx} \cosh, \sinh(c\,x); \tag{10.406}$$

*standard XI. Forcing by the product of an exponential and a circular cosine or sine (subsection 1.4.7):

$$B(x) = B e^{bx} \cos, \sin(a\,x); \tag{10.407}$$

*standard XII. Forcing by the product of an exponential by circular and hyperbolic cosines or sines (subsection 1.4.8):

$$B(x) = B e^{bx} \cosh, \sinh(c\,x) \cos, \sin(a\,x). \tag{10.408}$$

A. c. **Forced** (section 1.5) **Method of the Inverse Polynomial of Ordinary Derivatives**: $B(x) \neq 0$

*standard XIII. Forcing by a polynomial (subsections 1.5.1–1.5.7):

$$B(x) = \sum_{m=0}^{M} B_m\, x^m; \tag{10.409}$$

*standard XIV. Forcing by the product of an exponential by a smooth function (subsection 1.5.8):

$$J(x) \in \mathcal{D}^\infty(|R): \qquad B(x) = e^{bx} J(x); \tag{10.410a, b}$$

*standard XV. Forcing by the product of an exponential by a polynomial (subsections 1.5.9 and 1.5.13):

$$B(x) = e^{bx} \sum_{m=0}^{M} B_m\, x^m; \tag{10.411}$$

*standard XVI. Forcing by the product of a hyperbolic cosine or sine by a smooth function (subsections 1.5.9 and 1.5.14):

$$J(x) \in \mathcal{D}^\infty(|R): \qquad B(x) = J(x) \cosh, \sinh(c\,x); \tag{10.412a, b}$$

*standard XVII. Forcing by the product of an exponential by a hyperbolic cosine or sine and by a smooth function (subsections 1.5.9 and 1.5.16):

$$J(x) \in \mathcal{D}^\infty(|R): \qquad B(x) = e^{bx} J(x) \cosh, \sinh(c\,x); \tag{10.413a, b}$$

*standard XVIII. Forcing by the product of a circular cosine or sine by a smooth function (subsections 1.5.9 and 1.5.15):

$$J(x) \in \mathcal{D}^\infty(|R): \qquad B(x) = J(x)\cos,\sin(ax); \qquad (10.414\text{a, b})$$

*standard XIX. Forcing by the product of an exponential by a circular cosine or sines by a smooth function (subsections 1.5.9 and 1.5.17):

$$J(x) \in \mathcal{D}^\infty(|R): \qquad B(x) = e^{bx} J(x)\cos,\sin(ax), \qquad (10.415\text{a, b})$$

*standard XX. Forcing by the product of an exponential by a circular and a hyperbolic cosine or sine by a smooth function (subsections 1.5.9 and 1.5.18):

$$J(x) \in \mathcal{D}^\infty(|R): \qquad B(x) = e^{bx} J(x)\cosh,\sinh(cx)\cos,\sin(ax). \qquad (10.416\text{a, b})$$

A. d. Complete Integrals (subsection 1.5.19; E10.1.1)

B. Linear Ordinary Differential Equation with Homogeneous Coefficients

ℓ.o.d.e.h.c. (section 1.6.1.8)

$$\sum_{n=0}^{N} A_n x^n \frac{d^n y}{dx^n} = B(x), \qquad (10.417)$$

B. a. Unforced (section 1.6) $B(x) = 0$; roots of the characteristic polynomial:

$$0 = P_N(a) = \sum_{n=0} A_n a(a-1)\ldots(a-n+1), \qquad (10.418)$$

*standard XXI. Single root (subsections 1.6.2 and 1.6.4);
*standard XXII. Multiple root (subsections 1.6.3–1.6.4);
*standard XXIII. Two distinct real roots (subsection 1.6.6);
*standard XXIV. Pair of complex conjugate roots (subsection 1.6.6).

B. b. Forced—Direct Method (section 1.7) $B(x) \neq 0$

*standard XXV. Forcing by a power (subsection 1.7.1):

$$B(x) = x^a; \qquad (10.419)$$

*standard XXVI. Forcing by a hyperbolic cosine or sine of a logarithm (subsection 1.7.2):

$$B(x) = B\cosh,\sinh(c\log x). \tag{10.420}$$

*standard XXVII. Forcing by a circular cosine or sine of a logarithm (subsection 1.7.3):

$$B(x) = B\cos,\sin(a\log x); \tag{10.421}$$

*standard XXVIII. Forcing by a power multiplied by an hyperbolic cosine or sine of a logarithm (subsection 1.7.4):

$$B(x) = x^b\cosh,\sinh(c\log x). \tag{10.422}$$

*standard XXIX. Forcing by a power multiplied by a circular cosine or sine of a logarithm (subsection 1.7.5):

$$B(x) = x^b\cos,\sin(a\log x). \tag{10.423}$$

*standard XXX. Forcing by a power multiplied by hyperbolic and circular cosines and sines of a logarithm (subsection 1.7.6):

$$B(x) = x^b\cosh,\sinh(c\log x)\cos,\sin(a\log x). \tag{10.424}$$

B. c. Forced—Method of the Inverse Characteristic Polynomial (section 1.8):

$$B(x) \neq 0$$

*standard XXXI. Forcing by a polynomial of logarithms (subsections 1.8.3–1.8.4):

$$B(x) = \sum_{m=0}^{M} B_m \log^m x; \tag{10.425}$$

*standard XXXII. Forcing by the product of a power by a smooth function (subsections 1.8.6 and 1.8.7):

$$J(x) \in \mathcal{D}^\infty(|R): \qquad B(x) = x^b J(x); \tag{10.426a, b}$$

*standard XXXIII. Forcing by the product of a hyperbolic cosine or sine of a logarithm by a smooth function (subsections (1.8.6 and 1.8.8):

$$J(x) \in \mathcal{D}^{\infty}(|R): \qquad B(x) = \cosh, \sinh(c \log x) J(x); \qquad (10.427a, b)$$

*standard XXXIV. Forcing by the product of a power by the hyperbolic cosine or sine of a logarithm times a smooth function (subsections 1.8.6 and 1.8.10):

$$J(x) \in \mathcal{D}^{\infty}(|R): \qquad B(x) = x^b \cosh, \sinh(c \log x) J(x); \qquad (10.428a, b)$$

*standard XXXV. Forcing by the product of a circular cosine or sine of a logarithm by a smooth function (subsections 1.8.6 and 1.8.9):

$$J(x) \in \mathcal{D}^{\infty}(|R): \qquad B(x) = x^b \cos, \sin(a \log x) J(x); \qquad (10.429a, b)$$

*standard XXXVI. Forcing by the product of a power by a circular cosine or sine of a logarithm times a smooth function (subsections 1.8.6 and 1.8.11):

$$J(x) \in \mathcal{D}^{\infty}(|R): \qquad B(x) = x^b \cos, \sin(a \log x) J(x); \qquad (10.430a, b)$$

*standard XXXVII. Forcing by the product of a power by circular and hyperbolic cosines of sines of a logarithm times a smooth function (subsections 1.8.6 and 1.8.12):

$$J(x) \in \mathcal{D}^{\infty}(|R): \quad B(x) = x^b \cos, \sin(a \log x) \cosh, \sinh(c \log x) J(x). \qquad (10.431a, b)$$

B. d. Complete Integrals: (subsection 1.8.13: E10.1.2)

C. Linear Finite Difference Equation with Constant Coefficients -ℓ.f.d.e.c.c (section 1.9):

$$\sum_{k=0}^{N} A_n\, y_{n+k} = B_n. \qquad (10.432)$$

C. a. Unforced (subsections 1.9.3 and 1.9.5–1.9.7); $B(x) = 0$ roots of the characteristic polynomial (A.2):

*standard XXXVIII. Single root (subsection 1.9.3);
*standard XXXIX. Multiple roots (subsection 1.9.3);
*standard XL. Pair of complex conjugate roots (subsection 1.9.5).

C. b. Forced (subsections 1.9.4, 1.9.5, 1.9.8): $B_n \neq 0$

*standard XLI. Forcing by a power (subsection 1.9.4, E10.1.3):

$$B_n = b^n ; \tag{10.433}$$

*standard XLII. Forcing by the product of a power by a circular cosine or sine (subsection 1.9.5):

$$B_n = b^n \cos, \sin(n\phi). \tag{10.434}$$

*standard XLIII. Forcing by the product of a power by a hyperbolic cosine or sine (subsection 1.9.8):

$$B_n = B b^n \cosh, \sinh(n\psi); \tag{10.435}$$

*standard XLIV. Forced by the product of a power by circular and hyperbolic cosines and sines (subsection 1.9.8):

$$B_n = B b^n \cos, \sin(n\phi) \cosh, \sinh(n\psi). \tag{10.436}$$

D. Method of Variation of Parameters

*standard XLV. (notes 1.2–1.4; section 2.9; subsection 1.3.6; section 3.3) For a linear differential equation with variable coefficients:

$$L\left\{\left(\frac{d}{dx}\right)\right\} y(x) \equiv \sum_{n=0}^{N} A_n(x) \frac{d^n y}{dx^n} = B(x), \tag{10.437}$$

obtains a particular solution of the forced equation (10.437) as a linear combination (10.438c) of N linearly independent (10.438b) solutions of the unforced equation (10.438a):

$$L\left\{\left(\frac{d}{dx}\right)\right\} y_m(x) = 0, \quad W(y_1, y_2, \ldots, y_N) \neq 0: \quad y(x) = \sum_{m=1}^{M} C_m(x) y_m(x), \tag{10.438a–c}$$

with the coefficients not constant, but rather functions of the independent variable x, to be determined.

E. Influence or Green's Function

*standard XLVI. (notes 1.5–1.8; 2.10–2.11) Is the solution of a linear diferential equation (10.437) forced by a unit impulse or Dirac function (10.439):

$$\left\{L\left(\frac{d}{dx}\right)\right\}G(x;\xi)=\delta(x-\xi), \tag{10.439}$$

and specifies the solution (10.440b) for forcing of (10.437) by a continuous function (10.440a).

$$B\in C(a,b): \qquad y(x)=\int_a^b B(\xi)G(x;\xi)\,d\xi. \tag{10.440a, b}$$

F. Fourier Series—Discrete Spectrum

*standard XLVII. (notes 1.9–1.10 and 2.4): Forcing of a linear differential equation with constant coefficients (10.401) by a function of bounded fluctuation in a finite interval (10.441a) represented by its discrete spectrum (10.441b):

$$B\in C(-L,+L): \qquad \sum_{n=0}^{N} A_n\frac{d^n y}{dx^n}=B(x)\equiv\sum_{n=0}^{N} B_m \exp\left(i\frac{\pi m x}{L}\right). \tag{10.441a, b}$$

G. Fourier Integral/Transform—Continuous Spectrum

*standard XLVIII. (notes 1.11–1.14; 2.5–2.9 and 2.12–2.13): Forcing a linear differential equation with constant coefficients (10.401) by a function absolutely integrable (10.442a) and of bounded fluctuation (10.442b) on the real line represented by its continuous spectrum (10.442c):

$$B\in\mathcal{L}^1\cap\mathcal{F}(-\infty,+\infty): \qquad \sum_{n=0}^{N} A_n\frac{d^n y}{dx^n}=B(x)\equiv\int_{-\infty}^{+\infty}\tilde{B}(k)\,e^{ikx}\,dk. \tag{10.442a–c}$$

H. Laplace Transform—Initial Conditions

*standard XLIX. (notes 1.15–1.25): Forcing of a linear differential equation with constant coefficients (10.401) by a function absolutely integrable on the finite positive real line (10.443a) and of slow growth at infinity (10.443b) represented by its Laplace transform (10.443c):

$$B\in\mathcal{L}^1(0,L)\cap\underline{\mathcal{V}}(L,+\infty):\qquad \sum_{n=0}^{N} A_n\frac{d^n y}{dx^n}=B(x)=\int_0^\infty \bar{B}(s)\,e^{-sx}\,ds. \tag{10.443a–c}$$

I. First-Order Differential Equations (sections 3.1–3.7; examples 10.4–10.5):

$$y'\equiv\frac{dy}{dx}:\qquad F(x,y;y')=0 \tag{10.444a, b}$$

I. a. Solvable by Quadratures (sections 3.2–3.4; examples 10.4–10.5):

*standard L. separable (subsection 3.2.1 and example 10.4 and E10.9.1):

$$X,Y\in\mathcal{E}(|R):\qquad \frac{dy}{dx}=\frac{X(x)}{Y(y)}; \tag{10.445a, b}$$

*standard LI. linear unforced (subsection 3.2.2):

$$P\in\mathcal{E}(|R):\qquad y'=P(x)y; \tag{10.446a, b}$$

*standard LII. Linear forced (section 3.3; example 10.4):

$$P,Q\in\mathcal{E}(|R):\qquad y'=P(x)y+Q(x); \tag{10.447a, b}$$

*standard LIII. **Bernoulli** (1695) non-linear differential equation (section 3.4; example 10.4):

$$P,Q\in\mathcal{E}(|R):\qquad y'=P(x)y+Q(x)y^n. \tag{10.448a, b}$$

*standard LIV. Particular **Ricatti equation** (section 3.4):

$$P,Q\in\mathcal{E}(|R):\qquad y'=P(x)y+Q(x)y^2. \tag{10.449a, b}$$

I. b. Ricatti (1824) Equation (sections 3.5–3.6; example 10.4):

$$y' = P(x)y^2 + P(x)y + Q(x). \tag{10.450}$$

*standard LV. General integral involving two quadratures if one particular integral is known (subsection 3.5.2 and example 10.4);
*standard LVI, General integral involving one quadrature if two particular integrals are known (subsection 3.5.3);
*standard LVII. General integral involving no quadratures if three particular integrals are known (subsections 3.5.4–3.5.5).
*standard LVIII. Transformation to a linear second-order differential equation (subsections 3.6.1–3.6.2):

$$u'' + A\ u' + B\ u = 0. \tag{10.451}$$

*standard LIX. Reducible to a linear second-order differential equation with constant coefficients and distinct roots a, b of the characteristic polynomial (subsection 3.6.3):

$$y' = \frac{ab}{R(x)} + \left[A + B - \frac{R'(x)}{R(x)} \right] y + R(x)y^2; \tag{10.452}$$

*standard LX. As in the standard LIX with a = b double root (subsection 3.6.3):

$$y' = \frac{a^2}{R(x)} + \left[2a - \frac{R'(x)}{R(x)} \right] y + R(x)y^2; \tag{10.453}$$

*standard LXI. Reducible to a linear second-order differential equation with homogeneous coefficients and distinct roots a, b of the characteristic polynomial (subsection 3.6.4):

$$y' = \frac{ab}{x^2 R(x)} + \left[\frac{a+b-1}{x} - \frac{R'(x)}{R(x)} \right] y + R(x)y^2; \tag{10.454}$$

*standard LXII. As in the standard LXI with a double $a = b$ root (subsection 3.6.4):

$$y' = \frac{a^2}{x^2 R(x)} + \left[\frac{2a}{x} - \frac{R'(x)}{R(x)} \right] y + R(x)y^2. \tag{10.455}$$

*standard LXIII. Particular Ricatti equation (subsection 3.6.5):

$$a, b \in |R: \qquad y' = a x^{2\lambda} + \frac{\lambda}{x} y + b y^2. \qquad (10.456a–c)$$

I. c. Homogeneous Differential Equation (section 3.7):

*standard LXIV. Non-linear (subsections 3.7.1–3.7.3; section 4.1; examples 10.4 and 10.7):

$$y \in B(|R): \qquad y' = f\left(\frac{y}{x}\right); \qquad (10.457a, b)$$

*standard LXV. Linear (subsections 3.7.1–3.7.2):

$$y' = a\frac{y}{x} + b. \qquad (10.458)$$

J. Differentials (sections 3.8–3.9; notes 3.1–3.24)

J. a. First-Order Differential in Two Variables (section 3.8; examples 10.5, 10.6):

$$\vec{X} = \{X, Y\}: \qquad 0 = X(x,y)dx + Y(x,y)dy = \vec{X}.d\vec{x}. \qquad (10.459a–c)$$

*standard LXVI. Exact differential (10.460b) if the integrability condition (10.460a) is met (subsections 3.8.1–3.8.3; E10.6.1):

$$\Omega(x,y) \equiv \frac{\partial Y}{\partial x} - \frac{\partial X}{\partial y} = 0: \qquad X(x,y)dx + Y(x,y)dy = d\Phi(x,y); \qquad (10.460a, b)$$

*standard LXVII. Inexact differential (10.462a) for which an integrating factor (10.461b) always exists (subsections 3.8.4–3.8.6; E10.6.2–E10.6.3):

$$\Omega(x,y) \neq 0: \qquad X(x,y)\, dx + Y(x,y)dy = \lambda(x,y)d\Phi(x,y); \qquad (10.461a, b)$$

*standard LXVIII. Integrating factor (10.462b) depending only (10.462a) on the independent variable (subsection 3.8.7):

$$\frac{\Omega(x,y)}{Y(x,y)} \equiv f(x): \qquad X(x,y)\, dx + Y(x,y)dy = \exp\left(\int^x f(\xi)\, d\xi\right)d\Phi(x,y);$$

(10.462a, b)

*standard LXIX. Integrating factor (10.463b) depending only (10.463a) on the dependent variable (subsection 3.8.7; E10.6.2–E10.6.3):

$$\frac{\Omega(x,y)}{X(x,y)} \equiv g(y): \qquad X(x,y)\,dx + Y(x,y)dy = \exp\left(\int^{y} g(\eta)d\eta\right)d\Phi(x,y); \tag{10.463a, b}$$

*standard LXX. Integrating factor (10.464b) depending only (10.464a) on the sum of the variables (subsection 3.8.8; E10.6.2–E10.6.3):

$$\frac{\Omega(x,y)}{X(x,y)-Y(x,y)} \equiv h(x+y): \quad X(x,y)\,dx + Y(x,y)dy = \exp\left(\int^{x+y} h(z)\,dz\right)d\Phi(x,y); \tag{10.464a, b}$$

*standard LXXI. Integrating factor (10.465b) depending only (10.465a) on the product of the variables (subsection 3.8.9; E10.6.2–E10.6.3):

$$\frac{\Omega(x,y)}{xX(x,y)-yY(x,y)} \equiv j(xy): \quad X(x,y)dx + Y(x,y)dy = \exp\left\{\int^{x+y} j(u)\,du\right\}d\Phi(x,y); \tag{10.465a, b}$$

*standard LXXII. Integrating factor (10.466b) a homogeneous function (10.466a) depending only on the ratio of the two variables (subsection 3.8.10; E10.6.2–E10.6.3);

$$\frac{x^2\,\Omega(x,y)}{xX(x,y)-yY(x,y)} \equiv k\left(\frac{y}{x}\right): \quad X(x,y)dx + Y(x,y)dy = \exp\left\{\int^{x+y} k(v)dv\right\}d\Phi(x,y); \tag{10.466a, b}$$

*standard LXXIII. Other forms of integrating factor (10.467a) of (10.467b) an inexact differential (subsection 3.8.11):

$$\lambda = x^{a-1}y^{b-1}: \; a\,y\,d\,x + b\,x\,d\,y + x^{\alpha-a}y^{\beta-b}\left(\alpha\,y\,d\,x + \beta\,x\,dy\right) = \frac{1}{\lambda}d\left(x^a y^b + x^\alpha y^\beta\right). \tag{10.467a, b}$$

J. b. First-Order Differential in Three Variables (section 3.9):

$$\vec{X} = \{X, Y, Z\}: \qquad 0 = X(x,y,z)dx + Y(x,y,z)dy + Z(x,y,z)dz = \vec{X}.d\vec{x}. \tag{10.468a, b}$$

*standard LXXIV. **Exact differential** (10.469b) if the vector of coefficients is (10.469a) irrotational (subsection 3.9.1):

$$\vec{\Omega} \equiv \nabla \wedge \vec{X} = 0 \qquad \Leftrightarrow \qquad \vec{X}.d\vec{x} = d\Phi(\vec{x}); \tag{10.469a, b}$$

*standard LXXV. **Inexact differential** with integrating factor (10.470b) if (10.470a) the vector of coefficients has zero helicity (subsections 3.9.2–3.9.5):

$$H \equiv \vec{X}.\vec{\Omega} = 0 \qquad \Leftrightarrow \qquad \vec{X}.d\vec{x} = \lambda(\vec{x})d\Phi(\vec{x}); \tag{10.470a, b}$$

*standard LXXVI. **Pfaffian** (10.471b) if (10.471a) the vector of coefficients has non-zero helicity (subsections 3.9.5–3.9.7):

$$H \neq 0 \qquad \Leftrightarrow \qquad \vec{X}.d\vec{x} \neq \lambda(\vec{x})d\Phi(\vec{x}). \tag{10.471a, b}$$

J. c. Three-Dimensional Potentials (subsections 3.9.8–3.9.11):

*standard LXXVII. A continuously differentiable vector field (10.472a) is the gradient of a **scalar potential** (A10.472c) if (10.472b) is **irrotational** (subsections 3.9.8–3.9.10):

$$\vec{X} \in C^1(|R^2): \qquad \nabla \wedge \vec{X} = 0 \qquad \Leftrightarrow \qquad \vec{X} = \nabla\Phi, \tag{10.472a–c}$$

*standard LXXVIII. A continuously differentiable vector field (10.473a) is the curl of a **vector potential** (10.473c) if (10.473b) is **solenoidal** (subsection 3.9.9):

$$\vec{X} \in C^1(|R^3): \qquad \nabla.\vec{X} = 0 \qquad \Leftrightarrow \qquad \vec{X} = \nabla \wedge \vec{A}; \tag{10.473a–c}$$

*standard LXXIX. A continuously differentiable vector field (10.474a) is the sum (10.474b) of an irrotational (10.472b) [solenoidal (10.473b)] part that is the gradient (10.472c) [curl (10.473c)] of a scalar (vector) potential (subsections 3.9.8–3.9.9):

$$\vec{X} \in C^1(|R^3): \qquad \vec{X} = \nabla\Phi + \nabla \wedge \vec{A}; \tag{10.474a, b}$$

*standard LXXX. A continuously differentiable vector field (10.475a) is the sum (10.475b) of the gradient of a scalar potential with the outer product of the gradient of other two **Clebsch potentials** (subsections 3.9.8–3.9.9):

$$\vec{X} \in C^1\left(|R^3\right): \qquad \vec{X} = \nabla\Phi + \nabla\Xi \wedge \nabla\Psi. \qquad (10.475a, b)$$

*standard LXXXI. A continuously differentiable vector field (10.476a) is the sum (10.476b) of the gradients of two scalar potentials with the second multiplied by a third **Euler potential** (subsections 3.9.8–3.9.9):

$$\vec{X} \in C^1\left(|R^3\right): \qquad \vec{X} = \nabla\Phi + \Theta\nabla\Psi. \qquad (10.476a, b)$$

J. d. First-Order Differential in $N \geq 4$ Variables (notes 3.2–3.20):

$$n, m = 1, \dots, N: \qquad 0 = \sum_{n=0}^{N} X_n(x_m)\, dx_n. \qquad (10.477a, b)$$

*standard LXXXII. **Exact differential** (10.478b) if (10.478a) the curl bi-vector of coefficients is zero (notes 3.3 and 3.9):

$$\Omega_{mn} = \frac{\partial X_n}{\partial x_m} - \frac{\partial X_n}{\partial x_m} = 0 \quad \Leftrightarrow \quad \sum_{n=1}^{N} X_n(x_m)\, dx_n = d\Phi(x_m); \qquad (10.478a, b)$$

*standard LXXXIII. **Inexact differential** (10.479c) with integrating factor if the bi-vector (tri-vector) curl (10.479a) [helicity (10.479b)] is (is not) zero (notes 3.4, 3.5, and 3.10–3.12):

$$\Omega_{mn} = 0 \neq H_{m,ns} = \Omega_{mn} X_s + \Omega_{ns} X_m + \Omega_{ns} X_m: \quad \sum_{n=1}^{N} X_m(u_m) dx_n = \lambda(x_m)\, d\Phi(x_m);$$

(10.479a–c)

*standard LXXXIV. **Pfaffian** (10.480b) if the tri-vector helicity (10.480a) is nonzero (notes 3.6–3.10):

$$H_{mns} \neq 0 \quad \Leftrightarrow \quad \sum_{n=0}^{N} X_n(x_m) dx_n \neq \lambda(x_m)\, d\Phi(x_m). \qquad (10.480a, b)$$

*standard LXXXV. Reduction (10.481b) of the number of variables (10.481a) of a first-order differential (notes 3.11–3.15):

$$0 = \sum_{n=0}^{N} X_n(x_m)\, dx_n \quad \rightarrow \quad 0 = \sum_{m=1}^{N-1} Y_m(y_m)\, dy_n. \qquad (10.481a, b)$$

J. e. Homogeneous First-Order Differential in Two Variables: First-order differential in two variables (10.459c) with homogeneous coefficients (10.482a, b) of the same degree q (notes 3.17–3.20):

$$X(x,y) = x^q X\left(1, \frac{y}{x}\right), \qquad Y(x,y) = x^q Y\left(1, \frac{y}{x}\right); \tag{10.482a, b}$$

*standard LXXXVI. Integrating factor (10.483b) for inexact differential (10.483a):

$$\frac{\partial Y}{\partial x} \neq \frac{\partial X}{\partial y}: \qquad d\Phi(x,y) = \frac{X(x,y)dx + Y(x,y)\,dy}{xX(x,y) + yY(x,y)}; \tag{10.483a, b}$$

*standard LXXXVII. General integral (10.484c) for exact differential (10.484b) of degree distinct from minus unity (10.484a):

$$q \neq -1; \qquad \frac{\partial X}{\partial y} \equiv \frac{\partial Y}{\partial x}: \qquad xX(x,y) + yY(x,y) = C. \tag{10.484a–c}$$

J. f. Homogeneous First-Order Differential in *N* Variables (note 3.18): First-order differential in N variables (10.477a, b) whose coefficients (10.485a) are homogeneous functions (10.485b) of the same degree q:

$$m,n = 1,\ldots,N: \qquad X_n(x_1,\ldots,x_N) = (x_1)^q X\left(1, \frac{x_2}{x_1}, \ldots, \frac{x_N}{x_1}\right); \tag{10.485a, b}$$

*standard LXXXVIII. Inexact differential (10.486a) with integrating factor (10.486b):

$$\frac{\partial X_n}{\partial x_m} \neq \frac{\partial X_n}{\partial x_m}: \qquad \sum_{n=1}^{N} X_n(x_m)\,dx_n = \left\{\sum_{n=1}^{N} X_n(x_m)\,x_n\right\} d\Phi(x_m); \tag{10.486a, b}$$

*standard LXXXIX. General integral (10.487c) for exact differential (10.487b) of degree distinct from minus unity (10.487a):

$$q \neq -1; \qquad \frac{\partial X_n}{\partial x_m} = \frac{\partial X_n}{\partial x_m}: \qquad \sum_{n=1}^{N} X_n(x_m)\,x_n = C. \tag{10.487a–c}$$

J. g. Differential of Order *M* in *N* Variables (notes 3.21–3.22):

$$0 = \sum_{i_1,\ldots,i_M=1}^{N} X_{i_1 \ldots i_M}\, dx^{i} \ldots dx^{i_M}. \tag{10.488}$$

*standard XC. Second-order differential in two variables (note 3.21):

$$0 = A(x,y)(dx)^2 + B(x,y)(dy)^2 + D(x,y)dx\,dy. \tag{10.489}$$

*standard XCI. Second-order differential in three variables:

$$0 = A(dx)^2 + B(dy)^2 + C(dz)^2 + 2D\,dx\,dy + 2E\,dx\,dz + 2F\,dy\,dz, \tag{10.490a}$$

which is factorizable (notes 3.23–3.24) if:

$$ABC + 2DEF = AF^2 + BE^2 + CD^2. \tag{10.490b}$$

K. Special Integrals. Integrals not included in the general integral (sections 5.1–5.4; example 10.8):

K. a. C, p-discriminants and Special Points of First-Order Differential Equations (section 5.1):

*standard XCII. Envelope as a special integral (subsection 5.1.1);
*standard XCIII. C–discriminant: envelope, node, and cusp loci (subsection 5.1.2);
*standard XCIV. p–discriminant: envelope, tac, and cust loci (subsection 5.1.3);
*standard XCV. Classification of special curves (subsection 5.1.4);
*standard XCVI. Extension to special integral of differential equations of order higher than the first (subsection 5.1.5).

K. b. Quadratic Discriminants of First-Order Differential Equations (section 5.2):

*standard XCVII. First-order differential equation quadratic in the slope:

$$0 = L(x,y)\left(\frac{dy}{dx}\right)^2 + M(x,y)\frac{dy}{dx} + N(x,y); \tag{10.491}$$

*standard XCVIII. General integral of first-order differential equation quadratic in the arbitrary constant of integration C:

$$0 = P(x,y)\,C^2 + Q(x,y)C + R(x,y). \tag{10.492}$$

K. c. First-Order Differential Equations that Always Have Special Integrals (section 5.3):

*standard XCIX. **Clairaut** differential equation (10.493b) involving (10.493a) a differentiable function (subsections 5.3.1–5.3.2; E10.8.1)

$$h \in \mathcal{D}(R): \qquad y = x\frac{dy}{dx} + h\left(\frac{dy}{dx}\right); \qquad (10.493a, b)$$

*standard C. **D'Alembert** differential equation (10.494c) involving (10.494a, b) two differentiable functions (subsections 5.3.3–5.3.4; E10.8.1):

$$g, h \in \mathcal{D}(R): \qquad y = xg\left(\frac{dy}{dx}\right) + h\left(\frac{dy}{dx}\right). \qquad (10.494a–c)$$

K. d. First-Order Differential Equations Solvable for the Slope or a Variable (section 5.4):

*standard CI. First-order differential equation solvable for the dependent variable (10.495b) and involving (10.495a) a differentiable function (subsections 5.4.1–5.4.2):

$$h \in \mathcal{D}(|R^2): \qquad y = h\left(x, \frac{dy}{dx}\right); \qquad (10.495a, b)$$

*standard CII. First-order differential equation solvable for the independent variable (10.496b) and involving (10.496a) a differentiable function (subsections 5.4.1 and 5.4.3; E10.8.3):

$$g \in \mathcal{D}(|R^2): \qquad x = g\left(y, \frac{dy}{dx}\right). \qquad (10.496a, b)$$

*standard CIII. First-order differential equation of degree M in the slope (subsection 5.4.4):

$$0 = \sum_{m=0}^{M} A_m \left(\frac{dy}{dx}\right)^m. \qquad (10.497)$$

L. Transformation and Reduction of Differential Equations (sections 5.5–5.9)

L. a. Transformation of Differentials (section 5.5.1):

$$d\Phi = \sum_{m=1}^{N} X_n \, dx_n. \tag{10.498}$$

*standard CIV. Exchange of a variable and a coefficient (10.499b) via the **Legendre transformation** (10.499a):

$$\Psi(X_1, x_2, ..., x_N) = \Phi(x_1, x_2, ..., x_N) - x_1, X_1: \quad d\Psi = -x_1 d\, X_1 + \sum_{m=2}^{N} X_m \, dx_m. \tag{10.499a, b}$$

L. b. Dual First-Order Differential Equations (subsections 5.5.2–5.5.3):

*standard CV, General case:

$$0 = F\left(x; y, \frac{dy}{dx}\right) = F\left(\frac{dY}{dX}; X\frac{dY}{dX} - Y, X\right); \tag{10.500a, b}$$

*standard CVI. Special case:

$$0 = \Phi\left(x\frac{dy}{dx} - y\right) - x\Psi\left(\frac{dy}{dx}\right) = \Phi(Y) - \Psi(X)\frac{dY}{dX}. \tag{10.501a, b}$$

L. c. Second-Order Differential Equation Reduced to First-Order (section 5.6; E10.9.1–E10.9.2):

$$y' \equiv \frac{dy}{dx}, \quad y'' \equiv \frac{d^2y}{dx^2}: \qquad 0 = F(x; y, y', y''). \tag{10.502a–c}$$

*standard CVII. General case (subsection 5.6.1):

$$0 = F\left(x; y, y', y'\frac{dy'}{dy}\right). \tag{10.503}$$

*standard CVIII. Omitting the independent variable (subsection 5.6.2; E10.9.2):

$$0 = F(y, y', y'') = F\left(y, y', y'\frac{dy'}{dy}\right). \tag{10.504}$$

*standard CIX. Omitting both the independent variable and slope (subsection 5.6.3):

$$0 = F(y, y''); \tag{10.505}$$

*standard CX. Dependent variable missing (subsection 5.6.4):

$$z \equiv y': \qquad 0 = F(x, y', y'') = F(x; z, z'); \tag{10.506a, b}$$

*standard CXI. Missing both the slope and the dependent variable (subsection 5.6.4; E10.9.1):

$$0 = F(x; y''). \tag{10.507}$$

L. d. Depression of the Order of Differential Equations of Order $N > 2$, Higher than 2 (section 5.7; E10.9.3):

$$y^{(N)}(x) \equiv \frac{d^N y}{dx^N}: \qquad 0 = F\left(x; y; y', y'', \ldots. y^{(N)}\right). \tag{10.508a, b}$$

*standard CXII. Involving only the independent variable (subsection 5.7.1):

$$0 = F\left(x, y^{(N)}\right); \tag{10.509}$$

*standard CXIII. Involving only the independent variable and derivatives of order N and $N-1$ (subsection 5.7.2; E10.9.3):

$$z = y^{(N-1)}(x): \qquad 0 = F\left(x, y^{(N-1)}, y^{(N)}\right) = F(x; z, z'); \tag{10.510a–c}$$

*standard CXIV. Involving only the derivatives of orders $N-1$ and $N-2$ (subsection 5.7.3; E10.9.3):

$$w = y^{(N-1)}(x): \qquad 0 = F\left(y^{(N-1)}, y^{(N)}\right) = F(w, w'). \tag{10.511a–c}$$

*standard CXV. Involving only derivatives of orders $N-2$ and N (subsection 5.7.4):

$$u = y^{(N-2)}(x): \qquad 0 = F\left(y^{(N-2)}, y^{(N)}\right) = F(u, u''); \tag{10.512a–c}$$

*standard CXVI. Lowest-order derivative appearing is $N-P$ (subsection 5.7.5; E10.9.3):

$$z \equiv y^{(N-P)}(x): \qquad 0 = F\left(x, y^{(N-P)}, \ldots, y^{(N)}\right) = F\left(x; z, \ldots, z^{(P)}\right). \tag{10.513a–c}$$

L. e. Combinations of Differential Operators (section 5.8; E10.9.4–10.9.6):

*standard CXVII. **Factorizable** linear differential equation (subsection 5.8.1; E10.9.4):

$$\left\{P_N\left(\frac{d}{dx}\right)\right\}\left\{Q_M\left(\frac{d}{dx}\right)\right\} y(x)=0; \qquad (10.514)$$

*standard CXVIII. **Exact** differential equation (subsection 5.8.2 and E10.9.5):

$$0=F\left(x,y,y',\dots,y^{(N)}\right)=\frac{d^p}{dx^p}\left\{G\left(x;y,y',\dots,y^{(N-p)}\right)\right\}. \qquad (10.515)$$

L. f. Higher-Order Homogeneous Differential Equations (section 5.9):

*standard CXIX. **Homogeneous** differential equation of the **first kind** order N (subsection 5.9.1; E10.9.6):

$$0=F\left(\frac{y}{x},y',y'',\dots,y^{(N)}\right)=G\left(x,\frac{y'}{x},\frac{y''}{y},\dots,\frac{y^{(N)}}{y}\right); \qquad (10.516a, b)$$

*standard CXX. **Homogeneous** differential equation of the **second kind** and order N (subsections 5.9.2–5.9.3; E10.9.6):

$$0=F\left(y,y'x,y''x^2,\dots,y^{(N)}x^N\right). \qquad (10.517)$$

M. Simultaneous System of Differential Equations (sections 7.1–7.3):

*standard CXXI. Generalized autonomous system of differential equations (subsection 7.1.1):

$$m=1,\dots,M: \qquad \frac{dy_m}{dx}=Y_m\left(x;y_1,\dots,y_M\right); \qquad (10.518a, b)$$

*standard CXXII. General simultaneous system of M differential equations (subsection 7.1.2):

$$m,s=1,\dots,M;\ N_{m,s}\in|N: \qquad 0=F_s\left(x;y_m,y'_m,y''_m,\dots,y_m^{(N_{m,s})}\right); \qquad (10.519a–c)$$

*standard CXXIII. Implicit autonomous system of differential equations (subsections 7.2.1–7.2.4):

$$m, s = 1, \ldots, N: \qquad \frac{dx_n}{dt} = X_n(x_m); \qquad (10.520\text{a, b})$$

*standard CXXIV. Family of curves tangent to a vector field (subsections 7.2.1–7.2.4);
*standard CXXV. Hypersurfaces orthogonal to a vector field (subsection 7.2.5);
*standard CXXVI. Order of a simultaneous systems of differential equations (subsections 7.3.1–7.3.2);
*standard CXXVII. First integral of a system of simultaneous differential equations (subsection 7.3.4).

N. Simultaneous Linear System of Differential Equations with Constant Coefficients (sections 7.4–7.5):

*standard CXXVIII. Simultaneous linear system of differential equations (subsection 7.4.1):

$$m, s = 1, \ldots, M; \quad N_{m,r} \not\in| N: \qquad \sum_{m,r=1}^{M} \sum_{k=0}^{N_{m,r}} A_{m,r,k}(x) \frac{d^k y}{dx^k} = B_m(x), \qquad (10.521\text{a–c})$$

*standard CXXIX. Simultaneous linear system of differential equations with constant coefficients (subsections 7.4.1–7.4.2):

$$m = 1, \ldots, M; \quad N_{m,r} \not\in| N: \qquad \sum_{m,r=1}^{M} \sum_{k=0}^{N_{m,r}} A_{m,r,k} \frac{d^k y}{dx^k} = B_m(x); \qquad (10.522\text{a–c})$$

*standard CXXX. Simultaneous linear system of differential equations with homogeneous derivatives (subsection 7.4.1):

$$m = 1, \ldots, M; \quad N_{m,r} \not\in| N: \qquad \sum_{m,r=1}^{M} \sum_{k=0}^{N_{m,r}} A_{m,r,k}\, x^k \frac{d^k y}{dx^k} = B_m(x). \qquad (10.523\text{a–c})$$

N. a. Unforced (section 7.4): (10.522a–c) with $B_m(x) = 0$ and characteristic polynomial (subsections 7.4.2–7.4.3):

$$P_N(a) = \mathrm{Det}\{P_{m,r}(a)\}, \qquad P_{m,r}(a) \equiv \sum_{k=0}^{N_{m,r}} A_{m,r,k}\, a^k. \tag{10.524a, b}$$

*standard CXXXI. Degenerate and non-degenerate systems (subsections 7.4.3–7.4.4);
*standard CXXXII. Natural integrals for a single root of the characteristic polynomial (subsection 7.4.5);
*standard CXXXIII. Natural integrals for a multiple root of the characteristic polynomial (subsection 7.4.6);
*standard CXXXIV. General integral as a linear combination of natural integrals (subsections 7.4.7–7.4.10);
*standard CXXXV. Boundary conditions determining the arbitrary constants of integration (subsections 7.4.7–7.4.10);
*standard CXXXVI. Compatibility conditions determining the coefficients in the general integral (subsections 7.4.7–7.4.10);
*standard CXXXVII. Diagonal system for natural integrals corresponding to single roots of the characteristic polynomial (subsections 7.4.11 and 7.4.13);
*standard CXXXVIII. Two-banded diagonal system for the natural integrals corresponding to the same multiple root of the characteristic polynomial and block-banded diagonal system corresponding to distinct multiple roots of the characteristic polynomial (subsections 7.4.11–7.4.14).

N. b. Forced (10.522a–c) with $B_m(x) \neq 0$ (section 7.5):

*standard CXXXIX. Forcing by an exponential in non-resonant, resonant, and multiply-resonant cases (subsections 7.5.1–7.5.3):

$$P_m(x) = G_m\, e^{bx}; \tag{10.525}$$

*standard CXL. Forcing by the product of an exponential by a hyperbolic cosine or sine (subsection 7.5.4):

$$B_m(x) = G_m\, e^{bx} \cosh, \sinh(c\,x); \tag{10.526a, b}$$

*standard CXLI. Forcing by the product of an exponential by a circular cosine or sine (subsections 7.5.4–7.5.5):

$$B_m(x) = G_m\, e^{bx} \cos, \sin(g\,x); \tag{10.527a, b}$$

*standard CXLII. Forcing by the product of an exponential by a hyperbolic and a circular cosine or sine (subsection 7.5.4):

$$B_m(x) = G_m\, e^{bx} \cos, \sin h(cx) \cos, \sin(g\, x). \qquad (10.528a\text{–}d)$$

*standard CXLIII. Method of the inverse matrix of polynomials of ordinary derivatives (subsections 7.5.7–7.5.8);
*standard CXLIV. Complete integral of a forced coupled linear system of differential equations with constant coeffficients (subsection 7.5.9).

O. Simultaneous Linear System of Differential Equations with Homogeneous Derivatives (10.523a–c); (sections 7.6–7.7):

*standard CXLV. Alternative equivalent summation and matrix forms (subsection 7.6.2).

O. a. Unforced System: (10.523a–c) with $B_m(x) = 0$ (section 7.6):

*standard CXLVI. Characteristic polynomial (subsection 7.6.3):

$$Q_N(a) = \mathrm{Det}(Q_{m,r}), \qquad Q_{m,r}(a) \equiv \sum_{k=0}^{N_{m,r}} A_{m,r,k}\, a(a-1)\dots(a-k+1). \qquad (10.529a, b)$$

*standard CXLVII. Natural integrals corresponding to a single root of the characteristic polynomial (subsection 7.6.4);
*standard CXLVIII. Natural integrals corresponding to multiple roots of the characteristic polynomial (subsection 7.6.4);
*standard CXLIX. General integral for characteristic polynomial with single roots only (subsection 7.6.5);
*standard CL. General integral for characteristic polynomial with distinct multiple roots (subsection 7.6.5);
*standard CLI. Arbitrary constants and boundary conditions (subsections 7.6.5 and 7.6.7);
*standard CLII. Coefficients of the dependent variables and compatibility conditions (subsections 7.6.5–7.6.6);
*standard CLIII. Diagonal system for natural integrals corresponding to single roots of the characteristic polynomial (subsection 7.6.8);
*standard CLIV. Two-banded diagonal system for natural integrals corresponding to multiple roots of the characteristic polynomial (subsection 7.6.8);
*standard CLV. Block-banded diagonal system for several multiple roots of the characteristic polynomial (subsections 7.6.8–7.6.9).

O. b. Forced System (10.523a–c) with $B_m(x) \neq 0$ (section 7.7):

*standard CLVI. Comparison of simultaneous systems of linear differential equations with (α) constant coefficients; (β) homogeneous derivatives (subsections 7.7.2–7.7.5);
*standard CLVII. Forcing by a power in non-resonant, resonant, and multi-resonant cases (subsections 7.7.2–7.7.5):

$$B_m(x) = G_m\, x^b; \tag{10.530}$$

*standard CLVIII. Forcing by the product of a power by the hyperbolic cosine or sine of the multiple of a logarithm (subsection 7.7.6):

$$B_m(x) = G_m\, x^b \cosh,\, \sinh(c \log x); \tag{10.531a, b}$$

*standard CLIX. Forcing by the product of a power by a circular cosine or sine of the multiple of a logarithm (subsection 7.7.6):

$$B_m(x) = G_m\, x^b \cos,\, \sin(g \log x); \tag{10.532a, b}$$

*standard CLX. Forcing by the product of a power by a hyperbolic and a circular cosine or sine of a logarithm (subsections 7.7.6–7.7.7):

$$B_m(x) = G_m\, x^b \cosh,\, \sinh(c \log x) \cos, \sin(g \log x); \tag{10.533a–d}$$

*standard CLXI. Inverse matrix of polynomials of homogeneous derivatives (subsections 7.7.8–7.7.9);
*standard CLXII. Complete integral of a forced linear system of differential equations wih homogeneous derivatives (subsection 7.7.10).

P. Simultaneous System of Linear Finite Difference Equations with Constant Coefficients (sections 7.8–7.9):

$$m = 1,\ldots,M; \quad N_{m,r} \in |N: \qquad B_{m,\ell} = \sum_{m,=1}^{M} \sum_{k=0}^{N_{m,r}} A_{m,r,k}\, y_{r,k+\ell}; \tag{10.534a–c}$$

*standard CLXIII. The identity (10.534c) ≡ (10.535b) follows using (10.535a) forward finite diferences (subsections 7.8.1–7.8.2):

$$\Delta^k\, y_{r,\ell} = y_{r,\ell+k}: \qquad B_{m,\ell} = \sum_{m,=1}^{M} \sum_{k=0}^{N_{m,r}} A_{m,r,k}\, \Delta^k y_{r,k+\ell}; \tag{10.535a, b}$$

P. a. Unforced (section 7.8): (10.534c) ≡ (10.535b) with $B_{m,\ell} = 0$ and characteristic polynomial:

$$R_N(\Delta) = \mathrm{Det}\{R_{m,r}(a)\}, \qquad R_{m,r} = \sum_{k=0}^{N_{m,r}} A_{m,r,k}\,\Delta^k. \tag{10.536a, b}$$

*standard CLXIV. The roots of the characteristic polynomial specify the natural sequences (subsection 7.8.3);
*standard CLXV. Natural sequences corresponding to a single root of the characteristic polynomial (subsection 7.8.4);
*standard CLXVI. Natural sequences corresponding to a multiple root of the characteristic polynomial (subsection 7.8.4);
*standard CLXVII. General solution for characteristic polynomial with all roots distinct (subsection 7.8.5);
*standard CLXVIII. General solution for characteristic polynomial with distinct multiple roots (subsection 7.8.5);
*standard CLXIX. Arbitrary constants determined from starting conditions (subsections 7.8.5 and 7.8.7);
*standard CLXX. Coefficients of natural sequences determined from compatibility conditions (subsections 7.8.5–7.8.6);
*standard CLXXI. Diagonal system of natural sequences corresponding to single roots of the characteristic polynomial (subsections 7.8.8 and 7.8.10);
*standard CLXXII. Lower triangular system of natural sequences corresponding to multiple roots of the characteristic polynomial (subsection 7.8.8);
*standard CLXXIII. Block-lower triangular system of natural integrals corresponding to distinct multiple roots of the characteristic polynomial (subsection 7.8.9).

P. b. Forced (subsection 7.9): $B_{m,\ell} \neq 0$ in (10.535b):

*standard CLXXIV. Forcing by powers (subsections 7.9.2–7.9.4):

$$B_{m,\ell} = G_m\, b^\ell; \tag{10.537}$$

*standard CLXXV. Forcing by the product of a power by a hyperbolic cosine or sine of the multiple of an angle (subsections 7.9.5–7.9.6):

$$B_{m,\ell} = G_m\, b^\ell \cosh, \sinh(c\,\ell\,\phi); \tag{10.538a, b}$$

*standard CLXXVI. Forcing by the product of a power by a circular cosine or sine of a multiple angle (subsection 7.9.5):

$$B_{m,\ell} = G_m\, b^\ell \cos, \sin(g\,\ell\,\phi); \tag{10.539a, b}$$

*standard CLXXVII. Forcing by the product of a power by a hyperbolic and a circular cosine or sine of a multiple angle (subsection 7.9.5):

$$B_{m,\ell} = G_m\, b^{\ell} \cos h, \sin h\left(c\,\ell\,\phi\right)\cos, \sin\left(g\,\ell\,\phi\right); \qquad (10.540\text{a–d})$$

*standard CLXXVIII. Complete solution of a forced linear system of finite difference equations with constant coefficients (subsections 7.9.7–7.9.8).

Q. Generalized Isotropic Equation of a Mathematical Physics (notes 8.1–8.17):

$$\sum_{n=0}^{N} \frac{\partial^2 F}{\partial x_n^2} + \sum_{m=0}^{M} A_m \frac{\partial^2 F}{\partial t^m} = 0. \qquad (10.541)$$

Q. a. Reduction to a Helmholtz equation (notes 8.1–8.5):

$$\nabla^2 \equiv \sum_{n=1}^{N} \frac{\partial^2 F}{\partial x_n^2}: \qquad \nabla^2 \tilde{F} + k^2\, \tilde{F} = 0. \qquad (10.542\text{a, b})$$

*standard CLXXIX. Reduction of the generalized equation of mathematical physics (10.541) to a Helmholtz equation (10.542a, b) via (10.543b) a Fourier (10.442c)≡ (10.543a) transform (notes 8.1–8.2):

$$k^2 \equiv \sum_{m=0}^{M} A_m \left(-i\,\omega\right)^m: \qquad F\left(x_n, t\right) = \int_{-\infty}^{+\infty} \tilde{F}\left(x_n, t\right) e^{-i\omega t}\, d\omega. \qquad (10.543\text{a, b})$$

*standard CLXXX. Solution of the Helmholtz equation (10.542b) in N-dimensional (10.542a) Cartesian coordinates (note 8.3);
*standard CLXXXI. Cylindrical Bessel differential equation with integer order (note 8.4; sections 9.5–9.9);
*standard CLXXXII. Solution of the Helmholtz equation (10.542b) in cylindrical coordinates (note 8.4);
*standard CLXXXIII. Solution of the Helmholtz equation (10.542b) in polar coordinates (note 8.4);
*standard CLXXXIV. Associated Legendre differential equation (notes 8.5 and 9.21);

*standard CLXXXV. Spherical Bessel differential equation (note 8.5; subsections 9.5.23–9.5.26 and 9.6.6–9.6.8);
*standard CLXXXVI. Solution of the Helmholtz equation (10.542b) in spherical coordinates (note 8.5).

Q. b. Hyperspherical (Hypercylinderical) Coordinates (notes 8.6–8.8):

*standard CLXXXVII (CLXXXVIII). Transformation from N-dimensional cartesian coordinates to hyperspherical (hypercylindrical) coordinates (note 8.6);
*standard CLXXXIX (CXC). Inverse coordinate transformation from hyperspherical (hypercylindrical) coordinates to N-dimensional cartesian coordinates (note 8.7);
*standard CXCI (CXCII). Base vectors, scale factors, metric tensor, and its determinant in hyperspherical (hypercylindrical) coordinates (note 8.8).

Q. c. Helmholtz Equation (10.542b) Involving the Laplacian (10.542a) in Hyperspherical Coordinates:

*standard CXCIII (CXCIV). Helmholtz equation in hyperspherical coordinates in explicit form (nested form to facilitate the separation of variables) [note 8.9(8.10)];
*standard CXCV. Set of N ordinary differential equations arising from the solution of the Helmholtz equation (10.542a, b) in hyperspherical coordinates (standard CXCV) by separation of variables (note 9.11);
*standard CXCVI. Radial dependence (10.544c) of the solution of the Helmholtz equation (10.542a, b) in hyperspherical coordinates specified by (10.544a) in terms of Bessel and Neumann functions of order (10.544b; note 8.12):

$$y(x) = J_\nu(x), Y_\nu(x); \quad \nu^2 = a^2 + (N - 1/2)^2, \quad x^2 y'' + (N-1) x y' + \left(x^2 - a^2\right) y = 0; \tag{10.544a–c}$$

*standard CXCVII. Dependence on the co-latitudes (10.545b) of the solution of the Helmholtz equation (10.542a, b) in hyperspherical coordinates in terms of hyperspherical associated Legendre functions (10.545a) of degree n, order m, and dimension ℓ (note 8.13):

$$w(\theta) = P^m_{n,\ell}(\cos\theta), Q^m_{n,\ell}(\cos\theta): \; w'' + (1+\ell)\cot\theta\, w' + \left[n(n+1) - m^2 \csc^2\theta\right] w = 0; \tag{10.545a, b}$$

*standard CXCVIII. Solution of the Helmholtz equation (10.542a, b) in hyperspherical coordinates in four dimensions, which is next higher dimension than (standard CLXXXVI) spherical harmonics (note 8.14).

Q. d. Solution in Hypercylindrical Coordinates (notes 8.15–8.17):

*standard CXCIX. Solution of the Helmholtz equation (10.542a, b) in four dimensions in hypercylindrical instead of hyperspherical (standard CXCVIII) coordinates (note 8.15);
*standard CC. Solution of the generalized equation of mathematical physics (10.541) in N-dimensional hyperspherical coordinates as a superposition of hyperspherical harmonics (note 8.16);
*standard CCI. As for standard CC in hypercylindrical coordinates using a hypercylindrical coordinates using a superposition of hypercylindrical harmonics (note 8.17).

R. Existence, Unicity, Robustness, and Uniformity Theorems (section 9.1):

R. a. First-Order Differential Equation with Explicit Slope (subsections 9.1.1–9.1.14):

$$\frac{dy}{dx} = f(x,y;\lambda), \quad y(x_0) = y_0 + \varepsilon: \qquad y = y(x;y_0,\lambda,\varepsilon). \tag{10.546a–c}$$

*standard CCII. Transformation to an integral equation and application of the **Picard method** of successive approximations (subsections 9.1.2–9.1.3);
*standard CCIII. **Lipshitz condition** for one function of one variable and relation with bounded, continuous, and differentiable functions (subsections 9.1.4–9.1.5);
*standard CCIV. **Existence theorem** for the solution (10.546c) of the differential equation (10.546a) omitting the parameter λ with the boundary condition (10.546b) without perturbation $\varepsilon = 0$ (subsections 9.1.6–9.1.8);
*standard CCV. Rectangular region containing the successive approximations (standard CCII) to the (standard CCV) unique solution (subsection 9.1.9);
*standard CCVI. **Unicity theorem** for the solution (10.546c) of the differential equation (10.546a) omitting the parameter λ with the boundary condition (10.546b) without $\varepsilon = 0$ perturbation (subsection 9.1.10);
*standard CCVII. **Robustness condition** in which a small pertubation ε in the boundary condition (10.546b) leads to a small perturbation ε in the solution (10.546c) of the (10.546a) differential equation (subsections 9.1.11–9.1.13);
*standard CCVIII. **Robustness theorem** for the solution (10.546c) of the differential equation (10.546a) without parameter λ for a small perturbation ε of (10.546b) the boundary condition (subsections 9.1.12–9.1.13);

*standard CCIX. **Uniformity theorem** on the differentiability of the solution (10.546c) of the differential equation (10.546a) with regards to the parameter λ, with the unperturbed $\varepsilon = 0$ boundary (10.546b) condition (subsection 9.1.14).

R. b. Generalized Autonomous System of Differential Equations (subsections 9.1.15–9.1.17):

$$m, n = 1, \ldots, M: \quad \frac{dy_m}{dx} = f_m(x, y_n; \lambda), \quad y_m(x_0) = y_{m,0} + \varepsilon_m \, y = y(x; y_{0,m}, \lambda, \varepsilon_m). \tag{10.547a–d}$$

*standard CCX. Lipshitz condition (standard CCIII) extended to M functions of L variables (subsection 9.1.16);
*standard CCXI. Existence and unity of the solution (10.547d) of the autonomous system of differential equations (10.547a, b) without the parameter λ, with initial conditions (10.547c) without $\varepsilon_m = 0$ perturbations (subsections 9.1.15–9.1.17);
*standard CCXII. Robustness theorem for the solution (10.547d) of the autonomous system of differential equations (10.547a, b) in the absence of the parameter λ, for small perturbations ε_m of (10.547c) the boundary conditions (subsections 9.1.16–9.1.17);
*standard CCXIII. Uniformity theorem for the solution (10.547d) of the autonomous system of differential equations (10.547a, b) with the parameter λ, in the absence $\varepsilon_m = 0$ of perturbations of (10.547c) the boundary conditions (subsections 9.1.16–9.1.17).

R. c. Non-Linear Differential Equation of Order N (subsections 9.1.18 and 9.1.20):

$$n = 0, \ldots, N-1: \quad \frac{d^N y}{dx^N} = F\left(x; \frac{d^N y}{dx^N}; \lambda\right), \quad y^{(n)}(x_0) = y_0^{(n)} + \varepsilon_n, \; y = y\left(x; y_0^{(n)}, \lambda, \varepsilon_n\right). \tag{10.548a–d}$$

*standard CCXIV. Existence and unicity of solution (10.548d) of the N-th order differential equation (10.548a, b) without parameter λ, with boundary conditions (10.548c) without $\varepsilon_n = 0$ perturbations (subsections 9.1.18 and 9.1.20);
*standard CCXV. Robustness theorem for the solution (10.548d) of the non-linear N-th order differential equation (10.548a, b) without the parameter λ, and with small pertubations ε_n of the (10.548c) boundary condition (subsections 9.1.18 and 9.1.20);
*standard CCXVI. Uniformity theorem for the solution (10.548d) of the non-linear N-th order differential equation (10.548a, b) with parameter λ, and without $\varepsilon_n = 0$ perturbation of (10.548c) the boundary conditions (subsections 9.1.18 and 9.1.20).

R. d. Linear Differential Equation of Order *N* (subsections 9.1.19–9.1.20):

$$\sum_{n=0}^{N} A_n(x;\lambda)\frac{d^n y}{dx^n} = B(x;\lambda); \quad m = 0;\ldots,N-1: \tag{10.549a–d}$$

$$y^{(m)}(x_0) = y_0^{(m)} + \varepsilon_n, \quad y = y\left(x; y_0^{(m)}, \lambda, \varepsilon_m\right).$$

*standard CCXVII. Existence and unicity of solution (10.549d) of the linear *N*th order differential equation (10.549a) without parameter λ, and with unperturbed $\varepsilon_n = 0$ boundary (10.549b, c) conditions (subsections 9.1.19–9.1.20);
*standard CCXVIII. Robustness theorem for the solution (10.549d) of the linear *N*-th order differential equation (10.549a) without parameter λ, and with small perturbations ε_n of the (10.549b, c) boundary conditions (subsections 9.1.19–9.1.20);
*standard CCXIX. Uniformity theorem for the solution (10.549d) of the linear *N*-th order differential equation (10.549a) with parameter λ, without perturbations $\varepsilon_n = 0$ of the (10.549b, c) boundary conditions (subsections 9.1.19–9.1.20).

S. Stability of Equilibrium of a System (section 9.2)

S. a. Classification of Equilibrium and Related Concepts (subsections 9.2.1–9.2.3):

*standard CCXX. Seven cases of physical equilibrium consisting of indifferent, and stable (unstable) in a finite time, or asymptotically or an oscillatory evolution with time (subsection 9.2.1);
*standard CCXXI. Five cases of mathematical equilibrium consisting of indifferent, stable (unstable) for all time or only asymptotically (subsection 9.2.1);
*standard CCXXII. Classification of a function into positive (negative) definite or semi-definite or indefinite (subsection 9.2.2);
*standard CCXXIII. Extended positive (negative) definite function in the case of dependence on parameter(s) (subsection 9.2.2);
*standard CCXXIV. Five cases of zero force for a conservative system for which the force is specified by the gradient of a potential (subsection 9.2.2);
*standard CCXXV. Three cases of stability of the equilibrium for (standard CCXXIV) a conservative system (subsection 9.2.2);

*standard CCXXVI. Derivative (10.550b) following an (10.550a) autonomous system (subsection 9.2.3):

$$\dot{\vec{x}} = \vec{G}(\vec{x}): \qquad \frac{dH}{dt} = \frac{\partial H}{\partial \vec{x}} \cdot \frac{d\vec{x}}{dt} = \vec{G}.\nabla H; \qquad (10.550\text{a, b})$$

*standard CCXXVII. Derivative (10.551b) following a generalized (10.551a) or unsteady autonomous system (subsection 9.2.3):

$$\dot{\vec{x}} = \vec{F}(\vec{x},t): \qquad \frac{dH}{dt} = \frac{\partial H}{\partial t} + \frac{\partial H}{\partial \vec{x}} \cdot \frac{d\vec{x}}{dt} = \frac{\partial H}{\partial t} + \vec{F}.\nabla H; \qquad (10.551\text{a, b})$$

*standard CCXXVIII. Intermediate case between standards CCXXVI and CCXXVII for an asymptotically (10.552b) autonomous (10.552a) system (subsection 9.2.3):

$$\dot{\vec{x}} = \vec{F}(\vec{x},t): \qquad \lim_{t\to\infty} \vec{F}(x,t) = \vec{G}(\vec{x}). \qquad (10.552\text{a, b})$$

S. b. Stability of an Equilibrium Specified by an Liapunov Function (subsections 9.2.4–9.2.10):

*standard CCXXIX. First Liapunov theorem on stability, or asymptotic stability, or instability of an autonomous or generalized autonomous system (subsections 9.2.4–9.2.7);

*standard CCXXX. Stability of the linear damped oscillator (10.553) with constant mass m and friction coefficient $\mu(x)$ and the spring resilience $k(x)$ functions of position (subsection 9.2.8):

$$\left\{ m\frac{d^2}{dt^2} + \mu(x)\frac{d}{dt} + k(x) \right\} x(t) = 0; \qquad (10.553)$$

*standard CCXXXI. Stability of the linear damped oscillator (10.554) with constant mass m and friction coefficient $\mu(t)$ and the spring resilience $k(t)$ functions of time (subsection 9.2.9):

$$\left\{ m\frac{d^2}{dt^2} + \mu(t)\frac{d}{dt} + k(t) \right\} x(t) = 0; \qquad (10.554)$$

*standard CCXXXII. Particular case of the standard CCXXXI concerning the instability of the parametric resonance (10.555) of the linear undamped oscillator with natural frequency ω_0, and excitation frequency ω_e and amplitude h (subsection 9.2.10 and section 4.4):

$$\left\{ \frac{d^2}{dt^2} + \omega_0^2\left[1 + 2h\cos(\omega_e t)\right] \right\} x(t) = 0. \qquad (10.555)$$

S. c. Linear Differential Equation with Bounded Coefficients (subsections 9.2.11–9.2.14):

*standard CCXXXIII. Exponential positive upper (negative lower) asymptotic bounds for the solution of a single (simultaneous system of) linear differential equation(s) with constant coefficients (subsection 9.2.11);
*standard CLXXXIV. Second Liapunov theorem stating that there exist exponential positive upper (negative lower) asymptotic bounds for the solutions of an autonomous system of differential equations (10.556a, c) with bounded (10.556b) coefficients (subsection 9.2.12):

$$m,n=1,\dots,\ M; \qquad \left|A_{mn}(x)\right| \le B < \infty: \quad \frac{dy_n}{dx} = \sum_{m=1}^{M} A_{nm}(x)\,y_m(x), \qquad (10.556\text{a–c})$$

*standard CCXXXV. Existence of at least one eigenvalue for the linear autonomous system of differential equations (10.556a, c) with bounded (10.556b) coefficients (subsection 9.2.13);
*standard CCXXXVI. Existence of at least one eigenvalue (standard CCXXXV) or equivalently existence of exponential positive upper (negative lower) bounds (standards CCXXXIII–CCXXXIV) for the solution and first $N-1$ derivatives of a linear differential equation (10.557c) of order N with bounded (10.557a, b) coefficients (subsection 9.2.14):

$$m=0,\dots,N; \qquad \left|A_{mn}(x)\right| \le B < \infty: \quad \sum_{m=1}^{M} A_{nm}(x)\,\frac{d^n y}{dx^n} = 0. \qquad (10.557\text{a–c})$$

S. d. Stability of an Equilibrium Specified by an Autonomous Differential System (subsections 9.2.15–9.2.21):

*standard CCXXXVII. Solutions of a linear autonomous system (10.556a, c) with constant coefficients (subsection 9.2.15);
*standard CCXXXVIII. Third Liapunov theorem on the stability of the equilibrium (10.558c) of a twice-continuously differentiable (10.558b) autonomous (10.558a, d) system (subsections 9.2.16–9.2.20):

$$n,m=1,\dots,M; \qquad F_n(x_m) \in C^2\left(\left|\vec{x}\right| < \varepsilon\right), \qquad F_m(0)=0; \qquad (10.558\text{a–c})$$

$$\frac{dy_n}{dx} = F_n\left(x_m(t)\right), \quad \vec{x}_0 = \vec{x}(0), \qquad \vec{x} = \vec{x}\left(t;\vec{x}_0\right), \qquad (10.558\text{d–f})$$

*standard CCXXXIX. Upper bound for the solution (10.558f) of the autonomous differential system (10.558a–d) with the initial (10.558e) condition (subsections 9.2.16–9.2.20);

*standard CCXL. General integral of a linear autonomous differential system as a linear combination of fundamental solutions (subsection 9.2.17);
*standard CCXLI. Positive-definite quadratic form specifying a stability quadratic form (subsection 9.2.18);
*standard CCXLII. Upper and lower bounds for a quadratic form (subsection 9.2.18);
*standard CCXLIII. Upper bound for the gradient of a quadratic form (subsection 9.2.18);
*standard CCXLIV. Third Liapouvov theorem on the upper bound (standard CCXXXIX) for the solution (standard CCXXXVIII) of the autonomous (10.558a–f) differential system (subsection 9.2.20);
*standard CCXLV. Stability of an autonomous differential equation (10.559b) in which the independent variable does not appear explicitly and the function (10.559a) has continuous second-order derivative (subsection 9.2.21):

$$F \in C^2\left(|R^{N-1}\right): \qquad \frac{d^N y}{dx^N} = F\left(y, \frac{dy}{dx}, \frac{d^2 y}{dx^2}, \ldots, \frac{d^{N-1} y}{dx^{N-1}}\right). \qquad (10.559\text{a, b})$$

T. Linear Differential Equation with Periodic Coefficients (section 9.3):

$$n = 0, \ldots, N; \quad A_n(t) = A_n(t+\tau): \qquad \sum_{m=0}^{M} A_n(x) \frac{d^n x}{dt^n} = 0. \qquad (10.560\text{a–c})$$

T. a. Differential Equation of Arbitrary Order (subsections 9.3.1–9.3.4):

*standard CCXLVI. **Floquet theorem** on the existence of solutions for a linear differential equation (10.560a, c) with periodic coefficients (10.560b) in the case of single or multiple eigenvalues (subsections 9.3.1–9.3.3);
*standard CCXLVII. Four cases of stability of the solution of a linear differential equation (10.560a, c) with periodic coefficients (10.560b) based on the eigenvalues and exponents in (standard CCXLVII) the Floquet theorem (subsection 9.3.3);
*standard CCXLVIII. **Diagonal (banded diagonal)** system associated with single (multiple) eigenvalues (standard CCXLVI) linear differential equation (10.560a, c) with (10.560b) periodic coefficients (subsection 9.3.4);
*standard CCXLIX. Transformation into a **Jordan matrix** of the banded diagonal matrix (standard CCXLVIII) associated with multiple eigenvalues (standard CCXLVII) of a (standard CCXLVI) linear differential equation (10.560a, c) with (10.560b) periodic coefficients (subsection 9.3.4).

T. b. Second-Order Differential Equation in Invariant Form (10.561b; subsections 9.3.5–9.3.9):

$$I(t) = I(t+\tau): \qquad \left\{ \frac{d^2}{dt^2} + I(t) \right\} x(t) = 0. \qquad \text{(10.561a, b)}$$

*standard CCL. Stable (unstable) and monotonic (oscillatory) cases with equal or distinct eigenvalues of the linear second differential equation in invariant form (10.561b) with periodic coefficient (10.561a) (subsections 9.3.5–9.3.6);
*standard CCLI. General integral of a linear second-order differential equation (10.560c) of order N as a linear combination of N fundamental solutions (subsection 9.3.7);
*standard CCLII. Eigenvalues of the linear second-order differential equation (10.561b) in invariant form with periodic coefficients (10.561a) (subsection 9.3.8);
*standard CCLIII. Fourth Lyapunov theorem on the stability of solutions of the linear second-order differential equation (10.561b) in invariant form with periodic coefficients (10.561a) (subsection 9.3.9).

U. Linear Differential Equation with Analytic Coefficients (section 9.4; example 10.20):

$$n = 0,\ldots,N: \qquad A_n \in \mathcal{A}(|C): \qquad \sum_{n=0}^{N} A_n(x) \frac{d^n y}{dx^n} = 0. \qquad \text{(10.562a–c)}$$

U. a. Classification of Points of Functions of a Complex Variable (subsections 9.4.1–9.4.4):

*standard CCLIV. Convergence of the **Laurent series** of a function analytic in an annulus around an isolated singularity (subsection 9.4.1);
*standard CCLV. Classification of the points of a complex single-valued function in four classes: regular, simple poles, or multiple poles, and essential singularities (subsection 9.4.1);
*standard CCLVI. Convergence of the MacLaurin series of a function in a circle with a regular point at the centre (subsection 9.4.1);
*standard CCCVII. Calculation of the residue of a complex single-valued function at a simple pole or multiple pole (subsection 9.4.2);
*standard CCLVIII. Distinction between poles and essential singularities of a single-valued complex function of a complex variable (subsection 9.4.2);

*standard CCLIX. N branches of the multi-valued complex function N-th root, and associated Riemann surface, principal branch, branch-point, and discontinuity across the branch-cut (subsection 9.4.3);
*standard CCLX. As the standard CCLIX for the infinitely many branches of the many-valued function logarithm of a complex variable (subsection 9.4.4);
*standard CCLXI. Definition and modulus, and argument of the power with complex base and exponent (subsection 9.4.4);
*standard CCLXII. Classification of the power with complex base and exponent (standard CCLXI) into five cases: ordinary point, zero, pole, multi-valued, or many-valued branch point (subsection 9.4.4).

U. b. Classification of Points of a Linear Differential Equation (subsections 9.4.5–9.4.7):

*standard CCLXIII. Three cases of solution of a linear unforced first-order differential equation; analytic, regular, or irregular integrals (subsections 9.4.5–9.4.6);
*standard CCLXIV. Most general particular solution of a linear differential equation as a logarithmic irregular integral:

$$y(x) = x^a \sum_{\beta=0}^{\alpha-1} g_\beta \log^\beta x \sum_{n=-\infty}^{+\infty} c_{n,\beta} x^n, \tag{10.563}$$

involving the index a, its multiplicity α, the logarithmic factors g_β and the coefficients $c_{n,\beta}$ of the Laurent series (subsection 9.4.6);
*standard CCLXV. Classification of analytic, regular, and irregular integrals of an unforced linear first-order differential equation in the case of the point at infinity that is excluded from the standard CCLXII (subsection 9.4.7);
*standard CCLXVI. Upper bound in modulus for the exponential of a complex matrix whose elements are bounded in modulus (subsection 9.4.8);
*standard CCLXVII. – Existence of a solution bounded in modulus for a linear first-order autonomous system with integrable coefficients (subsection 9.4.8);
*standard CCLXVIII. Analytic, regular, and irregular integrals of a linear autonomous system of differential equations (subsection 9.4.8).

U. c. Methods of Solution of a Linear Differential Equation with Analytic Coefficients (subsections 9.4.9–9.4.11):

*standard CCLIX. Existence of solution of the linear differential equation (10.562c) with analytic coefficients (10.562a, b) as an analytic integral (10.563a) whose coefficients c_n coincide with those of (10.563b), a MacLaurin series (subsection 9.4.9):

$$y(x) = \sum_{n=0}^{\infty} c_n x^n = \sum_{n=0}^{\infty} \frac{x^n}{n!} y^{(n)}(0); \tag{10.563a, b}$$

*standard CCLX. Particular case of the standard CCLIX for a linear second-order differential equation in invariant form (10.564b) with analytic (10.564a) coefficient (subsection 9.4.9):

$$I(x) = \sum_{k=0}^{\infty} I_k\, x^k: \qquad \left\{\frac{d^2}{dx^2} - I(x)\right\} y(x) = 0; \qquad (10.564\text{a, b})$$

*standard CCLXI. First method of solution of the standard CCLIX, with the standard CCLX as example, specifying the MacLaurin series (10.563b) as the analytic integral (subsection 9.4.10);
*standard CCLXII. Second alternative and equivalent method of solution to the standard CCLXI specifying the recurrence formula for the coefficients c_n of the (10.563a) analytic integral (subsection 9.4.11).

U. d. **Application to the Generalized Hyperbolic and Circular Functions** (subsections 9.4.12–9.4.20):

*standard CCLXIII. General integral (10.565b) of the generalized hyperbolic differential equation (10.565a) as a linear combination with coefficients (c_0, c_1) of the generalized hyperbolic cosine and sine with parameter m (subsections 9.4.12–9.4.13):

$$y'' - x^m\, y = 0: \qquad y(x) = c_0 \cos h(x;m) + c_1 \sinh(x;m); \qquad (10.565\text{a, b})$$

*standard CCLXIV. Airy differential equation (10.566a) [functions (10.566b)] as the particular case of parameter unity $m = 1$ of the (standard CCLXII) generalized hyperbolic differential equation (10.565a) [cosine and sine (10.565b)] (subsection 9.4.14):

$$y'' - xy = 0: \qquad y(x) = c_0\, Ai(x) + c_1\, Bi(x); \qquad (10.566\text{a, b})$$

*standard CCLXV. Changing the sign in (10.565a) leads to the generalized circular differential equation (10.567a) whose general integral (10.567b) is a linear combination with arbitrary constants (c_0, c_1) of the generalized circular cosine and sine (subsection 9.4.15):

$$y'' + x^m\, y = 0: \qquad y(x) = c_0 \cos(x;m) + c_1 \sin(x;m); \qquad (10.567\text{a, b})$$

*standard CCLXVI. Extension of the general integral (10.565b) [(10.567b)] of the generalized hyperbolic (10.565a) [circular (10.567a)] differential equation as a linear combination of generalized hyperbolic (circular) cosines and sines from positive integer values [standard CCLXIII (CCLXV)] of the parameter m to all complex values of m other than negative integers; for negative integer values of m see the heading U. e., which follows (subsections 9.4.16–9.4.17);

*standard CCLXVII. Derivative of the generalized hyperbolic (circular) sine with complex variable (subsection 9.4.18);
*standard CCLXVIII. Derivative of the first and second Airy functions (subsection 9.4.18);
*standard CCLXIX. Derivative of the generalized hyperbolic (circular) sine with complex variable (subsection 9.4.18);
*standard CCLXX. Generalized hyperbolic and circular cosine and sine as increasing or decreasing functions of real variable and parameter (subsection 9.4.19);
*standard CCLXXI. Inequalities for the generalized hyperbolic and circular cosine, and sine of real variable and parameter (subsection 9.4.19);
*standard CCLXXII. Inequalities between hyperbolic and circular cosines (sines) with real variable and parameter (subsection 9.4.19);
*standard CCLXXXIII. Inequalities for the generalized hyperbolic and circular secant, cosecant, tangent, and cotangent with real variable and parameter (subsection 9.4.20);
*standard CCLXXXIV. Inequalities between the generalized hyperbolic and circular secant (cosecant) with real variable and parameter (subsection 9.4.20).

U. e. Generalized Hyperbolic (Circular) Differential Equation with Negative Integer Parameter (example 10.20):

$$m = -1, -2, \ldots, -p; \qquad p \in |N: \qquad y'' \pm x^m y = 0. \tag{10.568a–c}$$

*standard CCLXXXV. In the case $m = -1$ of a simple pole in the coefficient of (10.568c) the general integral integral is a linear combination of regular integrals of the first and second kinds (E10.20.1);
*standard CCLXXXVI. Elementary power solutions in the case of a double pole $m = -2$ in the coefficient of (10.568c) (E10.20.2);
*standard CCLXXXVII. In the case $m = -3$ of a triple pole in the coefficient of (10.568c), the general integral is a linear combination of regular asymptotic integrals of the first and second kinds (E10.20.3);
*standard CCLXXXVIII. In the cases $m = -4 - 5, \ldots,$ of pole of order higher than 3 the general integral is a linear combination of generalized hyperbolic (circular) cosines and sines of the asymptotic variable $1/x$ (E10.20.4);
*standard CCLXXXIX. In the particular case $m = -4$ ($m = -5$) of a quadruple (quintuple) pole of the coefficient of (10.568c) with ±[+] sign, the standard CCLXXXVIII simplifies to a general integral that is a linear combination of generalized hyperbolic (circular) cosines and sines [Airy functions of the first and second kinds] of the asymptotic variable $1/x$ (E10.20.5);
*standard CCXC. General integral of the generalized hyperbolic (circular) differential equation (10.568c) with $-(+)$ for all values of the parameter, combining the standards CCLXIII–CCLXVI and CCLXXXV–CCLXXXIX (subsections 9.4.12–9.4.17; E10.20.1–E10.20.5).

V. A Linear Differential Equation with Regular Singularities (section 9.5):

V. a. Linear Autonomous System of Differential Equations with a Regular Singularity (subsections 9.5.1–9.5.4):

$$m,n=1,\dots,N: \qquad P_{m,n} \in \mathcal{A}(|C): \qquad \frac{dy_m}{dx} = \sum_{n=1}^{N} \left[\frac{a_{m,n}}{x} + p_{m,n}(x) \right] y_n(x). \tag{10.569a–d}$$

*standard CCXCI. Solution of an autonomous linear system of differential equations (10.569a, b, d) with a regular singularity (10.569c) as a linear combination of regular integrals of the first kind (10.570b) with índex a and coefficients $c_n(a)$ to be determined and radius of convergence (10.570a) (subsections 9.5.1–9.5.2):

$$|x| < R: \qquad y(x) = x^a \sum_{n=0}^{\infty} x^n c_n(a), \tag{10.570a, b}$$

*standard CCXCII. Example of solution by two equivalent methods of a linear autonomous system of differential equations with a regular singularity (subsections 9.5.3–9.5.4).

V. b. Linear Differential Equation of Order *N* with a Regular Singularity (subsections 9.5.5–9.5.7).

$$n = 0,\dots,N; \qquad p_n \in \mathcal{A}(|C): \qquad \sum_{n=0}^{N} x^n p_n(x) \frac{d^n y}{dx^n} = 0. \tag{10.571a–c}$$

*standard CCXCIII. Linear differential equation (10.571c) of order N with a regular singularity (10.571a, b) whose solutions are all regular integrals (subsection 9.5.5);
*standard CCXCIV. General integral near a regular singularity (10.571a, b) of a linear differential equation (10.571c) of order N as a linear combination of regular integrals of two kinds (subsections 9.5.6–9.5.7).

V. c. Linear Second-Order Differential Equation with a Regular Singularity (subsections 9.5.8–9.5.12):

$$p, q \in \mathcal{A}(|C): \qquad x^2 \frac{d^2y}{dx^2} + x p(x) \frac{dy}{dx} + q(x) y(x) = 0. \tag{10.572a–c}$$

*standard CCXCV. General integral integral of (10.572a–c) as a linear combination of regular integrals of the first kind (10.570a, b) if the índices $a_\pm$, which are the roots of the índicial equation (10.573a, b), do not differ by an integer $|a_+ - a_-| \notin |N$ (subsection 9.5.8):

$$0 = a(a-1) + a p(0) + q(0) = (a - a_+)(a - a_-); \tag{10.573a, b}$$

*standard CCXCVI. As the standard CCXCV with coincident índices $a_+ = a_-$ so that the general integral is a linear combination of regular integrals of the first kind and of the second kind, first type (subsection 9.5.9);
*standard CCXCVII. As the standard CCXCV with índices differing by an integer $|a_+ - a_-| \in |N$ so that the general integral is a linear combination of regular integral integrals of the first kind and of the second kind, second type (subsection 9.5.10);
*standard CCXCVIII. Absolute (and uniform) convergence of the regular integrals of two kinds and two types (standards CCXCV–CCXCVII) in an annulus around the regular singularity extending up to the nearest singularity (subsection 9.5.11);
*standard CCXCIX. Wronskian (10.574c) of two particular integrals of a linear second-order differential equation (10.574a, b) in terms of (10.574d) the coefficient of the first derivative (subsection 9.5.12):

$$y''_{1,2} + P(x) y'_{1,2}(x) + Q(x) y_{1,2}(x) = 0, \qquad W(y_1, y_2) = y_1 y'_2 - y_2 y'_1,$$
$$W(x) = W(x_0) \exp\left\{ \int_{x_0}^{x} p(\xi)\, d\xi \right\}; \tag{10.574a–d}$$

*standard CCC. Two particular integrals (10.574a, b) of a linear second-order differential equation are linearly independent provided that the Wronskian (10.574c) ≡ (10.574d) does not vanish at one point (subsection 9.5.13);
*standard CCCI. Wronskian of the generalized Bessel differential equation (10.575e) with integrals (10.575a–d; subsection 9.5.13):

$$y(x) = J_\nu^\mu(x), Y_\nu^\mu(x), H_{\mu,\nu}^{(1,2)}(x): \quad x^2 y'' + x\left(1 - \frac{\mu}{2} x^2\right) y' + \left(x^2 - \nu^2\right) y = 0. \tag{10.575a–e}$$

V. d. **Generalized Bessel Function** (subsections 9.5.13–9.5.15):

*standard CCCII. Generalization of the factorial to complex values through the Euler integral of the first kind as the **gamma function**, which is meromorphic, that is, analytic in the whose complex plane except for poles (subsection 9.5.13);
*standard CCCIII. Symmetry formula for the gamma function derived from the Weierstrass infinite product (subsection 9.5.13);
*standard CCCIV. General integral of the generalized Bessel differential equation (10.575e) as a linear combination of Bessel functions (10.575a) of orders $\pm\nu$ and degree μ if ν is not integer (subsection 9.5.14);
*standard CCCV. Wronskian of the generalized Bessel functions (10.575a) of orders $\pm\nu$ and degree μ vanishes when ν is an integer, proving linear dependence, and failure of the general integral in the standard CCCIV (subsection 9.5.15);
*standard CCCVI. Linear relation between the generalized Bessel functions (10.575a) of degree μ and integer orders $\nu = \pm n$, in agreement with: (i) the vanishing of the Wronskian (standard CCCV); (ii) the breakdown of the general integral (standard CCCIV) (subsection 9.5.15).

V. e. **Generalized Neumann Function of Integer Order** (subsections 9.5.16–9.5.29):

*standard CCCVII. Properties of the **digamma function**, defined as the logarithmic derivative of the gamma function (standards CCCII–CCCIII), which is also meromorphic, including residues at the same poles and recurrence and symmetry formulas (subsection 9.5.16);
*standard CCCVIII. General integral of the generalized Bessel differential equation (10.575e) with degree μ and non-negative integer order $\nu = n \in |N_0$ as a linear combination of Bessel (10.575a) and Neumann (10.575b) function (subsections 9.5.17–9.5.19);
*standard CCCIX. Two alternative expressions for the generalized Neumann function (10.575b) of degree μ and non-negative integer order $\nu = n \in |N_0$ involving preliminary and complementary functions (subsections 9.5.17–9.5.19);
*standard CCCX. Non-zero Wronskian of the generalized Bessel (10.575a) and Neumann (10.575b) functions of degree μ and non-negative integer order $\nu = n \in |N_0$, confirming that: (i) they are linearly independent (standard CCCIX); (ii) their linear combination specifies (standard CCCVIII) the general integral of the generalized Bessel differential equation (10.575e) for non-negative integer order (subsection 9.5.20).

V. f. **Extension of the Generalized Neumann Function to Complex Order** (subsections 9.5.20–9.5.21):

*standard CCCXI. Lemma of the Wronskians states that if two Wronskians coincide and one function is common the other two functions differ by a multiple of the first function (subsection 9.5.20);

*standard CCCXII. Lemma related to the lemma of the Wronskians (standard CCCXI) states that adding a multiple of the first function to the second function does not change the Wronskian (subsection 9.5.20);
*standard CCCXIII. Extension of the generalized Neumann function (10.575b) of degree μ from non-negative integer order $\nu = n \in| N_0$ to arbitrary complex order $\nu =\in| C$(subsection 9.5.21);
*standard CCCXIV. General integral of the generalized Bessel differential equation (10.575e) as a linear combination of the generalized Bessel (10.575a) and Neumann (10.575b) functions without restrictions neither on the order (as the standards CCCIV and CCCVIII) nor on the degree (unrestricted in all cases) (subsection 9.5.21).

V. g. Cylindrical and Spherical Bessel Differential Equation (subsections 9.5.22–9.5.26):

*standard CCCXV. In the particular case of zero degree $\mu = 0$ in (10.575a–e) the integrals (10.576a–d) of the original cylindrical Bessel differential equation (10.576e) (subsection 9.5.22):

$$y(x) = J_\nu(x),\ Y_\nu(x),\ H_\nu^{(1,2)}(x):\quad x^2y'' + xy'' + y' + \left(x^2 - \nu^2\right)y = 0; \tag{10.576a–e}$$

*standard CCCXVI. In the further particular case of zero order $\nu = 0$ the integrals (10.577a–d) of the original Bessel differential equation (10.577e) of order zero (subsections 9.5.22);

$$y(x) = J_0(x),\ Y_0(x),\ H_0^{(1,2)}(x):\qquad xy'' + y' + xy = 0; \tag{10.577a–e}$$

*standard CCCXVII. Comparison of the cylindrical (10.576e) [spherical (10.578e)] Bessel differential equations and their integrals (10.576a–d) [(10.578a–d)] including cylindrical (spherical) Bessel (10.576a) [(10.578a)], Neumann (10.576b) [(10.578b)], and Hankel (10.576c, d) [(10.578c, d)] functions (subsection 9.5.23):

$$y(x) = j_n(x),\ y_n(x),\ h_n^{(1,2)}(x):\quad x^2y'' + 2xy' + \left[x^2 - n(n+1)\right]y = 0, \tag{10.578a–e}$$

*standard CCCXVIII. General integral of the spherical Bessel differential equation (10.578e) specified equivalently and alternatively by a linear combination of: (i) spherical Bessel functions (10.578a) of orders $\pm n$ corresponding to cylindrica Bessel functions (10.576a) of order $\nu = \pm(n + 1/2)$; (ii) spherical Bessel (10.578a) and Neumann (10.578b) functions of order n corresponding to cylindrical Bessel and Neumann functions of order $\nu = n + 1/2$ (subsection 9.5.23);

*standard CCCXIX. Power series expansions for the spherical Bessel (Neumann) functions (10.578a) [(10.578b)] of order n, which have a zero (pole) of order $n(n+1)$ at the origin (subsection 9.5.24);
*standard CCCXX. Six cases of regular integrals of a linear differential equation of second order (10.572c) with a regular singularity (10.572a, b) consisting of two analytic (four singular) cases of integrals, namely a zero of order n or finite value (a pole of order n, a power or logarithmic type of branch-point or their combination) (subsection 9.5.25);
*standard CCCXXI. Spherical Bessel (10.578a) [Neumann (10.578b)] functions expressed as derivatives involving the circular sines (cosine) (subsection 9.5.26);
*standard CCCXXII. The integrals of the generalized (10.575e), cylindrical (10.576e), and spherical (10.578e) Bessel differential equation around the regularity at the origin involve ascending power series, whereas around the point at infinity, which is an irregular singularity, there are irregular descending asymptotic expansions (next section W) (subsection 9.5.26).

W. Linear Differential Equation with Irregular Similarities (sections 9.6–9.7)

W. a. Existence of Regular Integrals Near an Irregular Singularity (subsections 9.6.1–9.6.3):

*standard CCCXXIII. Conditions for the existence of analytic, regular, and irregular integrals of a linear second-order differential equation with analytic coefficients (10.579c) in the neighborhood of an isolated singularity (10.579a, b; subsection 9.6.1):

$$P,Q \in \mathcal{A}\left(0<|x-x_0|<R\right): \qquad \frac{d^2y}{dx^2}+xP(x)\frac{dy}{dx}+Q(x)y=0; \qquad (10.579a, b)$$

*standard CCXXIV. Example of the existence of at most one regular integral near an irregular singularity (subsection 9.6.2).

W. b. Existence of Normal Integral(s) Near an Irregular Singularity (subsections 9.6.3 –9.6.5):

*standard CCCXXV. Conditions for the existence of two, one, or no normal integrals (10.580a, b) near an irregular singularity of a linear second-order differential equation (subsection 9.6.3):

$$\Omega\left(\frac{1}{x}\right)=\sum_{m=1}^{M}\frac{\Omega_m}{x^m}: \qquad y(x)=\exp\left[\Omega\left(\frac{1}{x}\right)\right]x^a\sum_{m=0}^{\infty}x^n c_n(a); \qquad (10.580a, b)$$

*standard CCCXXVI. Analytic, regular, and irregular integrals near the point at infinity of a linear second-order differential equation (subsection 9.6.4);
*standard CCCXXVII. Comparison of an asymptotic series with an asymptotic expansion (subsection 9.6.5);
*standard CCCXXVIII. Properties of asymptotic expansions including (i) the sum, (ii) the Cauchy rule for the product, (iii) term-by-term differentiation, and (iv) integration (subsection 9.6.5).

W. c. Asymptotic Integrals for the Cylindrical and Spherical Bessel Differential Equations (subsections 9.6.6–9.6.9):

*standard CCCXXIX. General integral of the spherical Bessel differential equation (10.578e) as a linear combination of spherical Hankel functions of two kinds (subsection 9.6.6);
*standard CCCXXX. Relations among the cylindrical Bessel (10.576a), Neumann (10.576b) and Hankel (10.576c) functions of two kinds (subsection 9.6.6);
*standard CCCXXXI. Leading asymptotic term for the cylindrical and spherical Hankel functions of two kinds (subsection 9.6.6);
*standard CCCXXXII. Asymptotic expansions for the spherical and cylindrical Bessel, Neumann, and Hankel functions of two kinds (subsections 9.6.7–9.6.8);
*standard CCCXXXIII. General integral of the cylindrical Bessel differential equation (10.576e) as a linear combination of Hankel functions (10.576c, d) of two kinds (subsection 9.6.8).

W. d. Asymptotic Integrals for the Generalized Bessel Differential Equation (subsections 9.6.9–9.6.11):

*standard CCCXXXIV. Generalized Hankel function of the first kind (10.575c) with order ν and non-zero degree $\mu \neq 0$ as a regular integral of the generalized Bessel differential equation (10.575e) near the point at infinity specified by an asymptotic expansion of descending powers (subsection 9.6.9).
*standard CCCXXXV. Generalized Hankel function of the second kind (10.575d) with order ν and non-zero degree $\mu \neq 0$ as a normal integral (10.580a, b) of the generalized Bessel differential equation (10.575e) near the point at infinity (subsections 9.6.10–9.6.11);
*standard CCCXXXVI. General integral of the generalized Bessel differential equation (10.575e) of order ν and non-zero degree $\mu \neq 0$ as a linear combination of generalized Hankel functions (10.575c) [(10.575d)] of the first (second) kind [standard CCCXXXIV (CCCXXXV)] (subsection 9.6.11);
*standard CCCXXXVII. Wronskian of the generalized Hankel functions of the first (10.575c) and second (10.575d) kinds with order ν and degree μ, showing they are linearly independent for non-zero degree $\mu \neq 0$, in agreement with the standard CCCXXXVI (subsection 9.6.11);

*standard CCCXXXVIII. General integral of the generalized Bessel differential equation (10.575e) as a linear combination of generalized Neumann functions (10.575b) of order μ and degrees $\pm\nu$ not integers $\nu \notin Z$ (subsection 9.6.11);
*standard CCCXXXIX. Equivalent and alternative forms of the general integral of the generalized Bessel differential equation (10.575e) involving the generalized Bessel (10.575a), Neumann (10.575b), and Hankel functions, the latter of first (10.575c) and second (10.575d) kind (subsection 9.6.11; table 9.5);
*standard CCCXL. Comparison of the generalized (10.575e) [cylindrical (10.576e)] Bessel differential equations and their integrals in terms of the generalized (cylindrical) Bessel (10.575a) [(10.576a)], Neumann (10.575b) [(10.576b)], and Hankel function of the first (10.575c) [(10.576c)] and second (10.575d) [(10.576d)] kinds (subsection 9.6.11; table 6.7).

W. e. Bifurcation of the Generalized Bessel Differential Equation at Infinity (subsections 9.6.12–9.6.15):

*standard CCCXLI. The generalized Bessel (10.575a) and Neumann (10.575b) [Hankel (10.575c, d)] functions do (do not) tend to the cylindrical Bessel (10.576a) and Neumann (10.576b) [Hankel (10.576c, d)] functions for zero degree because in the limit $\mu \to 0$ the singularity at the origin (infinity) remains regular (changes the degree of irregularity) (subsection 9.6.12);
*standard CCCXLII. There is no asymptotic solution of the generalized Bessel differential equation (10.575e) that tends to the cylindrical Hankel functions (10.576c, d) as the degree tends to zero $\mu \to 0$ (subsections 9.6.12–9.6.13);
*standard CCCXLIII. Alternate proof of the standard CCCXLII by reduction ad absurdum (subsection 9.6.13);
*standard CCCXLIV. Hopf-type bifurcation of the solution of the generalized Bessel differential equation (10.575e) at infinity for zero degree $\mu = 0$ when it reduces to the cylindrical Bessel differential equation (10.576e) (subsection 9.6.14);
*standard CCCXLV. The computation of the generalized (10.575a–d)/cylindrical (10.576a–d)/spherical (10.578a–d) Bessel (10.575a/10.576a/10.578a), Neumann (10.575b/10.576b/10.578b), and Hankel (10.575c, d/10.576c, d/10.578c, d) functions of two kinds for small (large) variable is performed more accurately using a few terms of the power series (asymptotic expansion) (subsection 9.6.15).

W. f. General Irregular Integrals of Two Kinds (subsections 9.7.1–9.7.6):

*standard CCCXLVI. Existence of eigenvalues and eigensolutions of a linear second-order differential equation whose coefficients have an isolated singularity (subsection 9.7.1);
*standard CCCXLVII. Distinct eigenvalues correspond to linearly independent eigenintegrals in the standard CCCXLVI (subsection 9.7.1);

*standard CCCXLVIII. The statement that linearly dependent particular integrals have the same eigenvalues in the standard CCCXLVI is equivalent to the standard CCCXLVII (subsection 9.7.1);
*standard CCCXLIX. The existence of at least one irregular integral of the first kind (10.581) of standard CCCXLVI consisting of a Laurent series (multiplied by a branch point) with coefficients (índex) to be determined (subsection 9.7.2):

$$y(x) = (x - x_0)^a \sum_{n=-\infty}^{+\infty} (x - x_0)^n c_n(a); \tag{10.581}$$

*standard CCCL. If the eigenvalues are distinct (standard CCCXLVII), that is the indices do not differ by an integer, there are two linearly independent irregular integrals of the first kind (standard CCCXLIX) and their linear combination specifies the general integral (standard CCCXLVI) (subsection 9.7.2);
*standard CCCLI. The general integral of a linear second-order differential equation with an isolated singularity (standard CCCXLVI) as a linear combination of irregular integrals of the first and second kinds when the eigenvalues coincide, that is the índices differ by an integer (subsection 9.7.3);
*standard CCCLII. The method alternative to standard CCCLI of obtaining the irregular integral of the second kind from the irregular integral of the first kind (subsection 9.7.4);
*standard CCCLIII. The derivation of the regular integrals of the second kind, first (second) type [standard CCXCVI (CCXCVII)] from the irregular integral of the second kind (standard CCCLI) by omitting the descending powers (subsection 9.7.5);
*standard CCCLIV. List of all possible solutions of a linear differential equation including: (i) analytic integrals near a regular point; (ii) regular integrals of the first kind, or second kind first or second type near a regular singularity; (iii) irregular integrals of the first and second kind, in particular, normal integrals, near an irregular singularity (subsection 9.7.6).

W. g. Infinite Determinants and Linear Systems (subsections 9.7.7–9.7.12):

*standard CCCLV. The irregular integral of a linear differential equation near an irregular singularity is specified by a Laurent series with a branch-point with: (i) coefficients satisfying an infinite linear system; (ii) índices the roots of an infinite determinant (subsection 9.7.8);
*standard CCCLVI. Classification of infinite determinants including (i) divergent, (ii) oscillatory, and (iii–viii) simply, conditionally, absolutely, uniformly, or totally convergent (subsection 9.7.9);
*standard CCCLVII. If the infinite product (double series) of diagonal (non-diagonal) elements is absolutely convergent the infinite determinant is convergent (subsection 9.7.10).

W. h. Multiple Parametric Resonance and Hill Differential Equation (subsections 9.7.11–9.7.16):

$$\frac{d^2 z}{d\theta^2} + \left[b_0 + \sum_{\ell=1}^{\infty} b_\ell \cos(2\ell\theta) \right] u(\theta) = 0. \tag{10.582}$$

*standard CCCLVIII. The parametric resonance (problems 90 to 95) of a harmonic oscillator excited at a fundamental applied frequency and all its harmonics leads to a generalization (note 9.33) of the Hill differential equation (10.582) (subsection 9.7.11);
*standard CCCLIX. The transformation of a linear second-order differential equation (problem 161) to the invariant form (problem 166) leads to the Hill differential equation (10.582) if the invariant is an even function of bounded fluctuation with period π (subsection 9.7.12);
*standard CCCLX. The irregular integral solution of the Hill differential equation with trignometric (10.582) [power (10.583)] coefficients valid in an upper-half-plane (circle) in the θ -plane (x-plane) (subsection 9.7.13):

$$0 = x^2 \frac{d^2 y}{dx^2} + x \frac{dy}{dx} - \left[b_0 + \sum_{n=1}^{\infty} b_n \left(x^n + x^{-n} \right) \right] y = 0. \tag{10.583}$$

*standard CCCLXI. Infinite linear system (determinant) specifying the coefficients (índices) of the irregular integral solutions of the Hill differential equation in trigonometric (10.582) [algebraic (10.583)] form (subsection 9.7.14);
*standard CCCLXII. Evaluation of the Hill infinite determinant whose roots are the índices that appear in the coefficients of the irregular integral solutions of the Hill differential equation in trigonometric (10.582) or algebraic (10.583) form (subsections 9.7.15–9.7.16).

X. Kernel and Path of the Solution by Integral Transforms (section 9.8)

X. a. Beta Function or Eulerian Integral of the Second Kind (subsections 9.8.1–9.8.4):

*standard CCCLXIII. Evaluation of integrals in terms of the **Euler beta function** (subsection 9.8.1);
*standard CCCLXIV. Properties of the beta function, including generalization of the permutation from positive integer to complex variables (subsections 9.8.1–9.8.2);

*standard CCCLXV. Relation between the gamma (standard CCCII) and beta (standard CCCLXIII) functions (subsection 9.8.3);
*standard CCCLXVI. Evaluation of integrals in terms of beta (standards CCCLIII–CCCLV) or gamma (standards CCCII–CCCIII) functions (subsection 9.8.4).

X. b. Generalized Laplace Transform Along a Path in the Complex Plane (subsections 9.8.5–9.8.11):

*standard CCCLXVII. Solution of a linear differential equation of order N whose coefficients are linear functions of the independent variable (10.584b) by a generalized Laplace transform (10.584a) along a path L in the complex plane (subsection 9.8.6):

$$y(x) = \int_L v(s)\, e^{sx}\, dx: \qquad \sum_{n=0}^{N} (p_n + q_n\, x) \frac{d^n y}{dx^n} = 0; \qquad (10.584a, b)$$

*standard CCCLXVIII. Solution of the linear first-order differential equation that specifies the transform $v(s)$ in (10.584a) for the standard CCCLXVII (subsection 9.8.6);
*standard CCCLXIX. In the case when the coefficients $A_n(x)$ of the linear differential equation (10.562c) of order N is a polynomial of degree M of the independent variable [instead of $M = 1$ in (10.584b)] the Laplace (10.584a) transform $\nu(s)$ satisfies a linear differential equation of order M (instead of $M = 1$) (subsection 9.8.7);
*standard CCCLXX. Depression of the degree of the cubic coefficients in the generalized Bessel differential equation (10.575e) to linear in (10.585c) via the changes of independent (10.585a) and dependent (10.585b) variable (subsection 9.8.7):

$$\eta = x^2, \quad y(x) = x^{\pm\nu}\, \Psi_\pm(x^2): \qquad \eta\, \Psi''_\pm + \left(1 \pm \nu - \frac{\mu\,\eta}{4}\right) \Psi'_\pm + \frac{2 \mp \mu\,\nu}{8} \Psi = 0; \qquad (10.585a–c)$$

*standard CCCLXXI. Choice of paths of integration $\Gamma_\pm$ for the generalized Laplace transform (10.584a) that satisties the generalized Bessel differential equation (10.575e) (subsections 9.8.8–9.8.9);
*standard CCCLXXII. Integral representation of the generalized Bessel function (10.575a) as a generalized Laplace (10.584a) parametric integral, but excluding the original Bessel function (standard CCCLXXIII) (subsection 9.8.9);
*standard CCCLXXIII. Integral representation for the Bessel function (10.576a) not included in the standard CCCLXXII (subsections 9.8.9–9.8.10).

X. c. Generalized Integral Transform and Adjoint Kernel Operator (subsections 9.8.12–9.8.16):

*standard CCCLXXIV. Solution of a linear differential equation (10.586a) has a general integral transform (10.586b) in which: (i) the kernel $k(x,s)$ satisfies a partial differential equation involving another linear differential operator M with s as the independent variable; (ii) the adjoint operator $\bar{M}$ specifies the integral transform $\nu(s)$; (iii) the path of integration Γ is such that the bilinear concomitant takes the same value at both ends (subsection 9.8.12):

$$\sum_{n=0}^{N} A_n(x)\frac{d^n y}{dx^n} = 0: \qquad y(x) = \int_\Gamma k(x,s)v(s)\,ds; \qquad \text{(10.586a–b)}$$

*standard CCCLXXV. Kernel $k(x,s)$, transform $\nu(s)$ and path of integration Γ in the general integral transform (10.586b) for the solution of the Bessel differential equation (10.576e) (subsection 9.8.13);
*standard CCCLXXVI. Integral representations for the Hankel functions of the first (10.576c) [second (10.576d)] kinds (subsection 9.8.14);
*standard CCCLXXVII. Integral representation for the Neumann (10.576b) function (subsection 9.8.15);
*standard CCCLXXVIII. Second Integral representation for the Bessel function (10.576a) distinct from the standard CCCLXXIII (subsection 9.8.16);
*standard CCCLXXIX. Integral representation for the Bessel coefficients, that is, Bessel functions (10.578a) of integer order, including zero (subsection 9.8.16).

Y. Solution of Linear Second-Order Differential Equations by Continued Fractions (section 9.9):

*standard CCCLXXX. Logarithmic derivative of the solution of a linear second-order differential equation (10.587a) as a continued fraction (10.587b) (subsections 9.9.1–9.9.2):

$$y = a_0 y' + b_1 y'': \qquad \frac{1}{a_0+}\frac{b_1}{a_1+}\frac{b_2}{a_2+}\frac{b_1}{a_{1+}}\frac{b_2}{a_{2+}}\cdots\frac{b_n}{a_n+r_n} = \frac{y'}{y} = \frac{d}{dx}(\log y); \qquad \text{(10.587a, b)}$$

*standard CCCLXXXI. Example of the rational solution of a linear second-order differential equation as a terminating continued fraction (subsection 9.9.3);
*standard CCCLXXII. Application of standard CCCLXXX to the confluent hypergeometric differential equation (10.588c) specifying the representation as a continued fraction of the logarithmic derivative of the confluent hypergeometric functions of the first (10.588a) and second (10.588b) kinds (subsection 9.9.4):

$$y(x) = F(\alpha;\gamma;x),\, G(\alpha;\gamma;x): \qquad xy'' + (\gamma - x)y' - \alpha y = 0; \qquad \text{(10.588a–c)}$$

*standard CCCLXXXIII. Convergence theorem for simple infinite continued fractions whose coefficients are real and positive (subsections 9.9.5–9.9.6);
*standard CCCLXXXIV. Theorem on the difference of successive continuants of a continued fraction (subsection 9.9.5);
*standard CCCLXXXV. Recurrence relations for the numerators and denominators of a continued fraction (subsection 9.9.5);
*standard CCCLXXXVI. The inverse continued fractions exchanging numerators and denominators (subsection 9.9.5);
*standard CCCLXXXVII. Convergence of the continued fraction for the logarithmic derivative of the confluent hypergeometric function (10.588a) for real positive variable x and parameters a, b (subsection 9.9.6);
*standard CCCLXXXVIII. General integral of the confluent hypergeometric differential equation (10.588c) as a linear combination of confluent hypergeometric functions of the first kind (10.588a) valid in the finite complex x-plane for γ not zero or a negative integer (subsection 9.9.8);
*standard CCCLXXXIX. Relation between the generalized Bessel function (10.575a) and the confluent hypergeometric function (10.588a) (subsection 9.9.9);
*standard CCCXC. Continued fraction for the logarithmic derivative of the generalized Bessel function (10.575a), not valid for the original Bessel function (10.576a) (subsection 9.9.9);
*standard CCCXCI. Differentiation and recurrence formulas for the cylinder functions (10.576a–d) (subsection 9.9.10);
*standard CCCXCII. Alternate proof of standard CCCXXI, concerning the Rayleigh formulas for spherical Bessel (10.578a) and Neumann (10.578b) functions (subsection 9.9.11);
*standard CCCXCIII. Convergent continued fraction for cylinder functions (subsection 9.9.12);
*standard CCCXCIV. Convergence theorem for special-limit periodic continued fractions (subsections 9.9.13–9.9.15);
*standard CCCXCV. Limit of the ratio of two cylinder functions of high order (subsection 9.9.12).

Z. Higher Transcendental Functions: Special and Extended (notes 9.7–9.47)

Z. a. Generalized Hypergeometric Differential Equation (notes 9.9–9.13):

$$\left\{\prod_{n=1}^{N}\left(x\frac{d}{dx}-a_n\right)-x\prod_{n=1}^{M}\left(x\frac{d}{dx}-b_m\right)\right\}y(x)=0; \qquad (10.589)$$

*standard CCCXCVI. General integral of the **generalized hypergeometric differential equation** (10.589) for $N > M$ as a linear combination of N generalized hypergeometric series convergent in the finite x-plane (note 9.9);
*standard CCCXCVII. Example of the solution of the generalized hypergeometric differential equation (10.589) in the case $3 = N > M = 2$ leading to the differential equation (10.590) (note 9.10):

$$\begin{aligned}&x^3 y''' + (3 - x - \alpha_1 - \alpha_2 - \alpha_3) x^2 y'' \\ &+\left[1 - \alpha_1 - \alpha_2 - \alpha_3 + \alpha_1\alpha_2 + \alpha_1\alpha_3 + \alpha_2\alpha_3 - x(1 - \beta_1 - \beta_2)\right] x y' \\ &-(\alpha_1\alpha_2\alpha_3 + \beta_1\beta_2 x) y = 0;\end{aligned} \tag{10.590}$$

*standard CCCXCVIII. General integral of the generalized hypergeometric differential equation (10.589) for $M > N$, which is opposite to the standard CCCXCVI, as a linear combination of generalized hypergeometric asymptotic series converging in the whole complex x-plane, including the point at infinity, and excluding only the origin (note 9.11);
*standard CCCXCIX. Example of the generalized hypergeometric differential equation (10.589) in the case $3 = M > N = 2$ opposite to the standard CCCXCVII, leading to the differential equation (10.591) (note 9.12);

$$\begin{aligned}&x^3 y''' + \left[(3 - \beta_1 - \beta_2 - \beta_3) x - 1\right] x^2 y'' \\ &+\left[(1 - \beta_1 - \beta_2 - \beta_3 + \beta_1\beta_2 + \beta_1\beta_3 + \beta_2\beta_3) x y' + \alpha_1\alpha_2 - 1\right] x y' \\ &-(\beta_1\beta_2\beta_3 x - \alpha_1\alpha_2) y = 0;\end{aligned} \tag{10.591}$$

*standard CD. Convergence of the ascending generalized hypergeometric series solutions (standard CCCXCVI) inside the unit disk and on the unit circle for the generalized hypergeometric differential equation (10.589) in the case $M = N$ (note 9.13);
*standard CDI. Convergence of the asymptotic generalized hypergeometric series solutions (standard CCCXCVIII) outside the unit disk and on the unit circle for the generalized hypergeometric differential equation (10.589) in the case $M = N$ (note 9.13);
*standard CDII. Existence of little or no overlap between the regions of validity [standard CD(CDI) of the inner (outer) solutions in ascending (descending) powers [standard CCCXCV (CCCXVIII)] of the generalized hypergeometric differential equation (10.589) in the case $M = N$ (note 9.13);
*standard CDIII. **Schwartz group** of six coordinates transformations that: (i) interchange between themselves the point $x = 0, 1, \infty$; (ii) these are the three regular singularities of the generalized hypergeometric differential equation (10.589) for $M = N$; (iii) hence the changes of coordinates (i) relate the generalized hypergeometric functions in distinct overlapping regions of the com plex x-plane and provide analytic continuation of the solutions (iii) (note 9.13).

Z. b. Gaussian Hypergeometric Differential Equation (notes 9.14–9.19):

$$y(x)=F(\alpha,\beta;\gamma;x),\ G(\alpha,\beta;\gamma;x):\quad x(1-x)y''+\left[\gamma-(\alpha+\beta+1)x\right]y'-\alpha\beta y=0, \tag{10.592a–c}$$

*standard CDIV. Derivation of the Gaussian hypergeometric differential equation (10.592c) from the Gaussian hypergeometric series (10.592a) (note 9.14);
*standard CDV. General integral of the Gaussian hypergeometric differential equation (10.592c) as a linear combination of Gaussian hypergeometric function of the first kind (10.592a) when γ is not an integer (note 9.15);
*standard CDVI. General integral of the Gaussian hypergeometric differential equation (10.592c) in the case of γ-positive integer, which is excluded from the standard CDV, when a Gaussian hypergeometric functions of the second kind (10.592b) appears (note 9.16);
*standard CDVII. Gaussian hypergeometric function of the second kind (10.592b) with $\gamma = n$, a positive integer, which appears in this case in the solution of the Gaussian hypergeometric differential equation (10.592a) (note 9.17);
*standard CDVIII. General integral of the Gaussian hypergeometric differential equation (10.592c) in the case when γ is zero or a negative integer, which is excluded from the standards CDV and CDVI, and unlike (like) the standard CDV(CDVI) involves a Gaussian hypergeometric function of the second kind (10.592b) (note 9.18);
*standard CDIX. Gaussian hypergeometric function of the second kind (10.592b), which appears in the general integral of the Gaussian hypergeometric differential equation (10.592c) when γ is zero or a positive integer (note 9.18);
*standard CDX. Particular case of the Gaussian hypergeometric function of the second kind (10.592b) for $\gamma = 1$ (note 9.19);
*standard CDXI. Simplification of the Gaussian hypergeometric function of the second kind (10.592b) when neither α nor β are negative integers (note 9.19);
*standard CDXII. Simplification of the Gaussian hypergeometric functions of the first kind (10.592a) or second kind (10.592b) when α or β is a negative integer (note 9.19);
*standard CDXIII. Summary of the general integrals of the Gaussian hypergeometric differential equation (10.592c) involving Gaussian hypergeometric functions of the first kind (10.592a) or second kind (10.592b) for all cases of values of the parameters (α,β,γ) (note 9.19).

Z. c. Legendre, Associated, Ultraspherical, and Hyperspherical Differential Equations (notes 9.20–9.25):

*standard CDXIV. Solution of the **Legendre differential equation** (10.593c) of degree ν as a linear combination of Legendre functions of the first kind (10.593a) and second kind (10.593b) (note 9.20):

$$y(x)=P_\nu(x),\quad Q_\nu(x):\qquad \left(1-x^2\right)y''-2xy'+\nu(\nu+1)y=0; \tag{10.593a–c}$$

*standard CDXV. Relation between the Legendre functions of the first (10.593a) [second (10.593b)] kind and the Gaussian hypergeometric functions of the first (10.592a) [second (10.592b)] kind (note 9.20);
*standard CDXVI. Solution of the Legendre differential equation (10.593c) finite in the unit circle $|x| \le 1$, which is proportional to the Legendre polynomial (10.593a) with non-negative integer degree (note 9.20);
*standard CDXVII. General integral of the **ultraspherical Legendre differential equation** (10.594d) of degree ν and dimension γ as a linear combination of ultraspherical Legendre functions of the first kind (10.594a) and second kind (10.594b) for $\lambda = 0, 2, 4, \ldots$ (note 9.21):

$$y(x) = P^{\nu,\lambda}(x),\, Q^{\nu,\lambda}(x),\, R^{\nu,\lambda}(x): \quad (1-x^2)y'' - (2+\lambda)xy' + \nu(\nu+1+\lambda)y = 0; \tag{10.594a–d}$$

*standard CDXVIII. General integral of the standard CDXVII for $\lambda \ne 0, \pm 2, +4, \ldots$ as a linear combination of ultraspherical Legendre functions of the first kind (10.594a, c) (note 9.21);
*standard CDXIX. General integral of the ultraspherical Legendre differential equation (10.594d) in the case $\lambda = -2, -4, \ldots$ excluded from the standards CDXVII and CDXVIII, and the convergence conditions in all three cases for all values of λ-(note 9.21);
*standard CDXX. Solution of the ultraspherical Legendre differential equation (10.594d) finite in the unit circle $|x| \le 1$, which is proportional to the ultraspherical Legendre polynomial (10.594a) with non-negative integer degree (note 9.21);
*standard CDXXI. General integral of the **associated Legendre differential equation** (10.595c) of degree ν and order μ as a linear combination of first (10.595a) and second (10.595b) associated Legendre functions of the first kind (note 9.22):

$$y(x) = P_\nu^\mu(x),\, R_\nu^\mu(x): \qquad (1-x^2)\, y'' - 2xy' + \left[\nu(\nu+1) - \frac{\mu}{1-x^2}\right] y = 0, \tag{10.595a–c}$$

*standard CDXXII. **Spherical harmonics** as the solution of the associated Legendre differential equation (10.595c) finite in the interval $|x| \le 1$, which is proportional to the first associated Legendre function of the first kind (10.595a), with integer degree $\nu = n$ larger $n > m$ than the integer order $\mu = m$ (note 9.22);
*standard CDXXIII. Invariance of the associated Legendre differential equation (10.595c) with regards to the change of sign of the order $\mu \to -\mu$, except for the convergence of solutions on the boundary of convergence (note 9.22);
*standard CDXXIV. General integral of the **hyperspherical-associated Legendre differential equation** (10.596c) of degree ν order μ and

dimension λ as a linear combination of the first (10.596a) and second (10.596b) hyperspherical-associated Legendre functions (notes 9.23–9.24):

$$y(x) = A^{\mu}_{\nu,\lambda}(x),\, B^{\mu}_{\nu,\lambda}(x):\quad \left(1-x^2\right)y'' - \left(2+\lambda\right)xy' + \left[\nu(\nu+1) - \frac{\mu^2}{1-x^2}\right]y = 0; \tag{10.596a–c}$$

*standard CDXXV. Particular cases $\lambda = 0\left(\lambda = 0 = \mu\right)$ of (10.596c) leading to the associated Legendre (10.595c) [Legendre (10.593c)] differential equation and functions (10.596a, b), which are linear combinations of (10.595a, b) [(10.593a, b)] (note 9.24);
*standard CDXXVI. Solution of the hyperspherical-associated Legendre differential equation (10.596c), which is finite in the unit circle $|x| \le 1$ and is proportional to the first hyperspherical-associated Legendre function (10.596a) (note 9.24);
*standard CDXXVII. General integral of the **hyperspherical Legendre differential equation** (10.597c) of degree ν and dimension λ as a linear combination of first (10.597a) [second (10.597b)] hyperspherical Legendre functions (note 9.25):

$$y(x) = P_{\nu,\lambda}(x),\, R_{\nu,\lambda}(x):\quad \left(1-x^2\right)y'' - \left(2+\lambda\right)xy' + \nu\left(\nu+1\right)y = 0; \tag{10.597a–c}$$

*standard CDXXVIII. Solution of the hyperspherical Legendre differential equation (10.597c), which is finite in the circle $0 \le |1-x| \le 2$ for $\mathrm{Re}(\lambda) > 0$ and is proportional to the first hyperspherical-associated Legendre function (10.597a) (note 9.25).

Z. d. Jacobi and Chebychev Functions of Two Kinds (notes 9.26–9.28):

*standard CDXXIX. Relation between the Jacobi function (10.598a) with degree ν and parameters (a, b) and the Gaussian hypergeometric function of the first kind (10.592a) (note 9.26);
*standard CDXXX. General integral of the **Jacobi differential equation** (10.598b) as a linear combination of (10.598a) Jacobi functions (note 9.26):

$$y(x) = I^{a,b}_{\nu}(x):\quad \left(1-x^2\right)y'' + \left[b - a - (a+b+2)x\right]y' + \nu\left(\nu+a+b+1\right)y = 0. \tag{10.598a, b}$$

*standard CDXXXI. Recurrence and differentiation formulas for the Chebychev functions of the first type (10.599a, b) (note 9.27);
*standard CDXXXII. Relation between the first (10.599a) [second (10.599b)] Chebychev functions of the first type and the Gaussian hypergeometric function (133a) of the first kind (note 9.27);

*standard CDXXXIII. General integral of the Chebychev differential equation of the first type (10.599c) as a linear combination of the first (10.599a) [second (10.599b)] Chebychev functions of the first type (note 9.27):

$$y(x) = T_\nu(x)\,,\ S_\nu(x): \qquad \left(1-x^2\right)y'' - xy' + \nu^2 y = 0; \qquad (10.599a\text{–}c)$$

*standard CDXXXIV. The solution of the **Chebychev differential equation of the first type** (10.599a), which is finite in the closed unit disk $|x| > 1$ is proportional to the first (10.599a) Chebychev function of the first type (note 9.27);
*standard CDXXXV. Recurrence and differentiational formulas for the Chebychev functions of the second type (10.600a, b) (note 9.28);
*standard CDXXXVI. Relation between the first (10.600a) [second (10.600b)] Chebychev function of the second type and the Gaussian hypergeometric function of the first kind (10.592a) (note 9.28);
*standard CDXXXVII. General integral of the **Chebychev differential equation of the second type** (10.600c) as a linear combination of the first (10.600a) and second (10.600b) Chebychev functions of the second type (note 9.28):

$$y = (x) = U_\nu(x),\ V_\nu(x): \qquad \left(1-x^2\right)y'' - 3xy' + \nu(\nu+2)y = 0; \qquad (10.600a\text{–}c)$$

*standard CDXXXVIII. The solution of the Chebychev differential equation of the second type (10.600c), which is finite in the closed unit disk $|x| \leq 1$ is proportional to the first (10.600a) Chebychev function of the second type (note 9.28);
*standard CDXXXIX. The Legendre functions (10.593a) and first Chebychev functions of the first (10.599a) [second (10.600a)] type with zero or positive integer degree $\nu = n$ are all distinct polynomials of degree n corresponding to terminating Gaussian hypergeometric series (10.592a) of the first kind (note 9.28).

Z. e. Confluent Hypergeometric, Laguerre, Associated, and Hermite Functions (notes 9.29–9.32):

*standard CDXL. Comparison of the Gaussian (10.592c) [confluent (10.588c)] differential equations and functions of the first kind (10.592a) [(10.588a)] (note 9.29);
*standard CDXLI. Comparison of the general integrals of the Gaussian (10.592c) [confluent (10.588c)] hypergeometric differential equations in the cases involving both functions of the first (10.592a) [(10.588a)] and second (10.592b) [(10.588b)] kinds (note 9.29);
*standard CDXLII. Relation between the Laguerre function of the first kind (10.601a) [second (10.601b) kind] and degree ν and the confluent hypergeometric function of the first (10.588a) [second (10.588b)] kind (note 9.30);

*standard CDXLIII. General integral of the **Laguerre differential equation** (10.601c) with degree ν as a linear combination of Laguerre functions of the first (10.601a) and second (10.601b) kinds (note 9.30):

$$y(x) = L_\nu(x), N_\nu(x): \qquad x y'' + (1 - x) y' + \nu y = 0. \qquad \text{(10.601a–c)}$$

*standard CDXLIV. The solution of the Laguerre differential equation (10.601c) finite at the origin is proportional to the Laguerre function of the first kind (10.601a) (note 9.30);
*standard CDXLV. Relation between the associated Laguerre function (10.602a) of degree ν and order μ and the confluent hypergeometric function of the first kind (10.588a) (note 9.31);
*standard CDXLVI. General integral of the **associated Laguerre differential equation** (10.602b) as a combination of associated Laguerre functions (10.602a) (note 9.31):

$$y(x) = L_\nu^\mu(x): \qquad x y'' + (1 + \mu - x) y' + \nu y = 0. \qquad \text{(10.602a, b)}$$

*standard CDXLVII. The solution of the associated Laguerre differential equation (10.602b) finite at the origin is proportional to one associated Laguerre function (10.602a) (note 9.31);
*standard CDXLVIII. Relation between the first Hermite function (10.603a) of degree ν and the confluent hypergeometric function of the first kind (10.588a) (note 9.32);
*standard CDXLIX. Relation between the second Hermite function (10.603b) of degree ν and the confluent hypergeometric function of the first kind (10.588b) (note 9.32);
*standard CDL. General integral of the **Hermite differential equation** (10.603c) of degree ν as a linear combination of the first (10.603a) and second (10.603b) Hermite functions (note 9.32):

$$y(x) = H_\nu(x),\ I_\nu(x): \qquad y'' - 2 x y' + 2 \nu y = 0. \qquad \text{(10.603a–c)}$$

Z. f. Sub- and Superhypergeometric Differential Equations
(notes 9.33–9.38):

*standard CDLI. Subhypergeometric differential equations that have three regular singularities (one regular singularity and one irregular singularity of degree one) like the Gaussian (confluent) hypergeometric (10.592c) [(10.588c)] differential equation [standards CCCXCV–CDXXXIX (CDXL-CDL)] (note 9.33);
*standard CDLII. Relation between the Bessel (10.576a) and Gaussian hypergeometric (10.592a) functions (note 9.33);

*standard CDLIII. Superhypergeometric differential equations that have (a) either more than three regular singularities or (b) two/one/zero regular singularities and one irregular singularity of degree at least one/two/three or (c) or two irregular singularities (note 9.34);
*standard CDLIV. Four alternative equivalent forms of the **generalized Hill differential equation** (10.604b) satisfied by (10.604a) the generalized Hill functions (note 9.34):

$$w = (\theta) = H(b_1, \ldots\ldots, b_M; \cos\theta): \qquad \frac{d^2 w}{d\theta^2} + \sum_{m=1}^{M} b_m \cos(m\theta) = 0. \tag{10.604a, b}$$

*standard CDLV. Relation between the generalized Hill function (10.604a) and the extended Gaussian hypergeometric function (10.606a) (note 9.35);
*standard CDLVI. Four equivalent forms of the **Mathieu differential equation** (10.605b) whose solutions are Mathieu functions (10.605a) (note 9.35):

$$y(x) = M(a, q; x): \qquad (1 - x^2)y'' - xy' - xy' + (a + 2q - 4qx^2)\, y = 0; \tag{10.605a, b}$$

*standard CDLVII. Relation between the Mathieu function (10.605a) and the extended Gaussian hypergeometric functions (10.606a) (note 9.35);
*standard CDLVIII. General integral of the **extended Gaussian hypergeometric differential equation** (10.606b) with upper (α, β), lower γ, and asymptotic $(A_1, \ldots, A_M)$ parameters as a linear combination of extended Gaussian hypergeometric functions of the first kind (10.606a) for γ not an integer (notes 9.35–9.36):

$$y(x) = F(\alpha, \beta; \gamma; A_1, \ldots, A_M; x):$$

$$x(1 - x)y'' + [\gamma - (\alpha + \beta + 1)x]y' - \left(\alpha\beta + \sum_{m=1}^{M} A_m\, x^m\right)y = 0. \tag{10.606a, b}$$

*standard CDLIX. General integral of the **extended confluent hypergeometric differential equation** (10.607b) in terms of (10.607a) extended confluent hypergeometric functions (note 9.37):

$$y(x) = F(\alpha, \beta; \gamma; A_1, \ldots, A_M; x): \quad xy'' + (\gamma - x)\, y' - \left(\alpha + \sum_{m=1}^{M} A_m\, x^m\right)y = 0; \tag{10.607a, b}$$

*standard CDLX. Singly- (doubly-) extended second-order linear differential equations, with coefficient of the dependent variable (its derivative) a polynomial of degree $M(L)$, for example (10.608b) doubly extending the (10.576e) cylindrical Bessel differential equation (note 9.38);
*standard CDLXI. The general integral of the **doubly-extended Bessel differential equation** (10.608b) is a linear combination of doubly-extended Bessel functions (10.608a) (note 9.38):

$$y(x) = J_{\pm\nu}\left(A_1,\ldots,A_M;B_1,\ldots,B_M;x\right):$$

$$x^2 y'' + x\left(1 + \sum_{\ell=2}^{L} B_\ell x^\ell\right) y' + \left(x^2 - \nu^2 + \sum_{m=1}^{M} A_m x^m\right) y = 0. \qquad (10.608a, b)$$

Z. g. Invariant and Self-Adjoint Linear Second-Order Differential Equations (notes 9.39–9.40):

*standard CDLXII. Transformation of a linear second-order differential equation (10.609a) through the **transformation factor** (10.609b) into a **self-adjoint** (10.610a) [**invariant** (10.610b, c)] **differential equation** (note 9.39):

$$y'' + P(x) y' + Q(x)\, y = 0, \qquad R(x) = \exp\left(\int^x p(\xi)\, d\xi\right): \qquad (10.609a, b)$$

$$\left(R y'\right)' + R Q y = 0; \qquad z = y\sqrt{R}: \qquad z'' + \left(Q - \frac{P'}{2} + \frac{P^2}{4}\right) z = 0. \qquad (10.610a–c)$$

*standard CDLXIII. Self-adjoint (10.611a, b) [invariant (10.612a, b)] form of the confluent hypergeometric differential equation (10.588c) (note 9.39):

$$y(x) = F(\alpha;\gamma;x): \qquad \left(e^{-x} x^\gamma y'\right)' - \alpha e^{-x} x^\gamma\, y = 0, \qquad (10.611a, b)$$

$$z(x) = e^{-x/2} x^{\gamma/2}\, F(\alpha;\gamma;x): \quad z'' - \left(\frac{1}{4} + \frac{\alpha}{x} - \frac{\gamma}{2x} - \frac{\gamma}{2x^2} + \frac{\gamma^2}{4x^2}\right) z = 0; \qquad (10.612a, b)$$

*standard CDLXIV. Relation between the confluent hypergeometric function of the first kind (10.588a) and the Whittaker function (10.613a) (note 9.40);
*standard CDLXV. General integral of the **Whittaker differential equation** (10.613b) with parameters (k,m) as a linear combination of Whittaker functions (10.613a) for 2m not an integer (note 9.40):

$$y(x) = W_{k,m}(x): \qquad y'' - \left(\frac{1}{4} - \frac{k}{x} + \frac{m^2}{x^2} - \frac{1}{4x^2}\right) y = 0; \qquad (10.613a, b)$$

*standard CDLXVI. Relation between the Whittaker (10.613a) and the generalized Bessel (10.575a) function (note 9.41);
*standard CDLXVII. Self-adjoint (10.614a, b) [invariant (10.615a, b)] form of the generalized Bessel differential equation (10.575e) (note 9.41):

$$y(x) = J_\nu^\mu(x): \quad \left[x \exp\left(-\frac{\mu x^2}{4}\right) y'\right]' + \left(x^2 - \nu^2\right) \exp\left(-\frac{\mu x^2}{4}\right) y = 0, \qquad (10.614\text{a, b})$$

$$z(x) = \sqrt{x} \exp\left(\frac{-\mu x^2}{2}\right) J_\nu^\mu(x): \qquad z'' + \left[1 - \frac{\nu^2}{x^2} + \frac{1}{4x^2} + \frac{\mu}{2}\left(1 - \frac{\mu x^2}{8}\right)\right] z = 0. \qquad (10.615\text{a, b})$$

*standard CDLXVIII. Self-adjoint (10.616a, b) [invariant (10.617a, b)] form of the Gaussian hypergeometric differential equation (10.592c) (note 9.44):

$$y(x) = F(\alpha, \beta; \gamma; x): \qquad \left[x^\gamma (1-x)^{\alpha+\beta+1-\gamma} y'\right]' - \alpha\beta x^\gamma (1-x)^{1+\alpha+\beta-\gamma} y = 0; \qquad (10.616\text{a, b})$$

$$z(x) = x^{\gamma/2} (1-x)^{(1+\alpha+\beta-\gamma)/2} F(\alpha, \beta; \gamma; x):$$

$$z'' + \left[\frac{\gamma(2-\gamma)}{4x^2} + \frac{1-(\alpha+\beta-\gamma)^2}{4\left(1-x^2\right)} + \frac{\gamma(1+\alpha+\beta-\gamma) - 2\alpha\beta}{2x(1-x)}\right] z = 0. \qquad (10.617\text{a, b})$$

*standard CDLXIX. Self-adjoint (10.618a, b) [invariant (10.619a, b)] form of the hyperspherical-associated Legendre differential equation (10.596c) (note 9.42):

$$y(x) = P_{\nu,\lambda}^\mu(x): \qquad \left[\left(1-x^2\right)^{1/2+\lambda} y'\right]' + \left(1-x^2\right)^{\lambda-1/2} \left(\nu(\nu+1) - \frac{\mu^2}{1-x^2}\right) y = 0; \qquad (10.618\text{a, b})$$

$$z(x) = \left(1-x^2\right)^{1/4+\lambda/2} P_{\nu,\lambda}^\mu(x):$$

$$z'' + \left[\frac{\nu(\nu+1) - 1 - \lambda/2}{1-x^2} + \frac{x^2(1+\lambda/2)(3+\lambda/2) - \mu^2}{\left(1-x^2\right)^2}\right] z = 0. \qquad (10.619\text{a, b})$$

*standard CDLXX. Self-adjoint (10.620a, b) [invariant (10.621a, b)] form of the ultraspherical Legendre differential equation (10.594d) (note 9.42):

$$y(x) = P^{\nu,\lambda}(x): \quad \left[\left(1-x^2\right)^{1/2+\lambda} y'\right]' + \nu(\nu+1+\lambda)\left(1-x^2\right)^{\lambda-1/2} y = 0; \qquad (10.620\text{a, b})$$

$$z(x)=\left(1-x^2\right)^{1/4+\lambda/2}P^{\nu,\lambda}(x):\quad z''+\left[\frac{\nu(\nu+1+\lambda)}{1-x^2}+\frac{x^2(1+\lambda/2)(3+\lambda/2)}{\left(1-x^2\right)^2}\right]z=0.$$

(10.621a, b)

*standard CDLXXI. Self-adjoint (10.622a, b) [invariant (10.623a, b)] form of the Jacobi differential equation (10.598b) (note 9.42):

$$y(x)=I_\nu^{a,b}(x):\quad \left\{\left(1-x^2\right)^{1+a/2+b/2}\exp\left[(b-a)\arg\tanh x\right]y'\right\}'$$

$$+\left(1-x^2\right)^{a/2+b/2}\exp\left[(b-a)\arg\tanh x\right]y=0;$$

(10.622a, b)

$$z(x)=\left(1-x^2\right)^{1/2+a/4+b/4}\exp\left(\frac{b-a}{2}\arg\tanh x\right)I_\nu^{a,b}(x):$$

$$z''-\left[\frac{(b-a)^2-2x(b-a)(4+a+b)-x^2(a+b+2)(a+b+6)}{4\left(1-x^2\right)^2}\right.$$ (10.623a, b)

$$\left.+\frac{a+b+2-\nu(\nu+a+b+1)}{1-x^2}\right]z=0.$$

*standard CDLXXII. Self-adjoint (10.624a, b) [invariant (10.625a, b)] form of the first Chebychev differential equation (10.599c) (note 9.43);

$$y(x)=T_\nu(x):\qquad \left(\sqrt{1-x^2}\,y'\right)'+\nu^2\sqrt{1-x^2}\,y=0;$$ (10.624a, b)

$$z(x)=\left(1-x^2\right)^{1/4}T_\nu(x):\qquad z''+\left[\frac{1/2+\nu^2}{1-x^2}-\frac{5}{4}\left(\frac{x}{1-x^2}\right)^2\right]z=0;$$ (10.625a, b)

*standard CDLXXII. Self-adjoint (10.626a, b) [invariant (10.627a, b)] form of the second Chebychev differential equation (10.600c) (note 9.43):

$$y(x)=U_\nu(x):\quad \left[\left(1-x^2\right)^{3/2}y'\right]''+\nu(\nu+2)(1-x)^{3/2}y=0;$$ (10.626a, b)

$$z(x)=\left(1-x^2\right)^{3/4}U_\nu(x):\quad z''+\left[\frac{3/2+\nu(\nu+2)}{1-x^2}-\frac{21/9}{\left(1-x^2\right)}\right]z=0;$$ (10.627a, b)

*standard CDLXXIV. Self-adjoint (10.628a, b) [invariant (10.629a, b)] form of the associated Laguerre differential equation (10.602b) (note 9.43):

$$y(x) = L_\nu^\mu(x): \qquad \left(e^{-x}x^{1+\mu}y'\right)' + \nu e^{-x}x^{1+\mu}y = 0; \tag{10.628a, b}$$

$$z(x) = e^{-x/2}x^{1/2+\mu/2}\,L_\nu^\mu(x): \qquad z'' + \left[\frac{1+\mu+\nu}{x} + \frac{1-\mu^2}{2x^2}\right]z = 0. \tag{10.629a, b}$$

*standard CDLXXV. Self-adjoint (10.630a, b) [invariant (10.631a, b)] form of the Hermite differential equation (10.603c) (note 9.43);

$$y(x) = H_\nu(x): \qquad \left[\exp\left(-x^2\right)y'\right]' + 2\nu\exp\left(-x^2\right)y = 0; \tag{10.630a, b}$$

$$z(x) = \exp\left(-\frac{x^2}{2}\right)H_\nu(x): \qquad z'' + \left(1+2\nu-4x^2\right)z = 0. \tag{10.631a, b}$$

Z. h. First Class of Transformed Generalized Bessel Differential Equations (note 9.44):

*standard CDLXXVI. Solution (10.632a) of the **first transformed generalized Bessel differential equation** (10.632b) (note 9.44);

$$y(x) = x^a J_\nu^\mu\left(cx^b\right): \quad x^2y'' + \left(1 - 2a - \frac{1}{2}\mu bc^2x^{2b}\right)xy' + \left[a^2 - b^2\nu^2 + b^2c^2x^{2b}\left(1 + \frac{\mu a}{2b}\right)\right]y = 0. \tag{10.632a, b}$$

*standard CDLXXVII. Particular case $a = 0, b = 1, c = i$ of (10.632a, b) leading to (10.633a, b):

$$y(x) = J_\nu^\mu(ix): \qquad x^2y'' + \left(1 + \frac{\mu x^2}{2}\right)xy' - \left(x^2 + \nu^2\right)y = 0. \tag{10.633a, b}$$

*standard CDLXXVIII. Particular case $a = 0, b = 1/2, c = 1$ of (10.632a, b) leading to (10.634a, b):

$$y(x) = J_\nu^\mu\left(\sqrt{x}\right): \qquad x^2y'' + \left(1 - \frac{\mu x}{4}\right)xy' + \frac{1}{4}\left(x^2 - \nu^2\right)y = 0. \tag{10.634a, b}$$

*standard CDLXXIX. Particular case $a=0,\, b=1/2, c=2i, \nu\to 2\nu$ of (10.632a, b) leading to (10.635a, b):

$$y(x)=J_{2\nu}^{\mu}\left(2i\sqrt{x}\right): \qquad x^2\, y''+\left(1+\mu\, x\right)x y' - \left(x+\nu^2\right)y=0. \qquad (10.635a, b)$$

*standard CDLXXX. Particular case $a=0, c=1, b=2$ of (10.632a, b) leading to (10.636a, b):

$$y(x)=J_{\nu}^{\mu}\left(x^2\right): \qquad x^2 y''+\left(1-\mu\, x^4\right)x y' + 4\left(x^4-\nu^2\right)y=0. \qquad (10.636a, b)$$

*standard CDLXXXI. Particular case $a=\nu=b, c=1$ of (10.632a, b) leading to (10.637a, b):

$$y(x)=x^{\nu}\, J_{\nu}^{\mu}\left(x^{\nu}\right):\; x^2 y''+\left(1-2\nu-\frac{\mu\,\nu}{2}x^{2\nu}\right)x y' + \nu^2\left\{1-\nu^2\left[1-x^{2\nu}\left(1+\frac{\mu}{2}\right)\right]\right\}y=0. \qquad (10.637a, b)$$

*standard CDLXXXII. Particular case $a=\nu, b=1=c$ of (10.632a, b) leading to (10.638a, b):

$$y(x)=x^{\nu}\, J_{\nu}^{\mu}(x): \qquad x y''+\left(1-2\nu-\frac{\mu\, x^2}{2}\right)y' + x^2\left(1+\frac{\mu\,\nu}{2}\right)y=0. \qquad (10.638a, b)$$

*standard CDLXXXIII. Particular case $a=1/2, b=1, c=i\sqrt{q}, \nu=p-1/2$ of (10.632a, b) leading to (10.639a, b):

$$y(x)=\sqrt{x}\, J_{p-1/2}^{\mu}\left(i x\sqrt{q}\right):\;\; x^2 y''+\frac{\mu q}{2}x^3 y' - \left[p(p-1)+q\left(1+\frac{\mu}{4}\right)x^2\right]y=0. \qquad (10.639a, b)$$

*standard CDLXXXIV. Particular case $a=1/2+p=\nu, b=1, c=i\sqrt{q}$ of (10.632b) leading to (10.640a, b):

$$y(x)=x^{1/2+p}\, J_{1/2+p}^{\mu}\left(i x\sqrt{q}\right):\;\; x y''-\left(2p-\frac{\mu q}{2}x^2\right)y' - q\left[1+\frac{\mu}{2}\left(p+\frac{1}{2}\right)\right]x y=0. \qquad (10.640a, b)$$

*standard CDLXXXV. Particular case $a=1/2,\, b=p, c=i\sqrt{q}/p, \nu=1/(2p)$ of (10.632b) leading to (10.641a, b):

$$y(x)=\sqrt{x}\, J_{1/(2p)}^{\mu}\left(i\frac{\sqrt{q}}{p}x^p\right):\; y''+\frac{\mu q}{2p}x^{2p-1}\, y' - q\left(1+\frac{\mu}{4p}\right)x^{2p-2}\, y=0. \qquad (10.641a, b)$$

*standard CDLXXXVI. Particular case $a=1/2, b=3/2, c=2/3, \nu=1/3$ of (10.632a, b) leading to (10.642a, b):

$$y(x)=\sqrt{x}\,J_{1/3}^{\mu}\left(\frac{2}{3}x^{3/2}\right): \qquad y''-\frac{\mu}{3}x^2\,y'+\left(1+\frac{\mu}{6}\right)x\,y=0. \tag{10.642a, b}$$

*standard CDLXXXVII. Particular case $\mu=0$ of (10.642a, b) leading to (10.643a, c), where (10.643c) is an Airy differential equation (10.566a) with variable $-x$, and thus, (10.643b) of Airy functions (10.566b) of the same variable:

$$y(x)=\sqrt{x}\,J_{1/3}\left(\frac{2}{3}x^{3/2}\right)=c_1\,Ai(-x)+c_2\,Bi(-x): \qquad y''+x\,y=0. \tag{10.643a–c}$$

Z. i. Second Class of Transformed Generalized Bessel Differential Equations (note 9.45):

*standard CDLXXXVIII. Solution (10.644a) of the **second transformed generalized Bessel differential equation** (10.644c) (note 9.45):

$$y(x)=f(x)J_\nu(g(x)): \qquad y''-\left(2\frac{f'}{f}+\frac{g''}{g'}-\frac{g'}{g}-\frac{\mu g'g}{2}\right)y'$$

$$+\left[\frac{f'}{f}\left(2\frac{f'}{f}+\frac{g''}{g'}-\frac{g'}{g}-\frac{\mu g'g}{2}\right)-\frac{f''}{f}+g'^2-\nu^2\frac{g'^2}{g^2}\right]y=0. \tag{10.644a–c}$$

*standard CDLXXXIX. Particular case $f=\sqrt{g/g'}$ of (10.644a, b) leading to (10.645a, b):

$$y(x)=\sqrt{\frac{g(x)}{g'(x)}}\,J_\nu^\mu(g(x)): \qquad y''+\frac{\mu g'g}{2}y'$$

$$+\left[\frac{g'''}{2g}+g'^2-\frac{3g''^2}{4g'^2}+\left(\frac{1}{4}-\nu^2\right)\frac{g'^2}{g^2}+\frac{\mu}{4}\left(g''g-g'^2\right)\right]y=0. \tag{10.645a, b}$$

*standard CDLXC. Particular case $f=g^a$ of (10.644a, b) leading to (10.646a, b):

$$y(x)=\left[g(x)\right]^a J_\nu^\mu(g(x)): \qquad y''+\left[\frac{g''}{g'}+(2a-1)\frac{g'}{g}-\frac{\mu g'g}{2}\right]y'$$

$$+\left[\left(a^2-\nu^2\right)\frac{g'^2}{g^2}+g'^2\left(1-\frac{\mu a}{2}\right)\right]y=0. \tag{10.646a, b}$$

*standard CDLXCI. Particular case (10.647a, b):

$$f(x)=x^a\exp\left(\alpha x^\beta\right),\qquad g(x)=c\,x^b,\qquad (10.647a, b)$$

of (10.644a, b) leading to (10.647c, d):

$$y(x)=x^a\exp\left(\alpha x^\beta\right)J_\nu^\mu\left(c\,x^b\right):\quad x^2y''+\left(1-2a-2\alpha\beta x^\beta-\frac{\mu b c^2}{2}x^{2b}\right)x\,y'$$

$$+\left[a^2-b^2\nu^2+b^2c^2\left(1+\frac{\mu a}{2b}\right)x^{2b}+\alpha\beta\left(2a-\beta\right)x^\beta+\alpha\beta x^\beta\left(\alpha\beta x^\beta+\frac{\mu b c^2}{2}x^{2b}\right)\right]y=0,$$

(10.647c, d)

which simplifies to (10.632a, b) for $\alpha=0$.
*standard CDXCII. Particular case $\beta=b$ in (10.647c, d) leading to (10.648a, b):

$$y(x)=x^a\exp\left(\alpha x^b\right)J_\nu^\mu\left(c\,x^b\right):\quad x^2y''+\left(1-2a-2\alpha b\,x^b-\frac{\mu b c^2}{2}x^{2b}\right)x\,y'$$

$$+\left[a^2-b^2\nu^2+\alpha b\left(2a-b\right)x^b+b^2\left(c^2+\alpha^2\right)x^{2b}+\frac{\mu b c^2}{2}\left(a+\alpha b\,x^b\right)x^{2b}\right]y=0.$$

(10.648a, b)

*standard CDXCIII. Particular case $\beta=b,\alpha=\pm ic$ of (10.647c, d), which is equivalent to $\alpha=\pm ic$ in (10.648a, b), leading to (10.648c, d):

$$y(x)=x^a\exp\left(\pm\,icx\right)J_\nu^\mu\left(c\,x^b\right):\quad x^2y''+\left(1-2a\mp 2ibc\,x^b-\frac{\mu b c^2}{2}x^{2b}\right)x\,y'$$

$$+\left[a^2-b^2\,\nu^2\pm ibc(2a-b)x^b+\frac{\mu b c^2}{2}\left(a\pm icb\,x^b\right)x^{2b}\right]y=0.$$

(10.648c, d)

*standard CDXCIV. Particular case $f=x^{-a},g=c\exp(bx)$ of (10.644a, b) leading to (10.649a, b):

$$y(x)=x^{-a}\;J_\nu^\mu\left(c\,e^{bx}\right):\quad x^2\,y''+\left(2a+\frac{\mu b c^2}{2}x\,e^{2bx}\right)x\,y'$$

$$+\left\{a(a-1)-b^2\left[\nu^2-c^2\,e^{2bx}\left(1+\frac{\mu a}{2b}\right)\right]x^2\right\}y=0.\qquad (10.649a, b)$$

*standard CDXCV. Particular case $f = x, g = \exp(1/x)$ of (10.644a, b) leading to (10.650a, b):

$$y(x) = x\, J_\nu^\mu\left(e^{1/x}\right): \quad x^4\, y'' - \frac{\mu\, x^2}{2}\, e^{2/x}\, y' + \left[\left(1 + \frac{\mu\, x}{2}\right) e^{2/x} - \nu^2\right] y = 0. \quad (10.650a, b)$$

*standard CDXCVI. Particular case $g = x$ of (10.644a, b) leading to (10.651a, b):

$$y(x) = f(x)\, J_\nu^\mu(x): \quad y'' + \left(\frac{1}{x} - 2\frac{f'}{f} + \frac{\mu\, x}{2}\right) y'$$
$$+ \left[1 - \frac{\nu^2}{x^2} + \frac{f'}{f}\left(2\frac{f'}{f} - \frac{1}{x} - \frac{\mu\, x}{2}\right) - \frac{f''}{f}\right] y = 0. \quad (10.651a, b)$$

*standard CDXCVII. Particular case of (10.651a, b) with $f = \left(x^2 - 1\right)^a$ leading to (10.652a, b):

$$y(x) = \left(x^2 - 1\right)^a J_\nu^\mu(x): x^2\left(x^2 - 1\right)^2 y'' + \left[(1 - 4a)\, x^2 - 1 + \frac{\mu\, x^2}{2}\left(x^2 - 1\right)\right] \neq x\left(x^2 - 1\right) y'$$
$$+ \left[\left(x^2 - \nu^2\right)\left(x^2 - 1\right)^2 + 4a\, x^2 - \mu\, a\, x^4\left(x^2 - 1\right)\right] y = 0.$$
(10.652a, b)

*standard CDXCVIII. Particular case $f = \sec x$ of (10.651a, b) leading to (10.653a, b):

$$y(x) = \sec x\, J_\nu^\mu(x): \quad x^2 y'' + \left(1 - 2x\tan x + \frac{\mu\, x^2}{2}\right) x y'$$
$$- \left[\nu^2 + x\tan x\left(1 + \frac{\mu\, x^2}{2}\right)\right] y = 0. \quad (10.653a, b)$$

*standard CDXCIX. Particular case $f = \csc x$ of (10.651a, b) leading to (10.654a, b):

$$y(x) = \csc x \, J_\nu^\mu(x): \quad x^2 y'' + \left(1 - 2x\cot x + \frac{\mu x^2}{2}\right) x y' - \left[\nu^2 + x\cot x\left(1 + \frac{\mu x^2}{2}\right)\right] y = 0. \tag{10.654a, b}$$

*standard D. Particular case (10.655a, b) of (10.651a, b) leading to (10.655c):

$$y(x) = \exp\left\{\int^x j(\xi)\,d\xi\right\} = y(x)\left[J_\nu^\mu(x)\right]^{-1}:$$

$$x^2 y'' + \left(1 - 2xj + \frac{\mu x^2}{2}\right) x y' + \left[x^2\left(1 + j^2 - j' - xj\right) - \nu^2 - \frac{\mu x^3 j}{2}\right] y = 0. \tag{10.655a–c}$$

Classification 10.2

500 Applications of Differential Equations to Physical and Engineering Problems

Classification 10.2 consists of the detailed application of differential equations to 500 physical and engineering problems leading to: (i) 100 distinct differential equations, all falling into at least one of the 500 standards of the recollection 10.1; (ii) 500 subcases of solutions depending on the specified application or combination of parameters. By detailed application is meant a three-stage process: (i) formulation of the model leading to a differential equation; (ii) solution of the differential equation with sufficient generality; (iii) interpretation of the results and assessment of practical consequences. The 500 problems in Classification 10.2 are divided in 26 sections A to Z, and form eight groups. The first group, consisting of section A and problems 1 to 69, concerns the linear second-order oscillator with damping or amplification and several types of forcing, including ordinary resonance. The second group, corresponding to section B and problems 70 to 89, concerns the calculation of trajectories and paths, which underlies other groups. The third group, corresponding to section C and problems 90 to 104, concerns the linear second-order oscillator with parameters depending on time including parametric resonance. The fourth group, consisting of sections D to H and problems 105 to 155, concerns non-linear second-order oscillators, including non-linear resonance, bifurcations, and chaotic motions. The consideration of second-order problems concludes with numerical and analytical approximate methods in the fifth group, consisting of sections I and J and problems 156 to 177.

The deformation and buckling of elastic bodies like bars, beams, and plates lead to fourth-order differential equations and are considered in the sixth group, consisting of sections K to Q and problems 178 to 338. The seventh group, consisting of sections R to T and problems 339 to 420, concerns linear and non-linear waves in inhomogeneous and unsteady media; the solutions are obtained for linear, steady, and inhomogeneous media, when the partial differential equations reduce to ordinary differential equations with variable coefficients. The eighth group, consisting of the sections U to Z and problems 421 to 500, concerns multidimensional oscillators with several degrees-of-freedom leading to simultaneous systems of ordinary differential equations describing combined oscillations and multiple resonance. Both the seventh and eighth groups concern waves and multidimensional oscillators, which involve several modes, infinite and finite in number. Four types of resonance are considered: simple, multiple, parametric, and non-linear, each with or without damping. The problems often have mechanical electric, acoustic, and other analogues. Classifications 10.1 and 10.2 provide a summary of the contents of this book and complement each other as a quick-look guide of where to find: (a) the solution of a specific differential equation among the 500 standards in Classification 10.1; (b) the indication of some contexts in which the differential equation arises and the interpretation and application of the solutions in Classification 10.2.

A. Linear, Attractive/Repulsive, Damped/Amplified, and Free/Forced Oscillator:

$$\frac{d^2x}{dt^2}+2\lambda\frac{dx}{dt}+\omega_0^2\,x=f(t). \tag{10.656}$$

*problem 1. Mechanical mass-damper-spring-force system (subsections 2.1.1–2.1.5):

$$m\ddot{x}+\mu\dot{x}+kx=F_m(x); \tag{10.657}$$

*problem 2. Electrical self-resistor-capacitor-battery circuit (subsections 2.1.6–2.1.13):

$$L\ddot{q}+R\dot{q}+\frac{1}{C}q=F_e(x). \tag{10.658}$$

A. a. Undamped and Unforced (section 2.2); $\lambda=0=f(t)$:

*problem 3. Harmonic oscillator (subsections 2.2.1–2.2.2; note 1.19); stable attractor: $\omega_0^2>0$;
*problem 4. Adiabatic invariant (subsection 2.2.3): $2\pi\,d\omega_0/dt<<\omega_0^2$;
*problem 5. Small oscillations of suspended pendulum (subsection 2.2.4): $\ell\ddot{\theta}=-g\theta$;
*problem 6. Monotonic instability of an inverted pendulum (subsections 2.2.4–2.25): $\ell\ddot{\theta}=g\theta$;
*problem 7. Unstable repeller (subsection 2.2.5): $\omega_0^2<0$.

A. b. Damped and Unforced (sections 2.3–2.4): $\lambda>0=f(x)$:

*problem 8. Critical damping (subsections 2.3.1–2.3.2; note 1.29): $\lambda=\omega_0$;
*problem 9. Supercritical damping (subsections 2.3.3–2.3.4; note 1.21): $\lambda>\omega_0$;

*problem 10. Subcritical damping (section 2.4, note 1.22, E10.2.1–E10.2.2); $\lambda < \omega_0$;
*problem 11. Weak damping (subsections 2.4.2–2.4.5; E10.1.4); $\lambda^2 << \omega_0^2$.

A. c. Amplified and Unforced (section 2.5):

*problem 12. Mechanical system on a conveyor belt (subsection 2.5.1):

$$\ddot{x} + (\lambda - \nu)\,\dot{x} + \omega_0^2\, x = 0. \tag{10.659}$$

*problem 13. Zero effective damping (subsection 2.5.2): $\lambda = \nu$;
*problem 14. Critical effective damping (subsection 2.5.2): $\lambda + \nu = \omega_0$;
*problem 15. Supercritical effective damping (subsection 2.5.2): $\lambda + \nu > \omega_0$;
*problem 16. Subcritical effective damping (subsection 2.5.2): $\lambda < \omega_0 + \nu$;
*problem 17. Weak effective damping (subsection 2.5.2): $\lambda\,(\lambda - 2\nu) << \omega_0^2 - \nu^2$;
*problem 18. Critical amplication (subsection 2.5.3): $\lambda = \nu - \omega_0 > 0$;
*problem 19. Supercritical amplification (subsection 2.5.3): $\lambda < \nu - \omega_0$;
*problem 20. Subcritical amplification (subsection 2.5.3): $\lambda > \nu - \omega_0$;
*problem 21. Froude pendulum suspended from a cam with frictional torque (subsection 2.5.4);
*problem 22. Electric circuit with valve (subsection 2.5.5).

A. d. Degenerate Cases (section 2.6):

*problem 23. Zero mass and damping (subsection 2.6.1): $m = 0 < \mu$;
*problem 24. Zero mass and amplification (subsection 2.6.1): $m = 0 > \mu$:
*problem 25. Zero mass and zero damping (subsection 2.6.1): $m = 0 = \mu$;
*problem 26. No spring and no damper (subsection 2.6.1): $k = 0 = \mu$;
*problem 27. Small mass (subsections 2.6.1–2.6.2): $mk << \mu^2$.

A. e. Undamped, with Sinusoidal Forcing (section 2.7):

$\lambda = 0$:
$$\ddot{x} + \omega_0^2\; x = f_a \cos(\omega_a t). \tag{10.660a, b}$$

*problem 28. Non-resonant forcing (subsections 2.7.1–2.7.2): $\omega_a \neq \omega_0$;
*problem 29. Resonant forcing (subsections 2.7.3–2.7.4, E10.2.3–E10.2.4): $\omega_a = \omega_0$;
*problem 30. Beats (subsections 2.7.5–2.7.6): $(\omega_0 - \omega_a)^2 << (\omega_0 + \omega_a)^2$.

A. f. Damped, with Sinusoidal Forcing (subsections 2.8.1–2.8.3):

$\lambda \neq 0$:
$$\ddot{x} + 2\lambda\,\dot{x} + \omega_0^2\, x = f_a \cos(\omega_a t). \tag{10.661a, b}$$

*problem 31. Non-resonant forcing (subsections 2.8.1–2.8.3): $\omega_a \neq \omega_0$;
*problem 32. Resonant forcing (subsection 2.8.2): $\omega_a = \omega_0$.

A. g. Simultaneous Forcing (10.662b) in Frequency and Damping (subsections 2.8.4–2.8.6) **for subcritical damping** (10.662a):

$$\lambda < \omega_0: \qquad \ddot{x} + 2\lambda\dot{x} + \omega_0^2 x = f_a \exp(-\lambda_a t)\cos(\omega_a t). \tag{10.662a, b}$$

*problem 33. Distinct applied and oscillation (10.662c) frequencies and distinct applied decay and natural damping (subsection 2.8.4): $\bar{\omega} \neq \omega_a, \lambda \neq \lambda_a$;

$$\bar{\omega} = \left|\omega_0^2 - \lambda^2\right|^{1/2}. \tag{10.662c}$$

*problem 34. Monotonically decaying forcing (subsection 2.8.4): $\omega_a = 0$;
*problem 35. Coincident applied and oscillation frequencies and distinct applied decay and natural damping (subsection 2.8.5): $\omega_a = \bar{\omega}$, $\lambda_a \neq \lambda$;
*problem 36. Distinct applied and oscillation frequencies and coincident applied decay and natural damping (subsection 2.8.5): $\omega_a \neq \bar{\omega}, \lambda_a = \lambda$;
*problem 37. Coincident applied and frequencies and applied decay equal to natural damping (subsection 2.8.5): $\omega_a = \omega_0$, $\lambda_a = \lambda$;
*problem 38. Resonance only if (i) the applied and oscillation frequencies coincide and (ii) the applied decay equals the natural damping (subsection 2.8.6): $\omega_a = \bar{\omega}$, $\lambda_a = \lambda$.

A. h. Forcing Involving a Power of Time (example 10.3):

$$\ddot{x} + 2\lambda\dot{x} + \omega_0^2 x = f_a t^n \cos(\omega_a t). \tag{10.663}$$

*problem 39. Undamped and non-oscillating (E10.3.1): $\lambda = 0 = \omega_a$;
*problem 40. Linear in time, undamped, oscillating, and non-resonant (E10.3.1): $n = 1, \lambda = 0 \neq \omega_a \neq \omega_0$;
*problem 41. Problem 40 but resonant (E10.3.1): $n = 1, \lambda = 0 \neq \omega_a = \omega_0$;
*problem 42. Linear in time, damped, non-oscillating (E10.13.2): $n = 1, \lambda \neq 0 = \omega_a$;
*problem 43. Linear in time, damped, oscillating (E10.13.2): $n = 1, \lambda \neq 0 \neq \omega_a \neq \omega_0$;
*problem 44. Problem 43 but resonant (E10.13.3): $n = 1, \lambda \neq 0 \neq \omega_a = \omega_0$.

A. i. Integrable Forcing Function (section 2.9): $f \in \mathcal{E}(|R)$ in (1):

*problem 45. Critical damping (subsections 2.9.1–2.9.3): $\lambda = \omega_0$;
*problem 46. Undamped (subsection 2.9.3): $\lambda = 0 \neq \omega_0$;
*problem 47. Supercritical damping (subsection 2.9.3): $\lambda > \omega_0$;
*problem 48. Subcritical damping (subsection 2.9.3); $\lambda < \omega_0$;
*problem 49. Constant forcing (subsection 2.9.4): $f(t) = f_0$;
*problem 50. Bounded forcing (subsection 2.9.5): $f \in B(|R)$.

A. j. Forcing by a Discrete Spectrum (10.664b) of a Function of Bounded Oscillation (10.664a) in a Finite Interval (10.664a) Represented by a *Fourier Series* (note 2.4):

$$f \in F(0,T): \qquad \ddot{x} + 2\lambda\dot{x} + \omega_0^2 x = \sum_{n=-\infty}^{+\infty} f_n \cos\left(\frac{n\pi t}{T}\right) \equiv f(t). \qquad \text{(10.664a, b)}$$

*problem 51. Undamped, non-resonant if no harmonic coincides with the natural frequency: $\lambda = 0, \omega T \neq n\pi$ for all n;
*problem 52. Undamped, resonant if one harmonic coincides with the natural frequency $\lambda = 0, \omega T = m\pi$ for one m;
*problem 53. Damped, non-resonant: $\lambda > 0$, $\omega T \neq n\pi$;
*problem 54. Damped, resonant: $\lambda > 0, \omega T = m\pi$.

A. k. Forcing by the Continuous Spectrum (10.665b) of a Function of Bounded Oscillation and Absolutely Integrable on the Real Line (10.665a) Represented by a *Fourier integral* (notes 2.5–2.8):

$$f \in F \cap L^1(-\infty,+\infty): \qquad \ddot{x} + 2\lambda\dot{x} + \omega_0^2 x = \int_{-\infty}^{+\infty} f(\omega) e^{i\omega t}\, d\omega \equiv f(t). \qquad \text{(10.665a, b)}$$

*problem 55. Undamped (note 2.5): $\lambda = 0$;
*problem 56. Critically damped oscillator (note 2.6): $\lambda = \omega_0$;
*problem 57. Supercritically damped oscillator (note 2.8): $\lambda > \omega_0$;
*problem 58. Subcritically damped oscillator (note 2.8): $\lambda < \omega_0$.

A. l. *Influence* or *Green Function* for Forcing by the Unit Impulse (notes 2.9–2.10):

$$G + 2\lambda\dot{G} + \omega_0^2 G = \delta(t). \qquad \text{(10.666)}$$

*problem 59. For the critically damped oscillator (note 2.9): $\lambda = \omega_0$;
*problem 60. For the subcritically damped oscillator (note 2.9): $\lambda < \omega_0$;
*problem 61. For the supercritically damped oscillator (note 2.9): $\lambda > \omega_0$;
*problem 62. For the undamped oscillator (note 2.9): $\lambda = 0$.

A. m. Forcing by a Continuous Function (note 2.11):

*problem 63. Using the *Green or influence function* (note 2.11): $f \in C(|R)$ in (1);
*problem 64. Undamped (note 2.11): $\lambda = 0$;
*problem 65. Subcritically damped (note 2.11): $0 < \lambda < \omega_0$;
*problem 66. Critically damped (note 2.11): $\lambda = \omega_0 > 0$;
*problem 67. Supercritically damped (note 2.11): $\lambda > \omega_0 > 0$.

A. n. Forcing by a Gaussian Function (notes 2.12–2.13):

*problem 68. Undamped forcing by Gaussian (note 2.12):

$$\ddot{x} + 2\lambda\dot{x} + \omega_0^2 x = f_a \exp\left(-\frac{b^2}{T^2}\right) \tag{10.667}$$

*problem 69. Undamped forcing by Gaussian random noise with mean μ and variance σ^2 (note 2.13):

$$\ddot{x} + 2\lambda\dot{x} + \omega_0^2 x = \frac{f_a}{\sigma\sqrt{2\pi}} \exp\left\{-\frac{(t-\mu)^2}{2\sigma^2}\right\}. \tag{10.668}$$

B. Motion Near a Stagnation Point

(sections 4.1–4.2; example 10.7):

B. a. Paths Near a Stagnation Point of the First Degree (section 4.1 and example 10.7):

$$ad \neq bc: \qquad \frac{dy}{dx} = \frac{cx + dy}{ax + by}. \tag{10.669a, b}$$

*problem 70. **Contact point** of inflexion of paths tangent to the principal line (subsection 4.1.4) for:

$$\Delta \equiv (a-d)^2 + 4cb = 0; \tag{10.670}$$

*problem 71. **Saddle point** through which pass two principal lines, to which the paths are asymptotically tangent (subsection 4.1.6): $\Delta > 0$, $bc > ad$;
*problem 72. **Nodal point** through which pass all paths tangent to a principal line (subsection 4.1.7): $\Delta > 0$ in (10.670) and:

$$\vartheta = 4\frac{ad - bc}{\left(a + d + \sqrt{\Delta}\right)^2} \neq 1, 0. \tag{10.671}$$

*problem 73. **Focal point** through which pass all straight paths (subsection 4.1.7): $\vartheta = 1$;
*problem 74. **Simple point** through which passes one of the set of parallel straight paths (subsection 4.1.7): $\vartheta = 0$;
*problem 75. **Common center** of elliptical paths (subsection 4.1.8): $\Delta < 0, a + d = 0$;
*problem 76. **Asymptotic point** as the limit of spiral paths (subsection 4.1.9): $\Delta < 0, a + d \neq 0$.

B. b. Paths Near a Stagnation Point of the Second Degree (example 10.7):

*problem 77. Paths tangent to the y-axis at the origin (E10.7.1):

$$\frac{dy}{dx} = \frac{y^2 - x^2}{xy}; \tag{10.672}$$

*problem 78. Paths with three asymptotes crossing at the origin with equal angles (E10.7.2):

$$2\frac{dy}{dx} = \frac{x^2 - y^2}{xy}. \tag{10.673}$$

B. c. Trajectories Near a Stagnation Point of First Degree (section 4.2):

$$\frac{dx}{dt} = ax + by, \qquad \frac{dy}{dt} = cx + dy. \tag{10.674a, b}$$

*problem 79. Equivalent damped (1) unforced $f = 0$ oscillator (subsections 4.2.1–4.2.3):

$$\lambda = -\frac{a+d}{2}, \qquad \omega_0^2 = ad - bc: \qquad \left\{\frac{d^2}{dt^2} - 2\lambda\frac{d}{dt} + \omega_0^2\right\} x, y(t) = 0, \tag{10.675a–c}$$

with (19a) damping $\lambda > 0$ (amplification $\lambda < 0$) and (19b) natural frequency $\omega_0^2 > 0$ (growth rate $\omega_0^2 < 0$) in (10.675c);
*problem 80. Critical damping corresponding to (problem 70) to a **contact point** of inflection (subsection 4.2.4): $\lambda = \omega_0$;
*problem 81. Supercritical damping corresponding to (problem 72) to a **nodal point** (subsection 4.2.5): $\lambda > \omega_0, 0 < rs \neq 0$:

$$r, s = -\lambda \pm \sqrt{\lambda^2 - \omega_0^2}; \tag{10.676a, b}$$

*problem 82. Supercritical damping corresponding (problem 73) to a **focal point** (subsection 4.2.5): $\lambda > \omega_0, r = 0 \neq s$;
*problem 83. Supercritical damping corresponding (problem 74) to a **simple point** (subsection 4.2.5): $\lambda > \omega_0, s = 0 \neq r$;
*problem 84. Supercritical damping corresponding to a **saddle point** (subsection 4.2.5): $\lambda > \omega_0.\ rs < 0$;
*problem 85. Subcritical damping corresponding (problem 76) to a spiral fall towards $\lambda > 0$ (exist from $\lambda < 0$) an **asymptotic point** (subsection 4.2.6): $\lambda \neq 0, |\lambda| < \omega_0$;
*problem 86. No damping corresponding (problem 75) to the **center** of elliptic or circular trajectories (subsection 4.2.6): $\lambda = 0$.

B. d. Two Orthogonal Undamped Oscillators (subsections 4.2.7–4.2.8):

$$x(t) = a\cos(\omega t), \qquad y(t) = b\cos(\omega t - \varphi). \tag{10.677a, b}$$

*problem 87. Straight path if in-phase (subsection 4.2.7): $\varphi = 0$;
*problem 88. Elliptic path aligned with the axis when out-of-phase (subsection 4.2.7): $\varphi = \pi/2$;
*problem 89. Elliptic path rotated relative to the axis for intermediate phases (subsection 4.2.8): $0 < \varphi < \pi/2$.

C. Parametric Resonance (section 4.3)

C. a. Undamped Oscillator with Coefficients Depending on Time (subsection 4.3.1):

*problem 90. Oscillator with mass and spring resilience a function of time:

$$\frac{d}{dt}\left[m(t)\frac{dx}{dt}\right] + k(t)x(t) = 0. \tag{10.678}$$

C. b. Parametric Resonance: Harmonic Oscillator with Support Oscillating in Time with Amplitude h and Excitation Frequency ω_e:

$$\frac{d^2x}{dt^2} + \omega_0^2\left[1 + 2h\cos(\omega_e t)\right]x(t) = 0. \tag{10.679}$$

*problem 91. Exact solution in terms of Mathieu functions (subsections 4.3.2–4.3.11):

$$w(\theta) \equiv x(t), \quad \theta \equiv \frac{\omega_e t}{2}, \quad a \equiv \left(\frac{2\omega_0}{\omega_e}\right)^2, \quad q \equiv -ha: \tag{10.680a–d}$$

$$\frac{d^2w}{d\theta^2} + \left[a - 2q\cos(2\theta)\right]w(\theta) = 0. \tag{10.680e}$$

C. c. Stability/Instability/Indifference of Solutions (subsections 4.3.3–4.3.6):

*problem 92. For linear unforced second-order differential equation (10.681e) with (10.681a, b) periodic coefficients (subsections 4.3.3–4.3.5):

$$n = 0, 1, 2: \qquad A_n(t) = A_n(t + \tau), \qquad \sum_{n=0}^{2} A_n(t)\frac{d^x x}{dt^n} = 0; \tag{10.681a–c}$$

*problem 93. For undamped harmonic oscillator (10.682b) with (10.682a) periodic "natural frequency" (subsection 4.3.6):

$$\omega(t)=\omega(t+\tau): \qquad \frac{d^2x}{dt^2}+\left[\omega(t)\right]^2 x(t)=0. \qquad (10.682a, b)$$

C. d. **Excitation Frequencies Leading to Parametric Resonance** (subsections 4.3.10–4.3.11):

*problem 94. Strongest parametric resonance for $\omega_e = 2\omega_0 + 2\varepsilon$ excitation frequency close to twice the natural frequency (subsection 4.3.10);
*problem 95. Weaker parametric resonance for excitation frequiency (10.683c) close to a multiple or submultiple (10.683a, b) of the natural frequency (subsection 4.3.11):

$$m,n=1,2,...: \qquad \omega_e^{\pm}=\frac{m\pm 1}{m}\left(\omega_0+\varepsilon\right), \qquad (10.683a–c)$$

including excitation frequency equal to the natural frequency $\left(n=1, m=2: \omega_e^{+}=\omega_0\right)$.

C. e. Undamped Parametric Resonance (subsections 4.3.12–4.3.15) by Approximate Solution of (10.679) to the Lowest Orders $O(h^n)$ in the Excitation Amplitude h:

*problem 96. Parametric resonance by excitation close to the first harmonic $\omega_e = 2\omega_0 + 2\varepsilon$ of the natural frequency to the lowest or the first *O(h)* order in the excitation amplitude (subsection 4.3.13);
*problem 97. Problem 96 to the next or second order in the excitation amplitude (subection 4.3.14);
*problem 98. Parametric resonance by excitation close to the natural frequency $\omega_e = \omega_0 + \varepsilon$ with the second $O\left(h^2\right)$ as the lowest order in the excitation amplitude (subsection 4.3.15).

C. f. **Parametric Resonance with Weak Damping (10.684a, b) for Several Excitation Frequencies** (subsections 4.3.16–4.3.18):

$$\lambda^2 << b^2 \equiv \left(\frac{\omega_0 h}{2}\right)^2: \quad \frac{d^2x}{dt^2}+2\lambda\frac{dx}{dt}+\omega_0^2\left[1+2h\cos(\omega_e t)\right]x(t)=0. \qquad (10.684a, b)$$

*problem 99. Strongest parametric resonance for excitation frequency $\omega_e = 2\omega_0 + 2\varepsilon$ close to twice the natural frequency (subsections 4.3.16–4.3.17);

*problem 100. Undamped $\lambda = 0$ parametric resonance due to excitation $2n\omega_e = \omega_0 + \varepsilon$ close to submultiples of the first harmonic of the natural frequency (subsection 4.3.18);
*problem 101. Problem 100 with weak (10.684a) damping (subsection 4.3.18).

C. g. Suspended Pendulum with Support Oscillating Vertically (10.685c) with Amplitude p Leading to Weakly Damped (10.685a) Small Amplitude (10.685b) Parametric Resonance (subsection 4.3.19):

$$\lambda^2 << \frac{g}{L}, \quad \theta^2 << 1: \qquad \frac{d^2\theta}{dt^2} + 2\lambda\frac{d\theta}{dt} + \frac{g}{L}\left[1 + \frac{8p}{L}\cos(\omega_e t)\right]\theta(t) = 0. \qquad (10.685a\text{–}c)$$

*problem 102. Undamped $\lambda = 0$ excitation at $\omega_e = 2\omega_0$ at twice the natural frequency;
*problem 103. Problem 102 with weak (10.685a) damping;
*problem 104. Problem 102 with weak damping and excitation $\omega_e = n\omega_0$ at a submultiple of the first harmonic of the natural frequency.

D. Non-Linear, Undamped, Unforced, Oscillator

(10.686a) hence, constant (10.686b) total energy (sections 4.4–4.5):

$$m\frac{d^2\theta}{dt^2} = F(x) = -\frac{d\Phi}{dx}: \qquad \frac{1}{2}m\left(\frac{dx}{dt}\right)^2 + \Phi(x) = E. \qquad (10.686a, b)$$

D. a. For general potential (subsections 4.4.2–4.4.3):

*problem 105. Paths in the phase plane and trajectories in the physical plane (subsection 4.4.2);
*problem 106. Separatrices between limit cycles and unstable regimes (subsection 4.4.3).

D. b. Bi-Quadratic Potential for a Soft/Hard Spring (subsections 4.4.5–4.4.15):

$$\Phi(x) = \frac{1}{2}kx^2\left(1 + \frac{\beta}{2}x^2\right), \qquad (10.687)$$

*problem 107. Non-linear hard $\beta > 0$ spring (subsections 4.4.4–4.4.6);
*problem 108. Non-linear soft $\beta < 0$ spring (subsections 4.4.6–4.4.8);
*problem 109. Exact solution for the position as a function of time in terms of the Jacobian elliptic sine (subsection 4.4.9);
*problem 110. Inverse solution with time as a function of position specified by a series of circular sines (subsections 4.4.10–4.4.11);
*problem 111. Inverse solution with time as a function of position specified by a series of Chebychev polynomials of the second kind (subsections 4.4.11–4.4.12);
*problem 112. Effect of non-linearity on the oscillation frequency (subsection 4.4.13);
*problem 113. Effect of non-linearity on the displacement and generation of harmonics (subsections 4.4.14–4.4.15).

D. c. Quartic Potential (10.688) Generalizing the Bi-Quadratic (10.687) Potential (section 4.5):

$$\Phi(x) = \frac{1}{2} k x^2 \left(1 + \frac{2}{3} \varepsilon \alpha x + \frac{1}{2} \varepsilon^2 \beta x^2 \right). \tag{10.688}$$

*problem 114. Method of parametric expansions for the displacement (10.689a) and frequency (10.689b) to second order (subsection 4.5.1):

$$x(t) = x_1(t) + \varepsilon x_2(t) + \varepsilon^2 x_3(t) + \dots, \qquad \omega = \omega_0 + \omega_1 \varepsilon + \omega_2 \varepsilon^2 + \dots; \qquad (10.689a, b)$$

*problem 115. First-order perturbation $0(\varepsilon)$ of displacement (subsection 4.5.2);
*problem 116. Second-order perturbation $0(\varepsilon^2)$ of displacement and oscillation frequency (subsections 4.5.3–4.5.4).

E. Resonance of a Non-Linear Oscillator

with (i) linear damping, (ii) non-linear restoring force corresponding to the quartic potential, and (iii) sinusoidal forcing with amplitude F_a and applied frequency ω_a (section 4.6):

$$m \frac{d^2 x}{dt^2} + \mu \frac{dx}{dt} + k x \left(1 + \varepsilon \alpha x + \varepsilon^2 \beta x^2 \right) = F_a \cos(\beta \omega_a t). \tag{10.690}$$

*problem 117. Non-linear resonance with applied frequency close to the natural frequency $\omega_a = \omega_0 + \varepsilon$ leading to the existence of amplitude jumps and hysterisis loop (subsections 4.6.1–4.6.3);
*problem 118. Problem 117 for subharmonic non-linear resonance with applied frequency close to half of the natural frequency $2\omega_a = \omega_0 + \varepsilon$ leading to smaller amplitude jumps and weaker hysteresis (subsections 4.6.4–4.6.5);
*problem 119. Non-linear resonance with applied frequency $\omega_a = 2(\omega_0 + \varepsilon)$ close to the first harmonic of the natural frequency leading to smooth amplitude variation, or amplitude jumps or suppressions of oscillations (subsections 4.6.6–4.6.7);
*problem 120. Non-linear resonance with applied frequency $\omega_e = 3(\omega_0 + \varepsilon)$ close to the second harmonic of the natural frequency leading to no oscillation, or suppression of oscillations or a threshold amplitude for the existence of oscillations (subsections 4.6.8–4.6.9);
*problem 121. Non-linear resonance at rational multiples of the natural frequency, that is, submultiples of harmonics of the natural frequencym (subsection 4.6.10).

F. Electromechanical Dynamo (subsections 4.7.1–4.7.9):

F. a. Electrical Dynamo:

$$L\frac{dJ}{dt} + RJ = \pm\frac{Z\Omega}{2\pi}J. \tag{10.691}$$

*problem 122. Counter-rotating electrical dynamo with – (minus) sign in (10.691) as a brake (subsection 4.7.2);
*problem 123. Co-rotating electrical dynamo with + (plus) sign in (10.691) with constant, decaying, or growing current (subsection 4.7.2).

F. b. Electromechanical Dynamo (10.692b) with small resistance (10.692a), compared with the mutual induction (subsections 4.7.3–4.7.4):

$$2\pi R << Z\Omega: \qquad L\dot{J} = -RJ \pm SJ^2. \tag{10.692a, b}$$

*problem 124. Exponential decay of electric current and angular velocity;
*problem 125. Linear decay if the first term on the r.h.s. of (10.692b) is omitted.

F. c. Exact Electromechanical Homopolar Dynamo (subsections 4.7.5–4.7.6):

$$\frac{d^2J}{dt^2}-\left(\frac{1}{J}\frac{dJ}{dt}\pm bJ\right)\frac{dJ}{dt}\mp bJ\left(\frac{R}{L}J+\frac{M}{aL}\right)=0. \tag{10.693}$$

*problem 126. Without driving torque $M=0$ the electric current and angular velocity decay to zero (subsection 4.7.5);
*problem 127. Balance of driving and Lorentz force torques $M\Omega=RJ^2$ leads to constant electric current and angular velocity (subsection 4.7.6).

F. d. Self-Excited Dynamo (subsection 4.7.7):

$$m\frac{dv_\pm}{dt}=\mp b\,v_\pm-a(v_\pm)^2. \tag{10.694}$$

*problem 128. For upper sign in (10.694) linear and quadratic damping leading to decay;
*problem 129. For lower sign in (10.694) linear amplification and quadratic damping leading to a steady state.

G. Circular Pendular Motion (subsections 4.7.10–4.7.18)

G. a. Large Motion without Damping (subsections 4.7.10–4.7.15):

$$\omega_0=\sqrt{\frac{g}{L}}: \qquad \ddot\theta+\omega_0^2\sin\theta=0. \tag{10.695a, b}$$

*problem 130. **Stopping point** at the highest position for $E=mgL$ (subsections 4.7.11–4.7.12);
*problem 131. **Circulatory motion** for $E>mgl$ (subsections 4.7.11–4.7.12);
*problem 133. **Oscillatory motion** with large amplitude for $E<mgL$ (subsections 4.7.11, 4.7.12).

G. b. Pendular Motion with Quadratic Damping (subsections 4.7.16–4.7.18):

$$\mu>0: \qquad mL\ddot\theta+\mu\dot\theta\left|\dot\theta\right|+mg\sin\theta=0. \tag{10.696a, b}$$

*problem 134. Decay of oscillations (subsection 4.7.18);

*problem 135. Start at the highest position (subsection 4.7.18);
*problem 136. Number of circulations before damping causes decay to oscillatory motion (subsection 4.7.18).

H. Bifurcations, Chaos, and Approximations

(sections 4.8–4.9; notes 4.1–4.13):

H. a. Bifurcations of Dynamical Systems (subsections 4.8.1–4.8.9):

$$\ddot{x} = f(x;q). \tag{10.697}$$

*problem 137. Stability and instability at boundaries (subsection 4.8.2).

H. b. Hopf Bifurcation: Gradient Dynamical System Perturbing a Spiral Flow (subsections 4.8.4–4.8.5):

$$\frac{dr}{dt} = r\left(q + \mu r^2\right). \tag{10.698}$$

*problem 138. Hopf subcritical bifurcation: $\mu < 0$;
*problem 139. Hopf supercritical bifurcation: $\mu > 0$.

H. c. Mixed Non-Linear Oscillator—van der Pol (subsections 4.8.6–4.8.7):

$$\frac{d^2x}{dt^2} + \gamma h(x)\frac{dx}{dt} + \omega_0^2 x = 0. \tag{10.699}$$

*problem 140. Weak $\gamma << 1$ damping (subsection 4.8.6);
*problem 141. Strong $\gamma >> 1$ damping (subsection 4.8.7).

H. d. Polynomial Potentials and Catastrophes (subsections 4.8.8–4.8.9):

*problem 142. **Fold catastrophe** (10.700b) **for** (10.700a) **a cubic potential** (subsection 4.8.8):

$$\Phi(x;a) = \frac{x^3}{3} - a\,x: \qquad \frac{d^2x}{dt^2} = -\frac{\partial\Phi}{\partial x} = a - x^2; \tag{10.700a, b}$$

*problem 143. **Cusp catastrophe** (10.701b) **for** (10.701a) **a quartic potential** (subsection 4.8.9):

$$\Phi(x;a) = -\frac{x^4}{4} + \frac{a\,x^2}{2} - b\,x: \qquad \frac{d^2x}{dt^2} = -\frac{\partial\Phi}{\partial x} = x^2 - a\,x + b. \tag{10.701a, b}$$

H. e. Chaotic Motions (subsections 4.8.10–4.8.14):

*problem 144. Poincaré maps and classification of singularities (subsection 4.8.10);
*problem 145. Passage from a deterministic to a choatic system (subsection 4.8.11);
*problem 146. Transition from a laminar to a turbulent flow (subsection 4.8.12);
*problem 147. Aircraft stall and departure into spin (subsections 4.8.13–4.8.14).

H. f. Limit Cycles (subsections 4.9.1–4.9.3):

*problem 148. Competing populations of preys and predators (subsections 4.9.1–4.9.2):

$$\frac{dx}{dt} = ax - bxy, \qquad \frac{dy}{dt} = -cy + dxy. \tag{10.702a, b}$$

*problem 149. Non-existence of a limit cycle (subsection 4.9.3):

$$\{u, v\} \equiv \left\{\frac{dx}{dt}, \frac{dy}{dt}\right\} \in C^1(D): \qquad \frac{\partial y}{\partial x} + \frac{\partial v}{\partial y} \neq 0. \tag{10.703a, b}$$

H. g. Stability of Orbits of Dynamical Systems (subsection 4.9.4):

*problem 150. General dynamical system:

$$u, v \in C^2(|R): \qquad \frac{dx}{dt} = u(x, y), \qquad \frac{dy}{dt} = v(x, y); \tag{10.704a–c}$$

*problem 151. Second-order system (10.656) with constant coefficients (10.705a, b):

$$\frac{dx}{dt} = v, \qquad \frac{dv}{dt} = -2\lambda v - \omega_0^2 x. \tag{10.705a, b}$$

H. h. Index of a Singularity (subsections 4.9.5–4.9.10):

*problem 152. Index of a domain with several singularities (subsection 4.9.6);
*problem 153. Dynamical system at infinity (subsection 4.9.7);
*problem 154. Index at infinity (subsection 4.9.8);
*problem 155. Classification of singularities by their índices (subsection 4.9.9);

I. Numerical Solution of Differential Equations (notes 4.1–4.13):

*problem 156. Discretization of derivatives of any positive integer order (note 4.8);
*problem 157. Transformation of a differential equation into a finite difference equation (note 4.9);
*problem 158. Comparison of the solutions of the differential and finite difference equations (notes 4.10–4.11);
*problem 159. Effect of step size on accuracy (note 4.12);
*problem 160. Comparison of truncation and discretization errors (note 4.13).

J. Optics and Acoustic Rays (notes 5.1–5.19)

J. a. Linear Second-Order Differential Equation (notes 5.3–5.5):

$$A_2(x)\frac{d^2y}{dx^2}+A_1(x)\frac{dy}{dx}+A_0(x)\,y(x)=B(x). \tag{10.706}$$

*problem 161. Non-singular form (note 5.3):

$$\frac{d^2y}{dx^2}+P(x)\frac{dy}{dx}+Q(x)y=f(x). \tag{10.707}$$

*problem 162. Given a particular integral (10.708a) of the unforced equation (10.706) with $B(x)=0$, find another (10.708b) linearly independent (10.708c) particular integral (notes 5.4–5.5):

$$y_1''+Py_1'+Qy_1=0: \qquad y_2''+Py_2'+Qy_2=0\wedge y_2(x)\neq Cy_1(x); \tag{10.708a–d}$$

*problem 162. Idem (10.708a) the general integral (10.709c) of the unforced (10.709a, b) equation (notes 5.4–5.5):

$$y_1''+Py_1'+Qy_1=0; \qquad B(x)=0: \qquad y(x)=C_1\,y_1(x)+C_2\,y_2(x). \tag{10.709a–c}$$

*problem 163. Idem (10.710a) the complete integral (10.710c) of the forced (10.710b) equation (notes 5.4–5.5):

$$y_1''+Py_*'+Qy_*=f, \qquad B(x)\neq 0: \qquad \bar{y}(x)=y(x)+y_*(x). \tag{10.710a–c}$$

J. b. Three Alternative Forms (notes 5.6–5.8):

*problem 164. Transformation to an **integro-differential equation** (note 5.6):

$$\frac{du}{dx}+u^2+Pu+Q=F(x)\ \exp\left\{-\int^x u(\xi)d\xi\right\}; \tag{10.711}$$

*problem 165. Transformation to a **self-adjoint form** (note 5.7):

$$\frac{du}{dx}\left[R(x)\frac{dy}{dx}\right]+Q(x)y=T(x); \tag{10.712}$$

*problem 166. Transformation to the **invariant form** (note 5.8):

$$\frac{d^2v}{dx^2}+I(x)v(x)=G(x); \tag{10.713}$$

*problem 167. Transformation of two distinct differential equations: (i) to the same invariant form (10.713); (ii) into each other (note 5.9).

J. c. Solutions of the Invariant Unforced Linear Second-Order Differential Equation (notes 5.10–5.12):

*problem 168. Constant positive, negative or zero invariant (note 5.10);
*problem 169. Variable invariant with change of sign (note 5.10);
*problem 170. Turning point for the **Airy differential equation** (note 5.11):

$$\frac{d^2\Psi}{dx^2}+\alpha^2(x-x_r)\Psi(x)=0. \tag{10.714}$$

J. d. Waves in a Refracting Medium (notes 5.13–5.15):

*problem 171. Classical wave equation in a refracting medium with non-unform propagation speed (note 5.13):

$$\frac{\partial^2\Phi}{\partial x^2}+\frac{\partial^2\Phi}{\partial y^2}+\frac{\partial^2\Phi}{\partial z^2}=\frac{1}{[c(x)]^2}\frac{\partial^2\Phi}{\partial t^2}. \tag{10.715}$$

*problem 172. Longitudinal wave propagation, evanescence or divergence (notes 5.14–5.16):

$$\frac{d^2\Psi}{dx^2}+\left\{\frac{\omega^2}{[c(x)]^2}-k^2\right\}\Psi(x)=0. \tag{10.716}$$

J. e. Light and Sound Rays (notes 5.16–5.20):

*problem 173. First-order ray approximation (notes 5.16–5.17);
*problem 174. Phase variation along ray paths (note 5.17);
*problem 175. Amplitude variation along ray tubes (note 5.17);
*problem 176. Second-order ray approximation (notes 5.18–5.19);
*problem 177. Validity of the ray approximation (note 5.20).

K. Buckling of Elastic Beams (sections 6.1–6.3; example 10.10)

K. a. General Equations (subsections 6.1.1–6.1.4):

*problem 178. Curvature of the elastica and tangential tension (subsection 6.1.1);
*problem 179. Shape of the elastica related to the shear stress and transverse force (subsection 6.1.2);
*problem 180. Non-linear buckling for a uniform beam (subsection 6.1.2);
*problem 181. Linear buckling, that is for small slope (subsection 6.1.3);
*problem 182. Linear buckling of a uniform beam (subsection 6.1.3);
*problem 183. Lowest-order non-linear correction to problem 182 (subsection 6.1.4).

K. b. Linear Buckling (subsections 6.1.5–6.1.9):

$$E\,I\,\frac{d^4\zeta}{dx^4} - T\,\frac{d^2\zeta}{dx^2} = 0. \tag{10.717}$$

*problem 184. Clamped at both ends (subsection 6.1.5);
*problem 185. Pinned at both ends (subsection 6.1.6);
*problem 186. Clamped at one end, pinned at the other end (subsection 6.1.7);
*problem 187. Non-linear and linear boundary conditions at a free end (subsection 6.1.8);
*problem 188. Cantilever beam, which is clamped at one end and free at the other end (subsection 6.1.9);
*problem 189. Comparison of critical buckling loads for four diferent combinations of supports (subsection 6.1.9).

K. c. Non-Linear Buckling to the Lowest Order (subsections 6.1.10–6.1.15):

*problem 190. Equation of the elastica (10.718a, c) in the lowest-order, non-linear (10.718b) approximation (subsection 6.1.10):

$$\zeta' \equiv \frac{d\zeta}{dx};\ \zeta'^3 << 1: \qquad \left\{\left(1-\frac{\zeta'^2}{2}\right)\left[\zeta''\left(1-\frac{3}{2}\zeta'^2\right)\right]'\right\}' + p^2\left[\zeta'\left(1-\frac{\zeta'^2}{2}\right)\right]' = 0. \tag{10.718a–c}$$

*problem 191. Cantilever beam (subsections 6.1.10–6.1.12 and 6.1.15);
*problem 192. Beam clamped or pinned at both ends (subsections 6.1.13–6.1.15);
*problem 193. Fundamental buckling mode plus first harmonic (subsection 6.1.15).

K. d. Buckling with a Point Translational Spring (subsections 6.2.1–6.2.5):

*problem 194. Boundary condition (10.719b) for a point translational spring at (10.719a) any position (subsection 6.1.1):

$$0 \le a \le L: \qquad k\zeta(a) = EI\zeta'''(a) - T\zeta'(a); \qquad (10.719a, b)$$

*problem 195. Cantilever beam with a point translational spring at the free end (subsection 6.2.2);
*problem 196. Clamped beam with a point translational spring in the middle (subsection 6.2.3);
*problem 197. Pinned beam with a point translational spring in the middle (subsection 6.2.4);
*problem 198. Clamped-pinned beam with a point translational spring in the middle (subsection 6.2.5).

K. e. Buckling with a Point Rotary Spring (subsections 6.2.6–6.2.10):

*problem 199. Boundary conditions (10.720b) for a point rotational spring at (10.720a) any position (subsection 6.2.6):

$$0 \le a \le L: \qquad -EI\zeta''(a) = \bar{k}\zeta'(a); \qquad (10.720a, b)$$

*problem 200. Cantilever beam with a point rotary spring at the free end (subsection 6.2.7);
*problem 201. Clamped beam with a point rotary spring in the middle (subsection 6.2.8);
*problem 202. Pinned beam with a point rotary spring in the middle (subsection 6.2.9);
*problem 203. Clamped-pinned beam with a point rotary in the middle (subsection 6.2.10).

K. f. Opposition to, or Facilitation of, Buckling (subsections 6.2.11–6.2.17):

*problem 204. Buckling loads and harmonics of all orders for a cantilever beam without point spring (subsection 6.2.12);
*problem 205. Fundamental and first two buckling harmonics for problem 204 (subsection 6.2.13);

*problem 206. Buckling loads of all orders for a cantilever beam with a point rotary spring at the free end (subsections 6.2.14–6.2.15);
*problem 207. Problem 206 with a point translational spring (subsections 6.2.14 and 6.2.16);
*problem 208. Buckled shape of a cantilever beam with a translational or rotary spring at the free end (subsections 6.2.14–6.2.17).

K. g. Bending of a Beam Continuously Supported on Springs (section 6.3):

*problem 209. Force balance equation for the linear deflection of an unforced uniform beam (subsections 6.3.1–6.3.2):

$$EI\frac{d^4\zeta}{dx^4} - T\frac{d^2\zeta}{dx^2} + k'\zeta = 0. \tag{10.721}$$

*problem 210. Pinned beam under traction $T > 0$ without $k' = 0$, spring support (subsection 6.3.3);
*problem 211. Pinned bar with attractive springs $k' > 0$ and $T = 0$, no axial tension (subsection 6.3.4);
*problem 212. Pinned bar supported on repulsive springs $k' < 0$ without $T = 0$, axial tension (subsection 6.3.5);
*problem 213. Pinned beam with balance $T^2 = 4EIk' > 0$ of axial compression $T < 0$ and attractive spring $k' > 0$ (subsection 6.3.6);
*problem 214. Pinned beam with balance $T^2 = 4EIk' > 0$ of axial traction $T > 0$ and attractive spring $k' > 0$ (subsection 6.3.7);
*problem 215. Pinned beam with predominance $T^2 > 4EIk'$ of axial traction $T > 0$ and $k' > 0$ attractive springs (subsection 6.3.8);
*problem 216. Pinned beam with predominance $T^2 > 4EIk'$ of axial compression $T < 0$ and $k' > 0$ attractive springs (subsection 6.3.9);
*problem 217. Pinned beam with predominance $T^2 > 4EIk'$ of axial tension over $k' < 0$ repulsive springs (subsection 6.3.10);
*problem 218. Pinned beam with predominance $0 < T^2 < 4EIk'$ of axial atractive springs $k' > 0$ over axial tension (subsection 6.3.11);
*problem 219. Extension of the problems 185 and 210–218 from pinned to cantilever, clamped and clamped-pinned beams using an effective axial tension (subsection 6.3.12);
*problem 220. To all problems 185 and 210–219, apply a combined tension-spring buckling load that does not affect the shape of the buckled elastica (subsection 6.3.13);
*problem 221. Extension of problem 219 to (10.722) to bending under own weight (subsection 6.3.14):

$$EI\frac{d^4\zeta}{dx^4} - |T|\frac{d^4\zeta}{dx^4} + |k'|\zeta = \rho g. \tag{10.722}$$

K. h. Linear Bending (10.723b) of a Beam Under Traction (10.723a) subject to shear stresses (example 10.10):

$$T > 0: \qquad EI\frac{d^4\zeta}{dx^4} - T\frac{d^2\zeta}{dx^2} = f(x). \qquad (10.723a, b)$$

*problem 222. Clamped beam (10.724a–d) with concentrated torque Q at (10.724e) the middle (E10.10.2):

$$\zeta(0) = 0 = \zeta'(0), \qquad \zeta(L) = 0 = \zeta'(L): \qquad f(x) = Q\delta'\left(x - \frac{L}{2}\right); \qquad (10.724a–e)$$

*problem 223. Pinned beam (10.725a–d) with concentrated force F at (10.725e) the middle (E10.10.3):

$$\zeta(0) = 0 = \zeta''(0), \qquad \zeta(L) = 0 = \zeta''(L): \qquad f(x) = F\delta'\left(x - \frac{L}{2}\right); \qquad (10.725a–e)$$

*problem 224. Clamped-pinned beam (10.726a–d) subject to (10.726e) own weight (E10.10.4):

$$\zeta(0) = 0 = \zeta'(0), \qquad \zeta(L) = 0 = \zeta''(L): \qquad f(x) = \rho g; \qquad (10.726a–e)$$

*problem 225. Cantilever beam (10.727a–d) subject to a shear stress, which is a linear function (10.727e) of the distance from the clamped support (E10.10.5):

$$\zeta(0) = 0 = \zeta'(0), \qquad \zeta''(L) = 0 = EI\zeta'''(L) - T\zeta'(L): \qquad f(x) = qx. \qquad (10.727a–e)$$

L. Axial Traction/Compression of a Straight Bar (section 6.4):

$$-F = (Eu')' = Eu'' + E'u'. \qquad (10.728a, b)$$

*problem 226. Analogy with the linear transvese deflection of an elastic string (subsection 6.4.1);
*problem 227. Analogy with one-dimensional steady heat conduction (subsection 6.4.2);
*problem 228. Strain and displacement for an inhomogeneous material (subsection 6.4.3);

*problem 229. Displacement, strain, and stress for an inhomogeneus rod with Young modulus (10.729b) subject to a (10.729a) constant longitudinal force (subsection 6.4.4):

$$F = const: \qquad E(x) = E_0 + (E_1 - E_0)\frac{x^2}{L^2}. \qquad (10.729a, b)$$

M. Plane Elastic Displacements, Strains, and Stresses (section 6.5):

*problem 230. Relation between the stress and strain tensors (subsection 6.5.1);
*problem 231. **In-plane stresses** and strains without out-of-plane stresses (subsection 6.5.2);
*problem 232. **Plane elasticity** without out-of-plane strains (subsection 6.5.3);
*problem 233. Transformation between in-plane stresses (plane elasticity) in the [problem 231 (232)] (subsections 6.5.3 and 6.5.8);
*problem 234. Differential equation (10.730) satisfied by the displacement vector (subsection 6.5.4):

$$0 = Eh\left[(1-\sigma)\nabla^2\vec{u} + (1+\sigma)\nabla(\nabla.\vec{u})\right] + 2(1-\sigma)\vec{f}; \qquad (10.730)$$

*problem 235. Bi-harmonic differential equation (10.731b) for (10.731a) the stress function (subsection 6.5.5):

$$\Theta \in \mathcal{D}^4\left(|R^2\right): \qquad 0 = \frac{\partial^4\Theta}{\partial x^4} + \frac{\partial^4\Theta}{\partial y^4} + 2\frac{\partial^4\Theta}{\partial x^2\,\partial y^2}; \qquad (10.731a, b)$$

*problem 236. Strains and stresses due to the drilling of a circular hole in an infinite thin elastic plate (subsection 6.5.6);
*problem 237. Stress concentration near a circular hole in an infinite plate with normal stresses at infinity (subsections 6.5.7–6.5.8);
*problem 238. In-plane deformations, strains, and stresses in a circular disk subject to a uniform pressure along the periphery (subsection 6.5.9).

N. Deflection of an Elastic Membrane under Anisotropic In-Plane Stresses (section 6.6):

*problem 239. Elastic strains and energy associated with the deflection of a membrane subject to anisotropic stresses (subsection 6.6.1);

*problem 240. Balance equation (10.732b) and boundary condition (10.732a) in the general non-linear anisotropic case and particular cases (subsection 6.6.2):

$$T_{\alpha\beta}\, N_\beta\, \delta\zeta_\alpha = 0: \qquad 0 = \frac{\partial}{\partial x_\alpha}\left(T_{\alpha\beta} \frac{\partial \zeta}{\partial x_\beta} \right) + f(x_\gamma); \tag{10.732a, b}$$

*problem 241. Transformation of the components of a vector or tensor by a rotation in the plane (subsection 6.6.3);
*problem 242. Green's function for (10.733) the plane anisotropic Laplace operator (subsection 6.6.4):

$$\left\{ T_{11} \frac{\partial^2}{\partial x_1\, \partial x_1} + T_{22} \frac{\partial^2}{\partial x_2\, \partial x_2} + 2T_{12} \frac{\partial^2}{\partial x_1\, \partial x_2} \right\} G(x_1, x_2) = \delta(x_1)\delta(x_2); \tag{10.733}$$

*problem 243. Characteristic lines of zero deflection for an infinite membrane under anisotropic stresses with no transverse force (subsection 6.6.5);
*problem 244. Linear deflection of a circular membrane under its own weight (subsection 6.6.6);
*problem 245. Linear deflection of an elliptic membrane under its own weight (subsection 6.6.6);
*problem 246. Deflection of an elastic membrane under anisotropic stresses for (10.734) arbitrary loading (subsection 6.6.7):

$$\left\{ T_{11} \frac{\partial^2}{\partial x_1^2} + T_{22} \frac{\partial^2}{\partial x_2^2} + 2T_{12} \frac{\partial^2}{\partial x_1\, \partial x_2} \right\} \zeta(x_1, x_2) = -f(x_1, x_2). \tag{10.734}$$

O. Weak Linear Bending of Elastic Isotropic Plates (section 6.7; example 10.11)

O. a. Transverse Displacement with Constant Bending Stiffness (subsections 6.7.1–6.7.6):

*problem 247. Curvature tensor and principal bending moments (subsection 6.7.2);
*problem 248. Curvatures and twist in axis rotated relative to the principal axis (subsection 6.7.3);
*problem 249. Stress and twist couples (subsection 6.7.4);
*problem 250. Elastic energy of weak linear bending (subsection 6.7.5);

*problem 251. Turning moments and linear weak deflection of an isotropic elastic plane (10.735b) with constant (10.735a) bending stiffness (subsection 6.7.6):

$$D \equiv \frac{Eh^3}{12\left(1-\sigma^2\right)} = \text{const:} \qquad \frac{f(x,y)}{D} = \frac{\partial^4 \zeta}{\partial x^4} + \frac{\partial^4 \zeta}{\partial y^4} + 2\frac{\partial^4 \zeta}{\partial x^2\, \partial y^2}. \qquad (10.735\text{a, b})$$

O. b. **Transverse Displacement with Non-Uniform Bending Stiffness** (subsections 6.7.7–6.7.11):

*problem 252. Displacement vector and strain, and stress tensor for weak linear bending (subsection 6.7.7);
*problem 253. Elastic energy for weak linear bending (subsection 6.7.8);
*problem 254. Elastic energy per unit volume or area and total elastic energy (subsection 6.7.9);
*problem 255. Analogy between the bending and deformation vectors (subsection 6.7.9);
*problem 256. Balance equation for the displacement with non-uniform bending stiffness (subsection 6.7.10);
*problem 257. Comparison of the weak linear bending of elastic bars and plates (subsection 6.7.11).

O. c. **Boundary Conditions for Isotropic Elastic Plates** (subsections 6.7.12–6.7.14):

*problem 258. Clamped, pinned, or supported, and free boundary conditions (subsection 6.7.12);
*problem 259. Displacement and slope for clamped or pinned boundary conditions (subsection 6.7.12);
*problem 260. Turning moment for free boundary conditions (subsection 6.7.13);
*problem 261. Polar coordinates as a particular case of orthogonal curvilinear coordinates (subsection 6.7.13);
*problem 262. Passage from polar to cartesian coordinates (subsection 6.7.13);
*problem 263. Stress couples for pinned or free boundary conditions (subsection 6.7.13);
*problem 264. Boundary conditions for rectangular, circular, and arbitrarily shaped plates (subsection 6.7.14);
*problem 265. Stress couples in polar coordinates (subsection 6.7.14).

O. d. **Weak Linear Bending of Isotropic Circular Plates** (subsections 6.7.15–6.7.19):

*problem 266. Concentrated force at the center and clamped at the boundary (subsections 6.7.15–6.7.16);

*problem 267. Problem 266 pinned or supported at the boundary (subsections 6.7.15–6.7.16);
*problem 268. Bending by a constant transverse force, such as the weight of a homogeneous plate with constant thickness (subsection 6.7.17);
*problem 269. Heavy uniform circular plate clamped at the boundary (subsection 6.7.18);
*problem 270. Problem 269 pinned or supported at the boundary (subsection 6.7.18);
*problem 271. Heavy circular plate hanging from the center with free boundary (subsection 6.7.19);
*problem 272. Circular plate with a concentric circular hole (example 10.11).

P. Linear Elastic Stability of a Stressed Orthotropic Plate (section 6.8; example 10.15)

P. a. Linear Strong Bending with Anisotropic In-Plane Stresses (subsections 6.8.1–6.8.2):

*problem 273. Balance equation (10.736) for the transverse displacement (subsection 6.8.1):

$$f = \nabla^2\left(D\nabla^2\zeta\right) - h\partial_\alpha\left(T_{\alpha\beta}\,\partial_\beta\zeta\right). \tag{10.736}$$

*problem 274. Comparison of elastic stressed plate and beam under tension (subsection 6.8.1);
*problem 275. Balance equation for the transverse displacement of a uniform stressed plate and beam (subsection 6.8.1);
*problem 276. Extreme cases of transverse deflection of a membrane and weak bending of an elastic plate (subsection 6.8.2).

P. b. Mechanics and Thermodynamics of Deformable Media (subsections 6.8.3–6.8.6):

*problem 277. **Momentum equation** balancing inertia and volume forces and stresses (subsection 6.8.3):

$$f_i + \partial_j T_{ij} = \rho a_i = \rho\frac{dv_i}{dt}; \tag{10.737a, b}$$

*problem 278. **Newton law (1686)** in the absence of stresses for mass independent of time (subsection 6.8.3);
*problem 279. **Balance of moments of forces** and symmetry of the stress tensor (subsection 6.8.4);

*problem 280. **Work** of the volume and surface forces (subsection 6.8.5);
*problem 281. **Internal energy,** including the work of deformation of the stresses on the strains (subsection 6.8.6).

P. c. Stress-Strain Relation for Elastic Materials (subsections 6.8.6–6.8.11):

*problem 282. Residual, elastic, and inelastic stresses (subsection 6.8.6);
*problem 283. Stiffness tensor and matrix, relating the strain and stress tensors in an anisotropic elastic material (subsection 6.8.7);
*problem 284. Stress-strain relation for an isotropic elastic material (subsection 6.8.8);
*problem 285. Relations between the two Lamé elastic moduli and the Young modulus and Poisson ratio (subsection 6.8.8);
*problem 286. **Hooke law (1678)** for an isotropic elastic material in terms of various elastic moduli (subsection 6.8.8);
*problem 287. Stiffness matrix for a homoclinic elastic material with x-plane of symmetry (subsection 6.8.9):
*problem 288. Stiffness matrix for an orthotropic elastic material with three orthogonal planes of systemetry (subsection 6.8.9);
*problem 289. Compliance matrix as the inverse of the stiffness amtrix (subsection 6.8.10);
*problem 290. Compliance matrix for an isotropic elastic material (subsection 6.8.10);
*problem 291. Stiffness and compliance matrices for an orthotropic elastic material (subsections 6.8.10–6.8.11);
*problem 292. Comparison of orthotropic and isotropic elastic materials (subsection 6.8.11).

P. d. Equation for the Transverse Displacement of a Pseudo-Isotropic Orthotropic Elastic Plate (subsections 6.8.12–6.8.16):

*problem 293. Elastic energy for a homogeneous anisotropic material (subsection 6.8.12);
*problem 294. Elastic energy for the weak linear deformation of an orthotropic plate (subsection 6.8.12);
*problem 295. Conditions for a pseudo-isotropic orthotropic elastic material (subsection 6.8.13);
*problem 296. Generalized bending stiffness (10.738) for (10.735b) a pseudo-isotropic orthotropic elastic plate (subsection 6.8.14):

$$D \equiv \frac{h^3}{12}\left[C_{11} - \frac{(C_{13})^2}{C_{33}}\right] = \frac{h^3}{12}\left[C_{22} - \frac{(C_{23})^2}{C_{33}}\right]. \tag{10.738}$$

*problem 297. Comparison of (i) anisotropic, (ii) orthotropic, (iii) pseudo-isotropic orthotropic, and (iv) isotropic elastic (a) materials and (b) plates (subsection 6.8.15).

P. e. Boundary Conditions for a Pseudo-Isotropic Orthotropic Plate (subsection 6.8.6; example 10.15):

*problem 298. General boundary condition for (i) isotropic and (ii) pseudo-isotropic orthotropic plates (subsection 6.8.16);
*problem 299. Particular case of constant first and second bending stiffnesses (subsection 6.8.16);
*problem 300. Relation (10.739) between the elastic energy per unit length of boundary of a plate and the stress couples and turning moment (subsection 6.8.16):

$$\tilde{E}_d = \frac{d\hat{E}_d}{ds} = -N_x\,\delta\zeta - M_n\,\delta(\partial_n\zeta); \tag{10.739}$$

*problem 301. Vanishing of the total elastic energy along the boundary of a (i) isotropic or (ii) pseudo-isotropic orthotropic plate (E10.15.1–E10.15.2);
*problem 302. Stress couple and turning moment for a pseudo-isotropic orthotropic plate of arbitrary shape (E10.15.3);
*problem 303. simplification of the stress couple and turning moment for a pinned plate of arbitrary shape (E10.15.3–E10.15.4);
*problem 304. Problem 303 for a clamped plate (E10.15.3–E10.15.4);
*problem 305. Comparison of (a) stress couple and (b) turning moment for (i) clamped or (ii) pinned plate of an (α) isotropic and (β) pseudo-isotropic orthotropic material (E10.15.5);
*problem 306. Boundary conditions for elastic plates: (i) of arbitrary, circular, or rectangular shape; (ii) with clamped, pinned, or free boundary; (iii) made of isotropic or pseudo-isotropic orthotropic elastic material (E10.15.6–E10.15.9).

P. f. Buckling of a Clamped Rectangular Plate with Normal Stresses (subsection 6.8.17):

*problem 307. Buckled shape of an elastic plate clamped on all four sides and subject to normal stresses only, that is, no shear stress;
*problem 308. Buckling conditions for two orthogonal compressions or one compression and a traction;
*problem 309. Comparison of buckling of a clamped rectangular plate and an elastic beam.

P. g. Buckling of a Clamped-Free Plate with Uniaxial Stresses (subsections 6.8.18–6.8.20):

*problem 310. Three cases distinguishing traction from two ranges of compression;
*problem 311. Buckling for weak compression below a threshold;
*problem 312. Buckling for strong compression in a range.

Q. Non-Linear Coupling of Strong Bending and In-Plate Stresses (section 6.9; example 10.16)

Q. a. Balance Equations for the Strong Bending of an Isotropic Elastic Plate (subsections 6.9.1–6.9.3):

*problem 313. Coupled non-linear fourth-order partial differential equations for the transverse displacement and stress function (subsection 6.9.1);

$$D\nabla^2\zeta - f - h\left[(\partial_{yy}\Theta)(\partial_{xx}\zeta) + (\partial_{xx}\Theta)(\partial_{yy}\zeta) - 2\partial_{yy}\Theta(\partial_{yy}\zeta)\right], \quad (10.740a)$$

$$\nabla^4\Theta = E\left[(\partial_{yy}\zeta)^2 - (\partial_{xy}\zeta)(\partial_{yy}\zeta)\right]; \quad (10.740b)$$

*problem 314. Degenerate linear case of weak bending (10.741a) of a (10.741b) stressed plate (subsection 6.9.1):

$$\nabla^4\zeta = -f, \qquad \nabla^4\Theta = 0; \quad (10.741a, b)$$

*problem 315. Exact strain tensor due to transverse and in-plane displacements of a plate (subsection 6.9.2);
*problem 316. Using the Hooke law and stress function to eliminate the in-plane displacements and keep the transverse displacement in (10.740b) (subsection 6.9.3).

Q. b. Extension of the Balance Equations to a Pseudo-Isotropic Orthotropic Plate (example 10.16):

*problem 317. Extension of the balance equation (10.740a) replacing the bending stiffness for isotropic plates by the generalized bending stiffness (10.738) pseudo-isotropic orthotropic plates;
*problem 318. Extension of complementary equation orthotropic plate with constant compliance matrix;
*problem 319. Extension of the complementary equation (10.740b) to an orthotropic plate in terms of generalized Young moduli, Poisson ratios, and shear moduli;
*problem 320. Two constraints additional to the problem 319 for pseudo-isotropic orthotropic plates.

Q. c. Boundary Conditions for the Transverse Displacement and Stress Function (subsections 6.9.4–6.9.5):

*problem 321. Force-stress balance equation in the absence of in-plane inertia force (subsection 6.9.4);

*problem 322. Boundary condition for the in-plane stress vector and displacement (subsection 6.9.4);
*problem 323. Principle of virtual work, including elastic energies of bending, deflection, and deformation (subsection 6.9.5);
*problem 324. Surface integral in problem 323 leading to (10.740a, b) the balance equations (subsections (subsection 6.9.5);
*problem 325. Boundary integral in problem 323 leading to the boundary conditions (subsection 6.9.5);
*problem 326. Second boundary condition from problem 325 involving the augmented turning moment (subsection 6.9.5);
*problem 327. Conditions for clamped, pinned, and free boundaries in the strong bending of an elastic plate (subsection 6.9.5).

Q. d. Deflection and Bending with an Elliptic Boundary (subsections 6.9.6–6.9.7):

*problem 328. Transverse deflection with an elliptic boundary satisfying the balance (10.740a) and complementary (10.740b) equations (subsection 6.9.6);
*problem 329. Incompatibility of the problem 328 with boundary conditions at low order of approximation (subsection 6.9.7).

Q. e. Perturbation Expansion to all Orders (subsections 6.9.8–6.9.11):

*problem 330. Perturbation expansion to all orders for the transverse displacement and stress function (subsection 6.9.8);
*problem 331. Balance and complementary equations, strains, and stresses, and stress couple and turning moment with axial symmetry (subsection 6.9.9);
*problem 332. The problem 330 simplified for the axisymmetric case, which is dependent only on the distance from the axis (subsection 6.9.10);
*problem 333. Particular integral of the axisymmetric bi-harmonic equation forced by a power (subsection 6.9.11);
*problem 334. Problem 333 extended to forcing by a polynomial or analytic function (subsection 6.9.11).

Q. f. Strong Non-Linear Bending of a Heavy Circular Plate Under Compression (subsections 6.9.12–6.9.17):

*problem 335. Transverse displacement and stress function to lowest non-linear order of approximation (subsections 6.9.12–6.9.13);
*problem 336. Problem 336 with the arbitrary constants determined for a clamped circular plate (subsection 6.9.14);
*problem 337. The displacements, strains, stresses, stress couple, and augmented turning moment for the problem 335 (subsections 6.9.14–6.9.17);
*problem 338. General method of solution for the strong non-linear bending with in-plane stresses, including the particular axisymmetric case (subsection 6.9.17).

R. Waves or Vibrations of Elastic Media (notes 6.1–6.23)

R. a. Non-Linear Waves in Inhomogeneous and Unsteady Media (notes 6.3–6.9):

*problem 339. Non-linear wave equation (10.742c) for the transverse displacement ζ of an elastic string with mass density per unit length ρ_1, tangential tension T, and shear stress f_a, which are all functions (10.742a, b) of position and time (note 6.3):

$$\zeta' \equiv \frac{\partial \zeta}{\partial x}, \dot{\zeta} \equiv \frac{\partial \zeta}{\partial t}: \qquad \left(\rho_1 \dot{\zeta}\right)^{\bullet} - \left\{T\zeta'\left|1+\zeta'^2\right|^{-1/2}\right\}' = f_a(x,t); \qquad (10.742a–c)$$

*problem 340. Non-linear wave equation (10.743) for the transverse displacement ζ of an elastic membrane with mass density ρ_1 and transverse applied force f_a per unit area and isotropic tangential tension T, which are all functions of position and time (note 6.4):

$$\left(\rho_2 \dot{\zeta}\right)^{\bullet} - \nabla.\left\{T\left|1+(\nabla\zeta.\nabla\zeta)\right|^{-1/2}\right\} = f_a(x,y,t). \qquad (10.743)$$

*problem 341. Linear torsional (10.744a) wave equation (10.744b) for the angle of rotation ϕ along a straight elastic rod with moment of inertia I and torsional stiffness of the cross-section C and applied axial torque or moment M_a, which are all functions of position and time (note 6.5):

$$\tau \equiv \dot{\phi}: \qquad \left(I\dot{\phi}\right)^{\bullet} - (C\phi')' = M_a(x,t); \qquad (10.744a, b)$$

*problem 342. Linear wave equation (10.745) for the longitudinal displacement u of a straight elastic rod with mass density per unit length ρ_1, Young modulus E and applied longitudinal force f_a, all depending on position and time (note 6.6).

$$\left(\rho_1 \dot{u}\right)^{\bullet} - (Eu')' = F_a(x,t); \qquad (10.745)$$

*problem 343. Non-linear wave equation (10.746) for the transverse displacement ζ of an elastic beam with mass density per unit length ρ_1, bending stiffness B, tangential tension T, and applied shear stress f_a, which are all functions of position and time (note 6.7):

$$\left(\rho_2 \dot{\zeta}\right)^{\bullet} - \left\{T\zeta'\left|1+\zeta'^2\right|^{-1/2}\right\}' + \left\{B\zeta'\left|1+\zeta'^2\right|^{-3/2}\right\}'' = f_a(x,y,t); \qquad (10.746)$$

*problem 344. Linear wave equation (10.747) for the transverse displacement ζ of an elastic stressed plate with mass density ρ_2 and transverse force f_a per unit area in-plane stresses $T_{\alpha\beta}$ and bending stiffness D, which are all functions of position and time (note 6.8):

$$\left(\rho_2 \dot{\zeta}\right)^{\bullet} - \partial_\alpha \left(T_{\alpha\beta}\, \partial_\beta \zeta\right) + \nabla^2 \left[D\left(\nabla^2 \zeta\right)\right] = f_a\left(x_1, x_2, t\right). \qquad (10.747)$$

R. b. Generalized and Analogous Wave Equations (notes 6.9–6.10):

*problem 345. Analogies of wave variables, inertia, restoring effect, wave speeds, and dispersion stiffness (note 6.9);
*problem 346. Linear general bending wave equation in one-dimension (10.748) for a wave variable ζ with mass density per unit length ρ_1, tangential tension T, bending stiffness B, friction coefficient μ, translational ν, and rotary ϑ spring resiliences, and shear stress f_a all depending on position and time (note 6.10):

$$\left(\rho_2 \dot{\zeta}\right)^{\bullet} - \left(T\zeta'\right)' + \left(B\zeta''\right)'' + \mu\dot{\zeta} + \nu\zeta + \vartheta\zeta' = f_a\left(x, t\right); \qquad (10.748)$$

*problem 347. Linear general bending wave equation in two dimensions (10.749) for the wave variable ζ with mass density per área ρ_2, in-plane stresses $T_{\alpha\beta}$, bending stiffness D, friction coefficient μ, translational spring resilience ν , vector rotary spring resilience ϑ, and transverse force per unit area f_a which are all functions of position and time (note 6.10):

$$\left(\rho_2 \dot{\zeta}\right)^{\bullet} - \partial_\alpha \left(T_{\alpha\beta}\, \partial_\beta \zeta\right) + \nabla^2 \left(D\nabla^2 \zeta\right) + \mu\dot{\zeta} + \nu\zeta + \vec{\vartheta}.\nabla\zeta = f_a\left(x, y, t\right); \qquad (10.749)$$

*problem 348. Particular case of problem 346 for the classical one-dimensional bending wave equation (10.750) for the wave variable ζ with damping χ, translational ω_t, and rotational ω_r natural frequencies, elastic wave speed, c_e and dispersion stiffness parameter b (note 6.10):

$$\ddot{\zeta} + 2\chi\dot{\zeta} + \omega_t^2\, \zeta + \omega_r^2\, \zeta' - c_e^2\, \zeta'' + b\, \zeta'''' = \rho_1^{-1}\; f_a\left(x, t\right); \qquad (10.750)$$

*problem 349. Particular case of problem 347 for the classic two-dimensional bi-dimensional bending wave equation (10.751) for the wave variable ζ, as in the one-dimensional case (10.750) with two wave speeds $c_{1,2}$ in the principal stress directions, a vector $\omega_{r1,2}$ natural frequency for the rotary spring and a dispersion stiffness parameter b (note 6.10):

$$\begin{aligned} &\ddot{\zeta} + 2\chi\dot{\zeta} + \omega_t^2\, \zeta + \omega_{r1}^2\, \partial_1 \zeta + \omega_{r2}^2\, \partial_2\, \zeta - c_1^2\, \partial_{11} \zeta \\ &\quad - c_2^2\, \partial_{22} \zeta + \bar{b}^2 \left(\partial_{11} + \partial_{22}\right)^2 \zeta = \rho_1^{-1}\; f_a\left(x, y, t\right). \end{aligned} \qquad (10.751)$$

R. c. Generalized Classical Bending Wave Equation in One-Dimension with Constant Coefficients (notes 6.11–6.13):

*problem 350. Solution by separation of variables of (10.752) the one-dimensional classical bending wave equation with constant coefficients and without forcing (note 6.11):

$$\rho_1 \ddot{\zeta} + \mu \dot{\zeta} + \nu \zeta + \vartheta \zeta' - T\zeta'' + B\zeta'''' = 0. \tag{10.752}$$

*problem 351. Fundamental and harmonics of the spatial modes specifying the wavelengths and wavenumbers (note 6.12);
*problem 352. Dispersion relation for linear transversal waves in an elastic beam with constant mass density per unit length, tangential tension, bending stiffness, and translational spring resilience (note 6.13);
*problem 353. Frequencies and periods of the fundamental mode and harmonics of a uniform elastic string (note 6.14).

R. d. Non-Dispersive and Dispersive Free Wave Propagation and Standing Modes (notes 6.14–6.17):

*problem 354. Phase and phase speeds of non-dispersive waves with a permanent waveform, which are solutions of the classical wave equation (note 6.14);
*problem 355. First-order permanent waveforms propagating in opposite directions and their superposition with the same amplitude in second-order standing modes (note 6.15);
*problem 356. Phase speed and group velocity for dispersive waves (note 6.16);
*problem 357. Dispersion relation, phase speed, and group velocity for transverse waves along an elastic beam (note 6.16);
*problem 358. Propagation of a non-dispersive or a dispersive wave packet (note 6.16);
*problem 359. General free wave field as a solution of the unforced wave equation specified by a superposition of eigenfunctions, corresponding to the eigenvalues with arbitrary amplitudes (note 6.17).

R. e. Wave Generation by Out-of-Equilibrium Initial Conditions and Forcing (notes 6.18–6.23):

*problem 360. Determination of the amplitudes of the eigenfunctions from the initial conditions, which in the case out-of-equilibrium specify wave generation (note 6.18);
*problem 361. Wave generation by forcing at an applied frequency with bounded fluctuation as a function of position (note 6.19);
*problem 362. Damped non-resonant forcing, which is with applied frequency distinct from the fundamental frequency and all its harmonics (notes 6.20–6.21);

*problem 363. Damped resonant forcing, which is with applied frequency equal to the fundamental frequency or equal to any of its harmonics (note 6.21);
*problem 364. Undamped non-resonant forcing, like problem 363 without damping (note 6.22);
*problem 365. Undamped resonant forcing, like problem 364 without damping (note 6.22).

S. Waves in Inhomogeneous Media (notes 7.1–7.21)

S. a. Classification of Wave Equations (notes 7.1–7.7):

*problem 366. One-dimensional non-linear waves in an unsteady inhomogeneous medium (note 7.3):

$$0 = F\left(x, t; \Phi, \frac{\partial \Phi}{\partial x}, \frac{\partial \Phi}{\partial t}, \frac{\partial^2 \Phi}{\partial x^2}, \frac{\partial^2 \Phi}{\partial t^2}, \frac{\partial^2 \Phi}{\partial x \, \partial t^2}, \ldots, \frac{\partial^{N+M} \Phi}{\partial x^N \, \partial t^M}\right); \tag{10.753}$$

*problem 367. One-dimensional forced linear waves in an unsteady inhomogeneous medium (note 7.3):

$$\sum_{n=0}^{N} \sum_{m=0}^{M} A_{nm}(x,t) \frac{\partial^{N+M} \Phi}{\partial x^N \, \partial t^M} = B(x,t); \tag{10.754}$$

*problem 368. One-dimensional forced linear waves in a steady homogeneous media (note 7.4): as (10.754) with constant coefficients A_{nm};
*problem 369. One-dimensional forced linear waves in a steady inhomogeneous media (note 7.5): as (10.754) with coefficients A_{nm} depending only on position x.

S. b. Quasi-One-Dimensional Waves in Inhomogeneous Media (notes 7.6–7.17):

*problem 370. Wave equation (10.755c) for the transverse displacement ζ in the free-linear (10.755a) vibrations of an **elastic string** under tangential tension T with mass density per unit length (10.755b) independent of time (notes 7.8–7.9):

$$\left(\frac{\partial \zeta}{\partial x}\right)^2 \ll 1, \quad \frac{\partial \sigma}{\partial t} = 0: \qquad \frac{\partial^2 \zeta}{\partial t^2} - \frac{1}{\sigma(x)} \frac{\partial}{\partial x}\left[T(x,t) \frac{\partial \zeta}{\partial x}\right] = 0; \tag{10.755a–c}$$

*problem 371. Wave equation (10.756d) for the **torsion** τ, which is the rate of rotation along the axis (10.756a), in the linear-free torsional oscillations of a straight elastic rod with moment of inertia I and torsional stiffness C of the cross-section that (10.756b, c) do not depend on time (note 7.10):

$$\tau \equiv \frac{\partial \phi}{\partial x}; \quad \frac{\partial I}{\partial t} = 0 = \frac{\partial C}{\partial t}: \qquad \frac{\partial^2 \tau}{\partial t^2} - \frac{1}{I(x)} \frac{\partial}{\partial x}\left[C(x)\frac{\partial \tau}{\partial x}\right] = 0; \tag{10.756a–d}$$

*problem 372. Wave equation (10.757c) for the longitudinal **displacement** u in the free-linear longitudinal oscillations of an elastic rod with mass density per unit length σ and Young modulus E that (10.757a, b) do not depend on time (note 7.11):

$$\frac{\partial \sigma}{\partial t} = 0 = \frac{\partial E}{\partial t}: \qquad \frac{\partial^2 u}{\partial t^2} - \frac{1}{\sigma(x)} \frac{\partial}{\partial x}\left[E(x)\frac{\partial u}{\partial x}\right] = 0; \tag{10.757a–c}$$

*problem 373. Wave equation (10.758e) for the transverse displacement ζ of the free-linear **surface waves** of an incompressible fluid (10.758a) in a uniform gravity field (10.758b) in a channel whose width b and depth h do not (10.758c, d) depend on time (notes 7.12–7.13):

$$\rho, g = const; \quad \frac{\partial b}{\partial t} = 0 = \frac{\partial h}{\partial t}: \qquad \frac{\partial^2 \zeta}{\partial t^2} - \frac{g}{b(x)} \frac{\partial}{\partial x}\left[h(x)b(x)\frac{\partial \zeta}{\partial x}\right] = 0; \tag{10.758a–e}$$

*problem 374. Wave equation (10.759e) for the electric field E of **electromagnetic waves** in a medium with di-electric permittivity ε and magnetic permeability μ independent of time (10.759c, d) in the absence of electric charges and currents (10.759a, b) involving the speed of light *in vacuo* c_0 (notes 7.14–7.15):

$$q = 0 = \vec{J}; \quad \frac{\partial \varepsilon}{\partial t} = 0 = \frac{\partial \mu}{\partial t}: \qquad \frac{\partial^2 E}{\partial t^2} - \frac{c_0^2}{\varepsilon(x)} \frac{\partial}{\partial x}\left[\frac{1}{\mu(x)}\frac{\partial E}{\partial x}\right] = 0; \tag{10.759a–e}$$

*problem 375. Wave equation (10.760c) for the acoustic pressure perturbation p of free-linear (10.760a) **sound waves**, which is with velocity perturbation v small compared with the sound speed c_s, in a **horn**, which is a duct with variable cross-sectional area A, which does not (10.760b) depend on time (notes 7.16–7.17):

$$\left(\frac{v}{c_s}\right)^2 << 1, \quad \frac{\partial A}{\partial t} = 0: \qquad \frac{\partial^2 p}{\partial t^2} - \frac{c_s^2}{A(x)} \frac{\partial}{\partial x}\left[A(x)\frac{\partial p}{\partial x}\right] = 0. \tag{10.760a–c}$$

S. c. Analogies among Six Types of Waves (notes 7.18–7.19):

*problem 376. Primal (10.761a) and dual (10.761b) **wave equations** (note 7.18):

$$\frac{\partial^2\Phi}{\partial t^2}-\left[c(x)\right]^2\left[\frac{\partial^2\Phi}{\partial t^2}+\frac{1}{L(x)}\frac{\partial\Phi}{\partial t}\right]=0, \tag{10.761a}$$

$$\frac{\partial^2\Phi}{\partial t^2}-\frac{\partial}{\partial x}\left\{\left[c(x)\right]^2\left[\frac{\partial\Psi}{\partial x}+\frac{\Psi}{L(x)}\right]\right\}=0, \tag{10.761b}$$

*problem 377. Primary wave variables (note 7.18);
*problem 378. Dual variables (note 7.18);
*problem 379. Inertia effects (note 7.19);
*problem 380. Restoring effects (note 7.20);
*problem 381. Phase speeds (note 7.20);
*problem 382. Lengthscales (note 7.20).

S. d. Duality Principles for Wave Variables (notes 7.21–7.22):

*problem 383. Duality principle for acoustic horns, problem 375 (note 7.20);
*problem 384. Duality principle for water waves in a channel, problem 373 (note 7.20);
*problem 385. Duality principle for electromagnetic waves in a dielectric, problem 374 (note 7.20);
*problem 386. Duality principle for the transverse oscillations of elastic strings, problem 370 (note 7.21);
*problem 387. Duality principle for the torsional oscillations of a rod, problem 371 (note 7.21);
*problem 388. Duality principle for the longitudinal oscillations of a rod, problem 372 (note 7.21).

T. Acoustics of Horns (notes 7.22–7.46)

T. a. General Properties (notes 7.22–7.27):

*problem 389. Horn wave equations for the acoustic pressure and velocity pertubation spectra (note 7.22);
*problem 390. Invariant form of the horn wave equation for the reduced acoustic pressure and velocity perturbation spectra (note 7.23);
*problem 391. Polarization relations between the acoustic pressure and velocity perturbation spectra in original and reduced form (note 7.24);

*problem 392. Classical wave equation for sound in a duct of constant cross-section (note 7.25);
*problem 393. Ray approximation for sound propagation in a horn with a wavelength short compared with the lengthscale of variations in cross-section (note 7.26).

T. b. Exact Elementary Solutions (notes 7.27–7.35):

*problem 394. The exponential horn as the only self-dual duct (note 7.28);
*problem 395. Filtering function as the solution of a filtering equation involving a cut-off frequency and leading to a reduced wavenumber (note 7.29);
*problem 396. Acoustic pressure and velocity perturbations in an exponential horn involving the filtering function (note 7.30);
*problem 397. Sound field in a catenoidal horn with a filtering function for the acoustic pressure perturbation spectrum (note 7.31);
*problem 398. Sound field in an inverse catenoidal horn with a filtering function for the acoustic velocity pertubation spectrum (note 7.32);
*problem 399. Imaginary change of lengthscale leading from the filtering to the transparency equation and function (note 7.33);
*problem 400. Sound field in a sinusoidal horn involving a transparency function for the acoustic pressure perturbation spectrum (note 7.33);
*problem 401. Sound field in an inverse sinusoidal horn involving a transparency function for the velocity perturbation spectrum (note 7.34);
*problem 402. Five shapes of horn for which the horn wave equation has exact solutions in terms of elementary functions (note 7.35).

T. c. Gaussian Horn and Displacement Amplifier (notes 7.36–7.38):

*problem 403. Exact solution of the wave equation in a Gaussian horn in terms of Hermite functions (note 7.36);
*problem 404. Acoustic pressure and velocity perturbation spectra in a Gaussian horn in terms of Hermite functions (note 7.36);
*problem 405. Frequencies of oscillation of an elastic rod with Gaussian cross-section for which the longitudinal displacement is specified by an Hermite polynomial (notes 7.37–7.38);
*problem 406. Fundamental frequency of Gaussian elastic rod used as a displacement amplifier for which the strain and stress are constant (note 7.38).

T. d. Power Law Horns and Cylindrical/Spherical Waves (notes 7.39–7.46):

*problem 407. Asymptotic scaling of the sound field in a power-law duct at large distance when the ray approximation holds (note 7.39);
*problem 408. Acoustic pressure and velocity perturbation spectra in a power-law horn in terms of Hankel functions (notes 7.40–7.41);
*problem 409. Cylindrical waves in a wedge due to a line-source at the edge (note 7.42);

*problem 410. Acoustic pressure and velocity perturbation spectra of cylindrical waves in the far-field (notes 7.42–7.43);
*problem 411. Spherical waves in a conical horn due to a point sound source at the vertex (note 7.44);
*problem 412. Acoustic pressure and velocity perturbation spectra for spherical waves in a conical horn that coincide as exact and asymptotic fields (note 7.44).

T. e. Reflection and Transmission at Interfaces (notes 7.47–7.55):

*problem 413. Impedance of a plane wave (note 7.47);
*problem 414. Locally-reacting boundary condition in terms of the specific impedance (note 7.47);
*problem 415. Reflection and surface adsorption coefficient for a plane wave incident normal to a locally reacting wall (note 7.48);
*problem 416. Wavelength and amplification or attenuation of standing modes trapped between walls with distinct specific impedances (notes 7.49–7.50);
*problem 417. Acoustic boundary conditions at the junction of two ducts with different cross-sections and containing fluids with distinct mass densities and sound speeds (note 7.51);
*problem 418. Reflection and transmission coefficients of sound waves at the junction of two tubes in terms of the overall impedance (note 7.52);
*problem 419. Scattering matrix for sound incident from either side at the junction between ducts with different cross-sections and containing distinct fluids (notes 7.53–7.54);
*problem 420. High (low) frequency limits of short (long) waves in the ray (scattering) approximations to the exact diffraction theory of wave refraction in inhomogeneous and/or unsteady media (note 7.55).

U. Oscillators with Several Degrees-of-Freedom (sections 8.1–8.2):

U. a. Equations of Motion and Energy Balance (section 8.1 and subsection 8.2.1):

*problem 421. Linear restoring and quadratic potential depending on the position (subsections 8.1.1–8.1.2);
*problem 422. Linear kinetic friction force and quadratic dissipation function depending on the velocity (subsections 8.1.1 and 8.1.3);
*problem 423. Equation of motion of a multi-dimensional linear oscillator, with inertia, restoring, friction, and external forces, in the case of coupled or decoupled degrees-of-freedom (subsections 8.1.1–8.1.4);

*problem 424. Energy balance equation the work of the external forces minus the dissipation by friction forces against the total energy, consisting of kinetic and potential energies (subsections 8.1.5–8.1.6);
*problem 425. Particular case of decoupled oscillators with (i) separate equations of motion and (ii)(iii) potential (dissipation) functions that involve only squares of position (velocity) and no cross-products (subsections 8.1.5–8.1.6);
*problem 426. Generalized equation of motion with explicit accelerations $\ddot{x}_r$, involving damping λ_{rs} and oscillations ω_{rs}^2 matrices, and reduced external forces $f_r(t)$ (subsection 8.2.1):

$$r = 1,\ldots,N: \qquad \frac{d^2 x_r}{dt^2} + \sum_{s=1}^{N}\left(2\lambda_{rs}\frac{dx_s}{dt} + \omega_{rs}^2\, x_s\right) = f_r(t). \qquad (10.762\text{a, b})$$

U. b. Simultaneous Multi-Dimensional Free Oscillations (subsections 8.2.2–8.2.8):

*problem 427. Modes of a multidimensional linear (10.762a, b) unforced (10.763a) oscillator as the roots (10.763c) of the determinant (10.763b) of the dispersion matrix (subsection 8.2.2):

$$F_r = 0: \qquad 0 = \mathrm{Det}\left(\delta_{rs}\xi^2 + 2\lambda_{rs}\xi + \omega_{rs}^2\right) = \prod_{n=1}^{2N}(\xi - \xi_n); \qquad (10.763\text{a–c})$$

*problem 428. Modal frequencies for free (10.763a) undamped $\lambda_{rs} = 0$ multidimensional oscillations around a position of stable equilibrium (subsections 8.2.3–8.2.4);
*problem 429. Modal frequencies and dampings for the free (10.763a) damped linear (10.762a, b) multi-dimensional oscillator (subsection 8.2.5);
*problem 430. Oscillation frequencies appearing in the modal coordinates of linear free (10.763a) multidimensional (10.762a, b) oscillators (subsection 8.2.6);
*problem 431. The transformation matrix relating the modal to the physical coordinates gives zero if multiplied by (problem 427) the dispersion matrix (subsection 8.2.7);
*problem 432. The transformation matrix is specified by the co-factors of the dispersion matrix evaluated at the modal frequencies and dampings (subsection 8.2.7);
*problem 433. Physical coordinates as functions of time for the free (10.763a) linear multidimensional oscillator (10.762a, b) satisfying the compatibility and initial conditions (subsection 8.2.8).

U. c. Multiple Resonance and Forced Motions (subsections 8.2.8–8.2.16):

*problem 434. Transformation from the physical to the modal coordinates: the inverse of the problem 431 (subsection 8.2.9);

*problem 435. Transformation between physical and modal forces (subsection 8.2.9);
*problem 436. Non-diagonal (diagonal) dispersion operators for the linear multidimensional oscillator with damping and reduced external physical (nodal) forces (subsection 8.2.10);
*problem 437. Diagonalization (10.764a, b) of the linearized forced multidimensional oscillator (10.762a, b), in terms of modal coordinates $q_\ell(t)$, reduced forces $g_\ell(\ell)$, frequencies ω_ℓ, and dampings λ_ℓ (subsection 8.2.11):

$$\ell = 1,\ldots,N: \qquad \frac{d^2 q_\ell}{dt^2} + 2\lambda_\ell \frac{d^2 q_\ell}{dt^2} + \omega_\ell^2 q_\ell = g_\ell(t); \tag{10.764a, b}$$

*problem 438. Solution of the equations of motion (10.762a, b) for the linear forced damped multidimensional oscillator via (10.764a, b) modal coordinates (subsections 8.2.11–8.2.12);
*problem 439. Modal matrix for the sinusoidal forcing of the (10.762a, b) linear damped multidimensional oscillator (subsection 8.2.13);
*problem 440. Sinusoidal forcing of (10.762a, b) the undamped $\lambda_{rs} = 0$ linear multidimensional oscillator (subsection 8.2.14);
*problem 441. Sinusoidal forcing, beats, and resonance of an undamped linear multidimensional oscillator, in terms of modal coordinates (subsection 8.2.15);
*problem 442. Sinusoidal forcing of a linear multidimensional damped oscillator, in terms of modal coordinates (subsection 8.2.16);
*problem 443. Diagonalization to a sum of squares of the potential and kinetic energies and dissipation function of a linear multidimensional oscillator (10.762a, b), using modal coordinates (subsection 8.2.16);
*problem 444. Three (four) cases of free (forced) oscillations of (10.764a, b) the linear multidimensional oscillator (subsection 8.2.16).

V. Coupled Two-Dimensional Oscillators (sections 8.3–8.5)

$$\begin{bmatrix} \dot{x}_1 \\ \ddot{x}_2 \end{bmatrix} + 2\begin{bmatrix} \lambda_{11} & \lambda_{12} \\ \lambda_{21} & \lambda_{22} \end{bmatrix}\begin{bmatrix} \dot{x}_1 \\ \dot{x}_2 \end{bmatrix} + \begin{bmatrix} \omega_1^2 & \omega_{12}^2 \\ \omega_{21}^2 & \omega_{22}^2 \end{bmatrix}\begin{bmatrix} x_1 \\ x_2 \end{bmatrix} = \begin{bmatrix} f_1(t) \\ f_2(t) \end{bmatrix}. \tag{10.765}$$

V. a. Mechanical and Electrical Analogues (section 8.3):

*problem 445. Modal frequencies for the undamped free oscillations of two masses connected by three springs between two fixed walls (subsection 8.3.1);

*problem 446. Modal frequencies for the undamped free oscillations of two coupled electrical circuits analogous to the two-dimensional mechanical oscillator in problem 445 (subsection 8.3.2);
*problem 447. Coupled vertical translational and rotational oscillations of a two-wheeled vehicle with distinct springs and dampers and choice of the moment of inertia and position of the center of mass (subsection 8.3.3);
*problem 448. Analogies among the variables, parameters, and forcing of the coupled electrical (mechanical) circuits in the problem(s) 446 (445 and 447), which satisfy a similar system of coupled linear differential equations (109) with constant coefficients (subsection 8.3.4);
*problem 449. Analogous modal matrices, consisting of mass, damping and resilience matrices, and analogous forcing vectors for problem(s) 446 (445 and 447) of electrical (mechanical) linear two-dimensional oscillators (subsection 8.3.5).

V. b. Translational and Rotational Free Oscillations of a Body (section 8.4):

*problem 450. Modal (natural) frequencies for the coupled (decoupled) free undamped rotational and translational oscillations of the two-wheeled vehicle in problem 447 (subsection 8.4.1);
*problem 451. Natural frequencies of translation and rotation for the decoupled case of two masses at fixed distance, like a diatomic molecule (subsection 8.4.2);
*problem 452. Extension to the coupled modal frequencies for the diatomic molecule (problem 451), which is a particular case of problem 447 ≡ 451 (subsection 8.4.3.);
*problem 453. Modal frequencies of the coupled oscillations of translation and rotation of a rod with center of mass in the middle, which is a particular case of problem 447 ≡ 451 (subsection 8.4.4);
*problem 454. Modal frequencies of the coupled translational and rotational frequencies of a homogeneous rod, which is a particular case of problem 453 (subsection 8.4.5);
*problem 455. Modal coordinates for the free undamped coupled translational and rotational oscillations of a homogeneous rod, specifying the points that oscillate only at one frequency (subsection 8.4.6);
*problem 456. Amplitudes and phases of the oscillations in problem 455, determined from initial conditions for the translational coordinate and velocity, and the rotation angle and angular velocity (subsection 8.4.7);
*problem 457. Method of application of initial conditions alternative to problem 456 (subsection 8.4.8);
*problem 458. Modal frequencies and dampings for the free coupled translational and rotational oscillations of a homogeneous rod in the case of subcritical damping (subsection 8.4.9);

*problem 459. Explicit natural frequencies and dampings for the free decoupled translational and rotational oscillations of a homogeneous rod, as a particular case of problem 458 (subsection 8.4.10);
*problem 460. Four exact relations satisfied by the modal frequencies and dampings of problem 458, for strong damping and coupling of translational and rotational motions (subsection 8.4.11);
*problem 461. Weak modal dampings and unchanged modal frequencies for problem 458 ≡ 460, in the case of weak damping (subsection 8.4.12).

V. c. Forced Oscillations, Beats, and Resonance of a Rod (section 8.5):

*problem 462. Non-resonant undamped forced coupled translational and rotational oscillations of a homogeneous rod (subsection 8.5.1);
*problem 463. As in problem 462, the resonant case when the applied frequency of the sinusoidal forcing coincides with one of the modal frequencies (subsection 8.5.2);
*problem 464. Forced coupled sinusoidal oscillations of an homogeneous rod in the non-resonant case in terms of modal coordinates (subsection 8.5.3);
*problem 465. As in problem 464, the resonant case of applied frequency of sinusoidal forcing coincident with one of the modal frequencies (subsections 8.5.3–8.5.4);
*problem 466. As in problem 464, in the case of beats, which is applied frequency close to a modal frequency (subsection 8.5.4);
*problem 467. Sinusoidal forcing with damping of the coupled translational and rotational oscillations of a inhomogeneous rod, both in the resonant and non-resonant cases (subsection 8.5.5).

W. Principle of the Vibration Absorber (section 8.6):

*problem 468. A **vibration absorber** is a secondary undamped unforced oscillator coupled to a primary damped forced oscillator (subsection 8.6.1);
*problem 469. The forced vibrations in the primary damped oscillator are transferred to the secondary damped oscillator if the natural frequency of the latter equals the frequency applied to the former (subsection 8.6.2);
*problem 470. Proof that the transient oscillations decay in both the primary and secondary circuits, due to damping in the former, assuming equal spring resiliences (condenser capacities) in the mechanical (electrical) case (subsection 8.6.3);
*problem 471. Natural frequencies of the undamped coupled vibration absorber, which coincide with the modal frequencies in the case of weak damping (subsection 8.6.4);

*problem 472. Modal dampings of the vibration absorber in the case of weak damping (subsection 8.6.4);
*problem 473. Operation of the vibration absorber, including application of the initial conditions (subsections 8.6.5–8.6.6).

X. Radioactive Disintegration Chain (section 8.7):

*problem 474. Radioactive disintegration chain in which the total mass is conserved and ultimately for long time is concentrated in the last element (subsection 8.7.1);
*problem 475. Decay with time of the mass of the first element of the radioactive disintegration chain (subsection 8.7.2);
*problem 476. Decay with time of the mass of the second element of the radioactive disintegration chain in the non-resonant case of distinct disintegration rates (subsection 8.7.2);
*problem 477. As in problem 476, the resonant case of coincidence of the first two radioactive disintegration rates (subsection 8.7.3);
*problem 478. Decay with time of the mass of the third element in the radioactive disintegration chain in the rotally non-resonant case when the three disintegration rates are distinct (subsections 8.7.4–8.7.5);
*problem 479. As in problem 478, the singly resonant case when the first two radioactive disintegration rates coincide and are distinct from the third (subsection 8.7.6);
*problem 480. As in problem 478, the doubly resonant case when all three disintegration rates coincide (subsection 8.7.7);
*problem 481. Decay with time of the mass of the third element of the radioactive disintegration chain in the single non-resonant (problem 478) and doubly resonant (problem 480) cases, plus three singly-resonant cases, of which problem 479 is one (subsection 8.7.7);
*problem 482. Decay of mass with time of the k-th element of the radioactive disintegration chain in the non-resonant extreme of all disintegration rates distinct (subsection 8.7.8);
*problem 483. As in problem 482, the opposite maximum resonance with all disintegration rates equal (subsection 8.7.8);
*problem 484. As in problems 482 and 483, in the intermediate case of multiple resonances due to the coincidence of some but not all disintegration rates (subsection 8.7.8);
*problem 485. Accumulation of the total mass of the radioactive disintegration chain towards the last element as a function of time (subsection 8.7.8);
*problem 486. Determination of all arbitrary constants in the mass as a function of time of k-th element of the radioactive disintegration chain from the initial masses of all the preceding elements (subsection 8.7.8).

Y. Sequence of Linked Oscillators (section 8.8):

*problem 487. Equations of motion for an N-dimensional forced damped oscillator, consisting of a sequence of oscillators (subsection 8.8.1);
*problem 488. Modal frequencies of an undamped unforced oscillator with three degrees-of-freedom associated with a sequence of three masses connected by four springs between two fixed walls (subsection 8.8.2);
*problem 489. Particular cases of problem 488, when the middle mass is much larger (smaller) than the other two leading to decoupling (strong coupling) (subsection 8.8.3);
*problem 490. Comparison of a radioactive disintegration chain with N elements with a sequence of mechanical (electrical) forced oscillators consisting of N masses (selfs) connected by $N + 1$ springs (capacitors) and dampers (resistors) with applied mechanical (electromotive) forces (subsection 8.8.4);
*problem 491. Modal frequencies and dampings of the unforced N-dimensional linear damped oscillator consisting of the sequence of N oscillators in problem 487 (subsection 8.8.5);
*problem 492. Modal coordinates for the N-dimensional oscillator in problem 487, with modal dampings and frequencies in problem 491, and amplitudes and phases determined by a sequence of continued fractions (subsection 8.8.6);
*problem 493. Determination of the modal amplitudes for three (four)-dimensional oscillators in problem 492 (subsection 8.8.7).

Z. Signals along a Transmission Line (section 8.9):

*problem 494 (495). Electrical (mechanical) impedance relating the electromotive (mechanical) force to the electric current (velocity) in a circuit (system) consisting of self (mass), resistor (damper), and capacitor (spring) elements (subsections 8.9.1–8.9.2);
*problem 496. Resistance (inductance) as the real (imaginary) part of the impedance, and relation with its inverse or admittance (subsection 8.9.2);
*problem 497. Five cases of operation of an infinite transmission line with two distinct sets of impedances in series and parallel (subsections 8.9.2–8.9.4);
*problem 498. Two sets of three cases of transmission lines depending on which of the self/resistance/capacitor lies in parallel or sequence (subsection 8.9.5);
*problem 499. Transmission line without dissipation, that is, without resistances (subsection 8.9.6);
*problem 500. Five regimes of signal passage along a non-dissipative infinite transmission line, including (a) signal reflection (b) frequency cut-off, and (c) lossless transmission in a frequency pass band above a cut-off frequency (subsections 8.9.6–8.9.7).

References

1678 Hooke, R. *De Potentia Restitutiva*. London, UK.

1686 Newton, I. *Principia*. Cambridge University Press, reprinted Dover 1934.

1691 Bernoulli, J. *Acta Eruditorium* 553 (*Opera* 1, 663).

1691 Bernoulli, J. *Differentialrechnung*. Manuscript found in 1921.

1695 Bernoulli, J. *Acta Erudita* **59–67**, 537–557.

1696 Leibnitz, G. W. *Acta Erudita* 145 (*Mathematische Werke* **5**, 329).

1696 L'Hôspital, G. F. A. *Annalyse des Infinitement Petits pour l'Intelligence des Courbes*. Paris.

1697 Bernoulli, J. "Problema pure Geometricum Eruditis Propofisum: De Conoitibus Spheroidibus Quadam." *Acta Evuditorium* 113–124.

1724 Ricatti, J. F. "Animadversiones in Equationes Diferentiales Secundi Gradus." *Acta Erudita Supplementa* **8**, 66–75.

1729 Euler, L. "Letter to Goldbach."

1734 Clairaut, A. C. "Solution de Plusieurs Problemes ou il s'agit de Trouver les Courbes dont la Proprieté Consiste dans une Certaine Relation entre les Branches Exprimée par Une Equation Donnée." *Histoire de l'Academic de Paris*, 196–215.

1743 Euler, L. *Miscelanea Berologica* **7**, 193 (*Institutiones Calculis Integralis* **2**, 375).

1748 D'Alembert, J. R. *Histoire de l'Académie de Berlin* **4**, 275.

1748 D'Alembert, J. R. "Suite des Recherches sur le Calcul Integral. Quatiéme Partie: Méthodes pour Intégrer Quelques Équations Differentielles." *Histoire de l'Académie de Berlin* **4**, 275–291.

1762 D'Alembert, J. R. *Miscelanea Turinesia*, 381.

1763 D'Alembert, J. R. *Histoire de l'Academie de Berlin*, 242.

1765 Lagrange, J. L. *Miscelanea Turinesia* **3**, 181 (*Oeuvres* **1**, 473).

1766 Euler, L. "De Motu Vibratorio Tympanorum." *Novi Commentari Academia Petropolitana* **10**, 243–260.

1769 Euler, L. *Institutiones Calculis Integralis* **2**, 483.

1771 Van der Monde, A. T. "Memoire sur la Resolutions des Équations." *Histoire de l'Académie des Sciences de Paris*, 365–416 (1774).

1772 Euler, L. *Novi Commentary Academia Scientarum Imperialis Petropolitana* **16**.

1772 Van der Monde, A. T. "Mémoire sur l'Elimination." *Histoire de l'Académie des Sciences de Paris*, 516–532 (1776).

1778 Euler, L. *Nova Acta Academia Scientarum Imperialis Petropolitana* **7**, 58.

1785 Legendre, A. M. "Sur l'Attraction des Spheroides." *Mémoires de Mathématique et Physique Presentées à l'Académie Royalle des Sciences par Divers Savants*, 10.

1807 Poisson, S. D. "Mémoire sur la Théorie du Son." *Journal de l'École Polytechnique* **7**, 367–390.

1812 Gauss, C. F. "Disquisitiones circam Seriem Infinitam ..." *Commentationes Societones Regiae Scientarum Göttensis Recentiores* (*Werke* **1**, 185).

1812 Hoene-Wronski, J. *Refutation de la Théorie des Fonctions Analytiques de Lagrange*. Paris.

1812 Laplace, P. S. *Théorie des Probabilités*. Gauthier-Villars, Paris.

1815 Cauchy, A. A. "Mémoire sur les Fonctions qui ne Peuvent Obtenir que Deux Valeurs." *Journal de l'École Polytechnique* **17**, 29–107 (*Oeuvres*, série 2, **1**, 91–169, Gaultier-Villars, 1905, Paris).

1818 Fourier, J. B. *Theorie Analytique de la Chaleur.* Reprinted Dover, New York, 1953.

1824 Bessel, F. W. "Untersuchung der Theils der Planetarischen Storungen Welchear aus des Bewegung der Sonne Entsteht." *Berliner Abhandlungen.*

1827 Cauchy, A. L. *Exercices Mathematiques* **2**, 159 (*Oeuvres* 7, 198).

1836 Kummer, E. E. "Ueber die Hypergeometrische Reihe." *Journal für die reine und angewandte Mathematik* **83**, 127–172.

1838 Airy, G. B. "On the Intensity of Light Near a Caustic." *Transactions of the Cambridge Philosophical Society* **6**, 379–402.

1850 Malmsten, C. J. "Théoremes sur l'Équation Differentielle." *Cambridge and Dublin Mathematical Journal* **5**, 180–182.

1853 Riemann, B. "Üeber die Darstellbarkeit einer Function durch eine Trignometrische Reihe." *Gescimmelte Mathematischan Werke* 227–271, reprinted Dover, New York.

1856 Weiertrass, K. T. W. "Theorie des Abel'schen Functionen." *Journal für Mathematik* **52**, 285–379.

1859 Chebychev, P. L. "Sur les Questions de Minima, qui se Ratachent à la Representation Approximative des Fonctions." *Mémoires de l'Académie Scientique de St. Petersbourg* **7**, 199–291 (*Oeuvres* **1**, 271–378).

1859 Jacobi, C. G. J. "Untersuchungen über die Differentialglechung der Hypergeometrischen Reihe." *Journal für die reine und angewandte Mathematik* **56**, 149–165.

1863 Maxwell, J. C. *Treatise of Electricity and Magnetism.* Clarendan Press, Oxford.

1864 Hermite, C. "Sur un Nouveau Development en Série de Fonctions." *Comptes Rendus de l'Académie des Sciences* **58**, 93–100, 266, 273 (*Oeuvres* **2**, 293–308, Gauthiers Villars, 1908).

1864 Lipshitz, R. "De Explicatione per Series Trignometricas Instituenda Functionum Unices Variablis Arbitrarium, et Praecipue Earum, qua per Variablis Spatium Finitum Valorum Maximum et Minimum Numerarum Habent Infinitum Disquisition." *Journal für die reine und angewandte Mathematik* **63**, 296–308.

1866 Fuchs, J. L. "Zur Theorie der Linearen Differentialgleichungen mit Verändlichen Koefflizienten." *Journal für die reine und angewandte Mathematik* **66**, 121–160; **68**, 354–385.

1867 Newmann, C. G. *Theorie der Bessel'schen Funktionen,* Teubner, Leipzig.

1868 Lommel, E. C. J. "Zur Theorie der Bessel'schen Functionen." *Mathematische Annalen* **14**, 510–536.

1869 Hankel, H. "Die Cylinderfunktionen Erster and Zweiter Art." *Mathematische Annalen* **1**, 467–501.

1873 Frobenius, G. "Ueber die Integration des Linearen Differentialgleichungen durch Reihen." *Journal für die reine und angewandte Mathematik* **76**, 214–235.

1873 Mathieu, E. *Cours de Physique Mathematique.* Gautiers-Villars, Paris.

1879 Laguerre, E. "Sur l'integrale $\int_x^{\infty} \xi^{-1} e^{-\xi} d\xi$." *Bulletin de la Societé Mathematique de France* **7**, 72–81 (*Oeuvres* **1**, 428–437, reprinted Chelsea, 1971).

1879 Lommel, E. C. J. *Studien über der Bessel'shen Functionen.* Teubner, Leipzig.

1880 Pearson, K. "On the Solution of Some Differential Equations by Bessel Functions." *Messenger* **9**, 127–131.

1881–6 Poincaré, H. "Mémoire sur les Courbes Définies par Une Equation Differentielle." *Journal de Mathematiques* **7**, 375–422; **8**, 251–296; **1**, 167–244; **2**, 151–217.

1883 Floquet, G. *Annales Scientifiques de l'École Normale Superieure* **12**, 47–88.

1883 Floquet, G. "Sur les Équations Differentielles à Coefficients Periodiques." *Annales Scientifiques de l'École Normale Supérieure* **12**, 14–88.

1883 Thomé, L. W. *Journal für Mathematik* **95**, 75.

1886 Hill, G. W. "On the Part of the Motion of the Lunar Perigee which is a Function of the Mean Motions of the Sun and the Moon." *Acta Mathematica* **8**, 1–36.

1886 Poincaré, H. "Sur les Integrales Irreguliéres des Equations Differentielles." *Acta Mathematica* **8**, 295–344.

1886 Poincaré, H. "Sur les Determinants d'Ordre Infini." *Bulletin de la Societé Mathematique de France* **14**, 77–90.

1892 Lyapunov, A. "The General Problem of Stability of Motion." *Communications of the Mathematical Society of Kharkov.*

1892 Poincaré, H. *Méthodes Nouvelles de la Mécanique Celeste.* Gauthier-Villars, Paris.

1892 von Koch, H. "Sur les Determinants Infinis et les Equations Differentielles Ordinaires." *Acta Mathematica* **16**, 217–295.

1893 Picard, E. "Sur l'Application de la Méthode des Approximations Sucessives à l'Étude de Certaines Équations Differentielles." *Journal de Mathématiques Pures et Appliqués* **9**, 217–272.

1896 Mellin, H. "Ueber die Fundamentale Wichtigkeit des Satzes ven Cauchy für die Theorie der Gamma und Hypergeometrischen Funktionen." *Acta Societarum Scientarum Fennica* **21**, 1–115.

1904 Rayleigh, J. W. S. "On the Acoustic Shadow of a Sphere." *Philosophical Transactions of the Royal Society* **A203**, 87–110 (*Scientific Papers* **5**, 149–171).

1904 Whittaker, E. T. "An Expression of Certain Known Functions as Generalized Hypergeometric Functions." *Bulletin of the American Mathematical Society* **10**, 125–134.

1907 Foppl, F. *Vorlesungen uber Technische Mechanik.* Teubner, Leipzig.

1907 Lyapunov, A. "Probléme General de la Stabilité du Mouvement." *Annales de la Faculté de Sciences de Toulouse* **9**, 203–469.

1909 Bateman, H. "The Solution of Linear Differential Equations by Means of Definite Integrals." *Transactions of the Cambridge Philosophical Society* **21**, 171–196.

1910 von Kármán, "Festigkeit Probleme in Machinenbau." *Enzyklopedie der Mathematischen Wissenschaften*, Springer, Berlin.

1916 Rayleigh, J. W. S. "On the Propagation of Sound in Narrow Tubes of Variable Cross-section." *Philosophical Magazine* **31**, 89–96.

1919 Webster, A. G. "Acoustical Impedance and the Theory of Horns and the Phonograph." *Proceedings of the National Academy of Sciences* **5**, 275–282.

1922 van der Pol, B. "On Oscillation Hysteresis in a Triode Generator with Two Degrees-of-Freedom." *Philosophical Magazine* **43**, 700–719.

1924 Jeffreys, H. "On Certain Approximate Solutions of Linear Differential Equations of the Second Order." *Proceedings of the London Mathematical Society* **23**, 428–436.

1926 Brillouin, L. "La Mécanique Ondulatoire de Schrödinger: Une Méthode Génerale de Solution por Approximations Successives." *Comptes Redus de l'Académie des Sciences de Paris* **183**, 24–26.
1926 Kramers, H. A. "Wellenmechanik und halbzahlige Quantisiering." *Zeitschrift für Physik* **39**, 828–840.
1926 Wentzel, G. "Eine Verallgemeinering der Quarterbedindungen für die Zwecke der Wellenmechanik." *Zeitschrift für Physik* **38**, 518–529.
1927 Ballantine, S. "On the Propagation of Sound in the General Bessel Horn of Infinite Length." *Journal of the Franklin Institute* **203**, 85–101.
1930 Olson, H. F. "A Sound Concentrator for Microphones." *Journal of the Acoustical Society of America* **1**, 410–417.
1931 Volterra, V. *Leçons sur la Theorie Mathematique de la Lute pour la Vie*. Gauthier-Villars, Paris.
1938 Kontorovich, M. I. and Lebedev, N. N. "A Method for the Solution of Problems in Diffraction Theory and Related Topics." *Journal of Experimental and Theoretical Physics* **8**, 1192–1206 (in Russian).
1943 Hopf, E. "Abzweigung einer periodischen Lösung von einer stationären Lösung eines Differentialsystems." *Akademie der Wissenschaten Leipzig, Mathematische – Naturwissenschaften Klasse* **95**, 3–22.
1946 Salmon, V. "A New Family of Horns." *Journal of the Acoustical Society of America* **17**, 212–218.
1947 Chebyshev, P. L. *Collected works*. Moscow. **2**, 25–51.
1953 Landau, L. D. and Lifshitz, E. F. *Fluid Mechanics*. Pergamon Press, Oxford.
1954 Lyapunov, A. *Collected works*. Moscow.
1962 Bies, D. A. "Tapering Bar of Uniform Stress in Longitudinal Oscillations." *Journal of the Acoustical Society of America* **34**, 1567–1572.
1966 Lyapunov, A. *Stability of Motion*, Academic Press, New York.
1967 Pyle, R. W. "Duality Principle for Horns." *Journal of the Acoustical Society of America* **37**, 1178A.
1971 Nagarkar, B. N. and Finch, R. D. "Sinusoidal Horns." *Journal of the Acoustical Society of America* **50**, 23–31.
1971 Ruelle, D. and Takens, F. "On the Nature of Turbulence." *Communications in Mathematical Physics* **20**, 167–192.
1972 Schwartz, H. A. "Beweis eines für die Theorie der trignometrischen Reihen in Betracht kommenden Hülfssatzes," *Gesammelte mathematischen Abhandlengen* 341–343, reprinted Chelsea, New York.
1984 Campos, L. M. B. C. "On Some General Properties of the Exact Acoustic Fields in Horns and Baffles." *Journal of Sound and Vibration* **95**, 177–201.
1985 Campos, L. M. B. C. "On the Fundamental Acoustic Mode in Variable Area Low Mach Number Nozzles." *Progress in Aerospace Sciences* **22**, 1–27.
1986 Campos, L. M. B. C. "On Waves in Gases. Part I: Acoustics of Jets, Turbulence, and Ducts." *Reviews of Modern Physics* **58**, 117–182.
2000 Campos, L. M. B. C. "On the Singularities and Solutions of the Extended Hypergeometric Equation." *Integral Transforms and Special Functions* **9**, 99–120.
2001 Campos, L. M. B. C. "On the Derivation of Asymptotic Expansions for Special Functions from the Corresponding Differential Equations." *Integral Transforms and Special Functions* **12**, 227–236.

2001 Campos, L. M. B. C. "On the Extended Hypergeometric Equation and Functions of Arbitrary Degree." *Integral Transforms and Special Functions* **11**, 233–256.

2001 Campos, L. M. B. C. "On Some Solutions of the Extended Confluent Hypergeometric Differential Equation." *Journal of Computational and Applied Mathematics* **137**, 177–200.

2012 Campos, L. M. B. C. and Cunha, F. S. R. P. "On Hyper-spherical Legendre Polynomials and Higher Dimensional Multipole Expansions." *Journal of Inequalities and Special Functions* **3**, 1–28.

2014 Campos, L. M. B. C. and Marta, A. C. "On the Prevention or Facilitation of the Buckling of Beams." *International Journal of Mechanical Sciences* **79**, 95–104.

Index